CLINICAL FLOW CYTOMETRY – EMERGING APPLICATIONS

Edited by **Ingrid Schmid**

Clinical Flow Cytometry – Emerging Applications
Edited by Ingrid Schmid

Published by InTech

Janeza Trdine 9, 51000 Rijeka, Croatia

Publishing Process Manager Martina Blecic

Technical Editor Teodora Smiljanic

Cover Designer InTech Design Team

Additional hard copies can be obtained from orders@intechopen.com

Clinical Flow Cytometry – Emerging Applications, Edited by Ingrid Schmid
p. cm.
ISBN 978-953-51-0575-6

For EU product safety concerns:
IN TECH d.o.o., Prolaz Marije Krucifikse Kozulić 3, 51000 Rijeka, Croatia,
info@intechopen.com or visit our website at intechopen.com.

Meet the editor

Mag. Schmid is an Academic Research Specialist in the Department of Medicine, Division of Hematology-Oncology, at the University of California at Los Angeles and the technical director of the UCLA Flow Cytometry Shared Resource. Mag. Schmid received her degree in the Pharmaceutical Sciences from the University of Vienna, Austria. She immigrated to the United States of America in 1981 and joined the UCLA laboratory of Dr. John Fahey, a noted immunologist, in 1983. She started working in flow cytometry at that time, and in 1989, working with Dr. Janis Giorgi, a well-known HIV researcher, she established the UCLA Flow Cytometry Core Facility. Mag. Schmid published twenty-seven peer-reviewed, first author papers, reviews, and book chapters and has co-authored an additional twenty-eight papers and two chapters. Her present interests include the development of accurate methods for the flow cytometric assessment of circulating epithelial progenitor cells as biomarkers of cardiovascular disease as well as the formulation of documents that provide guidance to the flow cytometry community at large for creating Standard Operating Procedures for cell sorting that contain appropriate safeguards.

Contents

Preface

Advances in patient management have often been closely linked to the development of critical quantitative analysis methods. Flow cytometry is such an important methodology. It can be applied to individual cells or organelles allowing investigators interested in obtaining information about the functional properties of cells to assess the differences among cells in a heterogeneous cell preparation or between cells from separate samples. It is characterized by the use of a select wavelength of light (or multiple ones) to interrogate cells or other particles one at a time providing statistically relevant, rapid correlated measurements of multiple parameters with excellent temporal resolution. These intrinsic attributes, as well as advances in instrumentation and fluorescent probes and reagents, have contributed to the tremendous growth of clinical applications of flow cytometry and to the world-wide expansion of laboratories which use this technology since its inception in the late 1960s.

This publication reflects these facts as indicated by the global author panel and the wide range of sample types, assays, and methodologies described. Openly accessible, the book is intended to introduce novices to this powerful technology and also provide experienced professionals with valuable insights and an opportunity to refresh or update their knowledge in various subject areas of clinical flow cytometry.

Ingrid Schmid, Mag. Pharm.
Department of Medicine
Division of Hematology-Oncology
University of California, Los Angeles
USA

1

Effect of Monocyte Locomotion Inhibitory Factor (MLIF) on the Activation and Production of Intracellular Cytokine and Chemokine Receptors in Human T $CD4^+$ Lymphocytes Measured by Flow Cytometry

Sara Rojas-Dotor
Unidad de Investigación Médica en Inmunología, Instituto Mexicano del Seguro Social
México

1. Introduction

The supernatant of Axenically cultured Enatamoeba *histolytica* (*E. histolytica)* produces a thermostable factor that was purified and characterized by high resolution chromatography (HPLC) and mass spectrometry (MS-MS), supplemented by the methods of Edman (Edman & Begg, 1967). This revealed a pentapeptide with a molecular weight of 583 Daltons and established the aminoacid sequence (Met - Gln - Cys - Asn - Ser), which was termed Monocyte Locomotion Inhibitory Factor (MLIF). MLIF has powerful and selective anti-inflammatory properties, which were established *in vitro* by Boyden chamber studies. MLIF inhibits locomotion, both random chemokinetic and chemotactic, of mononuclear phagocytes (PM) from normal human peripheral blood but not of neutrophils toward various attractants, such as C5a-Desargues lymphokine and Lymphocyte-derived chemotatic factor (LDCF) (Kretschmer et al., 1985). This factor also depresses the respiratory burst of monocytes and neutrophils activated with zymosan *in vitro*, as measured by chemiluminescence (Rico et al., 1992), and nitric oxide production in mononuclear phagocytes and human polymorphonuclear neutrophils (PMNs) (Rico et al., 2003). Such effects were not accompanied by changes in expression of CD43, a ligand critical in the initial activity of phagocytes, in the membrane of these cells, and did not affect the viability of phagocytes (Kretschmer et al., 1985). In contrast, MLIF does not affect either locomotion or the respiratory burst of zymosan-activated human PMNs (Rico et al., 1998). *In vivo*, MLIF delays the arrival of mononuclear leukocytes in Rebuck chambers applied to the skin of healthy human volunteers (Kretschmer et al., 1985), inhibits cutaneous delayed contact hypersensitivity to 1-chloro-2-4-dinitrobenzene (DNCB) in guinea pigs (Giménez-Scherer et al., 1997) and decreases expression of the adhesion molecules VLA-4 on monocytes and VCAM-1 in the vascular epithelium (Giménez-Scherer et al., 2000). MILF inhibits the expression induced in inflammatory proteins such as MIP-1α and MIP-1β in U-937 cells, which are NF-κB pathway-regulated proteins (Utrera-Barillas et al., 2003). The p65–p50 heterodimer comprises the most abundant form of NF-κB in a PMA-induced system. Temporary studies showed that MLIF induces p50 translocation, which may be explained by the ability of MLIF to induce AMPc synthesis and protein kinase A phosphorylation in NF-κB and IκB followed by NF-κB translocation (Kretschmer et al., 2004). This may also explain the atypical inflammation observed in invasive amoebiasis, in which there is decreased chemotaxis and disequilibrium in cytokine production. This is supported by *in vivo* observations that MLIF notably decreased cellular infiltration and inflammatory cytokine expression.

The selective actions of MLIF upon a variety of cell types suggest that it disrupts an organism's pro- and anti-*inflammatory* network (Giménez-Scherer et al., 1987; Kretschmer et al., 1985, 2001; Rojas-Dotor et al., 2006). A pentapeptide with the same amino acids but in a different sequence, termed a MLIF scramble (Gln-Cys-Met-Ser-Asn), showed no anti-inflammatory properties (Giménez-Scherer et al., 2004). The observed effects of MLIF could be attributed to the chemical activity of the peptide. Ongoing studies in quantum chemistry have revealed that a pharmacophore group in the MLIF sequence, Cys-Asn-Ser, could be responsible for most of the anti-inflammatory properties of the molecule (Soriano-Correa et al., 2006) Figure 1.

It is possible that MLIF is derived from a larger peptide or protein synthesized by the amoeba, which is then degraded by proteases present in the cytoplasm. The lysate of amoebae material, washed and processed according to the method of Aley (Aley et al., 1980), maintains the inhibitory activity, suggesting that the MLIF is produced by the amoeba through de novo synthesis and not due to a complex-degradation process of ingestion and regurgitation of a product present in axenic medium (Rico et al., 1997).

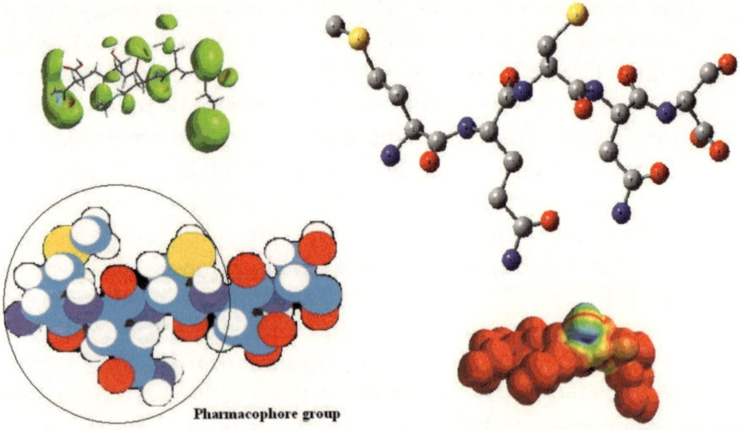

Fig. 1. Molecular Structure of Monocyte Locomotion Inhibitory Factor (Met-Gln-Cys-Asn-Ser). The pharmacophore site, Cys-Asp-Ser, is highlighted (Soriano-Correa et al., 2006)

MLIF seems to be exclusively produced by E *histolytica* and other related amebas, *E. invadens* and *E. moshkovski*, but it is absent in *E. dispar*, as we corroborated through the gene bank in which we only found the MLIF genetic sequence in the E *histolytica*, and not in any other parasites. Infections caused by E *histolytica* induce a transitory cell-mediated immunity-suppressed state in early inflammatory stages in the amebic hepatic abscess (AHA), and a complex cytokine signaling system is activated due to invasion of the parasite (Chadee & Meerovitch, 1984).

2. Inflammation

Inflammation is the body's reaction against invasion by an infectious agent, an antigenic stimulus or even just physical injury. This response induces the infiltration of leukocytes and plasma molecules into regions of infection or injury. Its main effects include increased blood flow to the region, increased vascular permeability allowing the passage of large serum molecules such as immunoglobulin and leukocyte migration through the vascular endothelium toward the inflamed area. Inflammation is controlled by cytokines, factors produced by mast cells, platelets and leukocytes, chemokines and plasma enzyme systems such complement, coagulation and fibrinolysis. Cytokines stimulate the expression of adhesion molecules by endothelial cells, and these adhesion molecules bind to leukocytes and initiate their attraction to areas of infection. Microbial products, such as peptides with N-formilmetionil, chemokines, and peptides derived from complement such as C5a, and leukotrienes (B4), act on leukocytes to stimulate their migration and their microbicidal abilities. The composition of cells involved in inflammatory processes changes with time and goes from neutrophil rich to mononuclear cell rich, reflecting a change in the leukocytes attracted (Roitt, 1998; Abbas & Lichtman, 2004). Macrophages attracted to the site of infection are activated by microbial products and interferon-gamma (IFN-γ) which cause them to phagocytose and kill microorganisms (Figure 2).

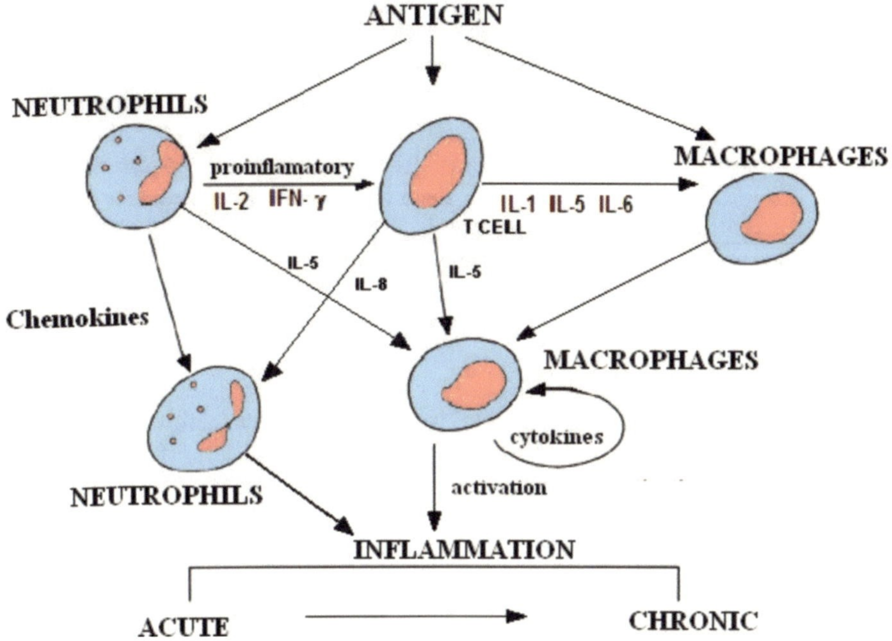

Fig. 2. Cytokines play an important role in the development of acute or chronic inflammatory responses. Interleukin 1 (IL-1), IL-6, tumor necrosis factor alpha (TNF-α) and IL-12, in addition to cytokines and chemokines, have redundant and pleiotropic effects, which together contribute to the inflammatory response. If the antigen is eliminated, inflammatory cells become apoptotic or return to the circulation. If the antigen persists for several days, it will induce chronic inflammation, recruit mast cells, eosinophils, lymphocytes and macrophages, and induce the production of antibodies and cytokines. These cells are often found in damaged tissue. (Luscinskas & Gimbrone, 1996)

Chemokines are small polypeptides that activate and direct the migration of monocytes, neutrophils, eosinophils and activated T lymphocytes from the bloodstream to sites of infection. They also regulate pro-inflammatory signals by binding to specific receptors belonging to the superfamily of seven trans-membrane domain alpha protein-coupled G (such as trimeric guanosine triphosphate (GTP)), and these can also be used as markers to differentiate chemokines and their receptors can also be used as markers of differentiation of helper T cell populations, pro-inflammatory (Th1) or anti-inflammatory (Th2) (Mosmann & Fong, 1989). Th1 cells express on their cell surface CCR5 chemokine receptor but not CCR3, whereas Th2 cells express the chemokine receptor CCR3 but not CCR5 (Sallusto et al., 1998). It has been shown that several inflammatory chemokine receptors, such as CCR1, CCR2, CCR3, CCR5 and CXCR3, are expressed shortly after signaling through the T cell receptor (TCR) in Th1 and Th2 cells. In contrast to CCR7, CCR4 and CCR8, which are over-expressed after activation through the TCR, these changes in chemokine receptor expression can be used to modify the migratory behavior of activated Th cells, and to establish the hierarchy of action between the different chemokine receptors (Loetscher et al., 1998; Zingoni et al., 1998).

2.1 Cytokines, soluble mediators

Cytokines are small peptide proteins with hormone-like activity that play a central role in communication between cells of the immune system. They are soluble mediators and regulators of innate and specific immunity. Additionally, cytokines promote growth and differentiation of leukocytes and blood cell precursors. Cytokines are key mediators of inflammation in many diseases, such as rheumatoid arthritis, lupus erythematosus, asthma and allergies (Ruschpler & Stiehl, 2002; Ivashkiv, 2003, D'Ambrosio et al., 2002, 2003). The host defenses against infectious pathogens are highly cytokine-dependent mechanisms mediated by humoral or cellular immunity. Each mechanism preferentially acts against intra or extracellular pathogens, viruses or worms. These host defense responses are strictly regulated by cytokines secreted by T helper populations, Th1 and Th2 (Kawakami, 2002). Cytokines have autocrine activity, increasing the proliferation, differentiation and effector functions of their own cell subset, and may additionally have far ranging effects on other cell types. T helper lymphocytes, the main orchestrators of the immune response, are subdivided into T_{helper} 1 (Th1) and T_{helper} 2 (Th2) subsets by the range of cytokines they secrete. Th1 cells mainly secrete the cytokines that promote cellular immunity and the inflammatory process, such as Interleukin-2 (IL-2) and Interferon-gamma (IFN-γ). (Mosmann, 1997). In contrast, Th2 cells secrete IL-4, IL-5 and IL-10, which direct the immune response toward a more humoral (antibody-mediated) response and impair differentiation toward the Th1 phenotype (Figure 3).

In the case of several infectious diseases, like-Leishmaniasis and HIV, the development of Th1-dependent immunity protects against the infectious agent. The development of Th2 dependent immunity, in contrast, was determined to protect the parasite or virus. Down-regulation of the immune response is a frequent parasitic strategy. Monitoring the immune response polarization toward a Th1- or Th2-type response is important for the development of effective vaccines. Because of the interplay between cytokines and the cells that respond to them, looking at changes in levels of soluble cytokines, changes in cell surface cytokine receptor expression and expression of intracellular cytokines by individual cell subpopulations is crucial to the understanding of cytokine biology. (Clark at al., 2011; Campanelli et al., 2010).

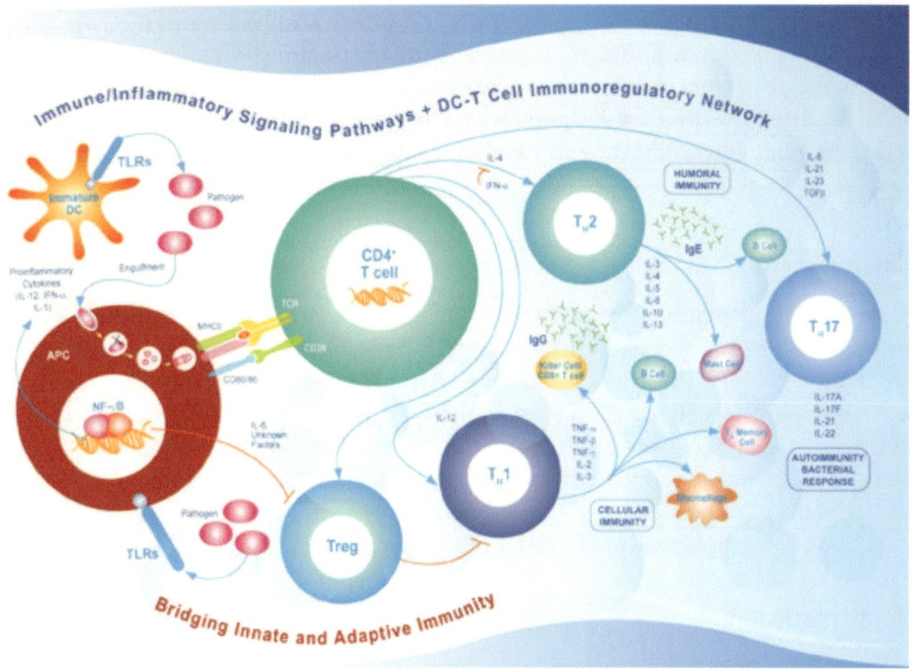

Fig. 3. Antigen-presenting cells (APCs) communicate with two types of helper T cells, Th1 and Th2. They first produce cytokines, such as IFN-γ, TNF-α and IL-2, which are responsible for inflammation, and Th2 cells produce cytokines involved in the production of antibodies. The balance of activation of between Th1 and Th2, maintained by IFN-γ and IL-10, determines the nature of an immune response. Th17 cells are another recently identified subset of CD4+ T helper cells. They are found at the interfaces between the external environment and the internal environment, such as the in the skin and the lining of the gastrointestinal tract. Regulatory T cells respond to the presence of IL-2 by rapid proliferation. Because IL-2 is secreted by effector T cells, this provides a negative-feedback mechanism, in which inflammatory T-cell activity (e.g., by Th1 cells) is restrained by the resulting expansion of regulatory T cells (Image taken from www.imgenex.com)

Lymphocyte activation, as measured early on by mitogenic assay, was used as an indicator of immune function. Mitogenic assays measure the proliferative response of isolated mononuclear cells to *in vitro* stimulation with mitogenic lectins (Phytohaemagglutinin, Concanalin A, and Pokeweed Mitogen) or certain specific antigens (Streptokinase, PPD). The proliferative index of activation is a proportion determined by the relative uptake of radiolabel nucleotides (^{3}H-thimidine) by the mitogen-stimulated culture compared to a basal nonstimulated culture. Actively proliferating cells incorporate more radionucleotides than weakly proliferating cells. Non-proliferating cells should have little or no incorporation of radionucleotides. These assays are often 48-72 hours in length and require licensing, storage and disposal of radioactive waste. A similar flow cytometry-based assay utilizes the uptake of the non-radioactve nucleotide bromo-deoxyuridine (BrdU) and detection with a fluorescent anti-BrdU antibody. These assays are somewhat non-specific and provide little information regarding cytokine production or cell communication. These tests have recently been supplanted with flow cytometry-basad assays for measuring changes in cells surface markers and assays for measuring the expression of intracellular cytokine. Flow cytometers are laser-based cell counters that are capable of distinguishing 3, 4, 5 or more (depending of flow cytometer), different fluorescence emissions, each associated with a particle identified by its light scatter proprieties. Fluorescence dyes with distinct fluorescence emissions are attached to monoclonal antibody that recognizes distinct cell surface antigens.

Traditionally, cytokines have been measured by radioimmunoassay (RIA) and enzyme-linked immunosorbent assay (ELISA). Unfortunately, these techniques are limited by their detection range and an inability to simultaneously measure multiple analytes (García, 1999).

Using extremely sensitive multiparameter flow cytometers, Multiplexed Cytokine Immunoassay Kits overcome both of these limitations. Multiplexing is the simultaneous assay of many analytes in a single sample. Applications for flow cytometry are diverse, ranging from simple cell counting and viability to more complex studies of immune function, apoptosis and cancer, stem cells, separation of cells populations such as monocytes and T and B lymphocytes, measuring changes in cell surface markers, cell cycle analysis, cellular activation, and measuring the expression of intracellular cytokines (Collins et al., 1998; McHugh, 1994; Spagnoli,et al., 1993; Trask et al., 1982).

3. Cell activation

Activation of lymphocytes is a complex yet finely regulated cascade of events that results in the expression of cytokine receptors, the production and secretion of cytokines and the expression of several cell surface molecules, eventually leading to divergent immune responses. Parasite-specific immune responses are regulated by cytokines and chemokines. They modulate and direct the immune response, but may also contribute to an infection induced by the pathogenesis and parasite persistence (Talvani et al., 2004). Parasitic infections frequently result in highly polarized $CD4^+$ T cell responses, characterized by Th1 or Th2 cytokine dominated production profiles. Although it was previously thought that these infections were strictly dependent on signaling by cytokines, such as IFN-γ, IL-12 and IL-4, recent data indicate that this polarization may be primarily directed by a series of different factors intrinsic to the pathogen–antigen-presenting-cell interaction that directs T cell priming, and that all of this is influenced by the local environment (Katzman et al., 2008). The infection caused by the *E. histolytica* parasite is associated with an acute inflammatory response (Chadee & Meerovitch, 1984). However, it is not completely clear how *E. histolytica* triggers the host inflammatory response or how host-parasite interactions start, modulate, and eventually turn off the inflammatory response.

During inflammation, leukocytes are orchestrated and regulated by the mononuclear leukocyte Thl/Th2 derived cytokine network. Thus, it was interesting for us to evaluate the effects of MLIF on lymphocyte activation and Thl/Th2 cytokine production. Additionally, it has been suggested that *E. histolytica* invasion occurs within a territory where the Thl response can be inhibited, this is, in an unbalanced environment where Thl < Th2. In this experiment, we evaluated the *in vitro* effect of MLIF on the activation and production of Thl/Th2 intracellular cytokines (IL-1β, IL-2, INF-γ IL-4, and IL-10) and the relation with the chemokine receptors CCR4 and CCR5 in human $CD4^+$ T cells. Peripheral blood samples were obtained from healthy, nonsmoking adult volunteer donors of both sexes. The peripheral blood mononuclear cells were obtained by Ficoll-Hypaque (Sigma Chemical Co.,

Louis, MO) and CD4+ T lymphocytes were obtained by negative selection technique (MACS® Reagents, Kit isolation, Human cell T CD4+). The purity of lymphocytes was analyzed by flow cytometry. The flow cytometry measures and analyzes the optical properties of individual cells pass through a laser beam. Depending on how cells interact with the laser beam, the cytometer measures five parameters for each cell: size (forward scatter, FSC), complexity (side scatter, SSC) and three fluorescence emissions (FL-1, FL-2 and FL -3). An electro-optical system converts the voltage signals, which is translated into a digital value which is stored in a computer, the data are then retrieved and analyzed with the software that combines information from different cells in statistical charts, which measure individual parameters (histograms) or two parameters at a time (dot plot, density or contour). For our study, purified lymphocytes were analyzed in a dot plot of SSC vs. FSC marking the region corresponding to lymphocytes, excluding debris and dead cells. In a dot plot is compensated for fluorescence with anti CD3-FITC and anti-CD4-PE (cluster of differentiation (CD) and marker for T lymphocytes CD4+).

Test samples of at least 10.000 events were acquired under these conditions. With this procedure, we obtained a population of CD4+ lymphocytes with 96% purity. (Figure 4)

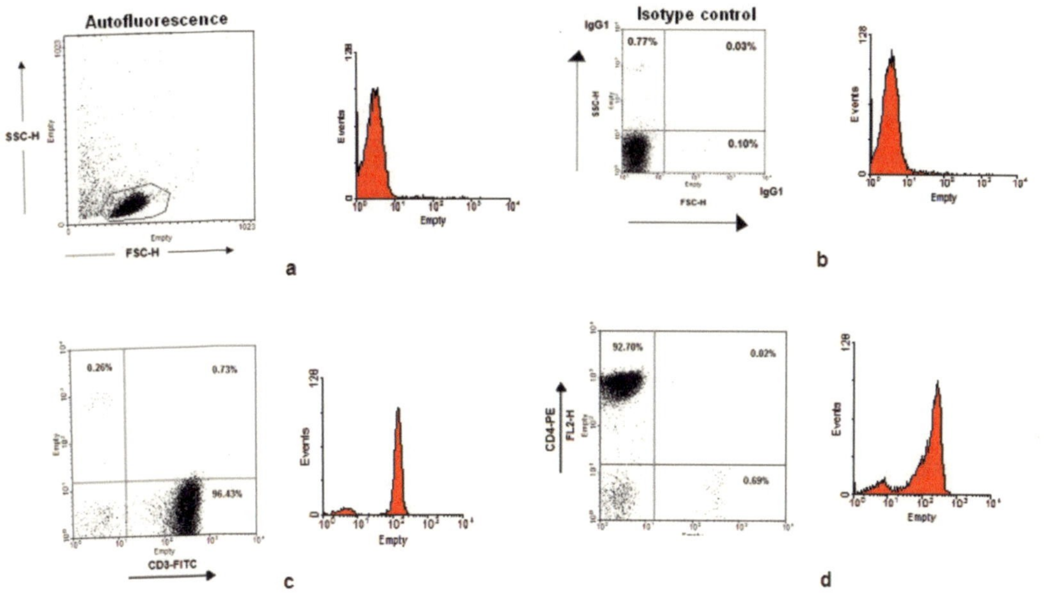

Fig. 4. Simple analysis of CD4+ T cells obtained from healthy individuals by flow cytometry. The X-axis shows staining with fluorescein isothiocyanate (FITC), and the Y-axis shows staining for phycoerythrin (PE). a) Autofluorescence; b) Isotype control, staining with mouse IgG1-FITC; c) Staining for subpopulations of CD3 coupled to FITC; d) Staining for subpopulations of CD4 coupled to PE. All stains show simple representation of the histogram and are an example of 6 experiments ± SE

The presence or absence of chemokine receptors on cell surfaces also provides information regarding the cell's state of activation. Chemokine receptors can by analyzed by flow cytometry using fluorescently labeled anti-receptor antibodies or fluorescently-labeled chemokines. Combining these reagents with antibodies against the activation marker CD69 enables analysis of cell activation within specific cell population. Figure 5 shows that the best activation was obtained with 50 ng of phorbol 12-myristate 13-acetate (PMA) and 50 μg of MLIF.

CD69 is a cell surface activation marker expressed on T cells, B cells, and activated NK cells. MLIF is able to induce expression of this marker, suggesting that it activates CD4+ T lymphocytes. T-lymphocyte activation is also associated with an up-regulation of cell surface chemokine receptors. (Figure 5)

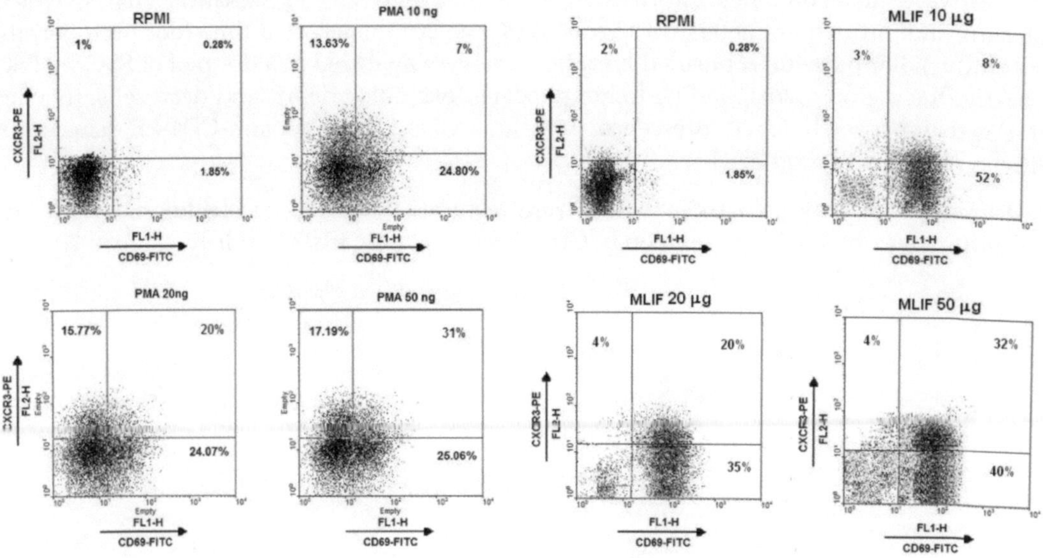

Fig. 5. Expression of the chemokine receptor CXCR3 and the activation marker CD69

Cell surface expression of the chemokine receptor CXCR3 and the activation marker CD69 on $CD4^+$ T cells after 24 hours of treatment with RPMI medium alone or activation with PMA and MLIF at different concentrations. The cell population positive for both CXCR3 and CD69 were identified using a FITC-labeled anti-CD69.

4. Cell surface molecules

Cellular activation may modify the expression of chemokines and chemokine receptors, which are essential for leukocyte recruitment during inflammation. Once activated, T lymphocytes acquire different migratory capacities and are necessary for efficient immune response regulation (Mackay, 1993; Katakai et al., 2002). CCR5 is a receptor that regulates normal activation, and it was expressed along with the tested Th1 cytokines. However, MLIF exposure inhibited these cells and induced significant decreases in production of IFN-γ and IL-1β. IFN-γ exerted a strong influence on Th1/Th2 polarization, and also affected chemokine receptor expression. MLIF induced an increase in CCR5 and CCR4 expression; however, this increase was only significant for the first. The observed CCR5 increase was greater in CCR4+ cells than in CCR4- cells (31% vs. 7%). The increases in CCR5 expression cannot be considered as a pro-Th1 response. The chemokine receptors, which are key factors in immune regulation, are influenced by MLIF. Th2 cells exhibited high CCR4 expression levels in response to MLIF and, when co-expressed, the increase was even greater, demonstrating that MLIF possessed an additive effect on these markers (Figure 6) (Rojas-Dotor et al., 2009).

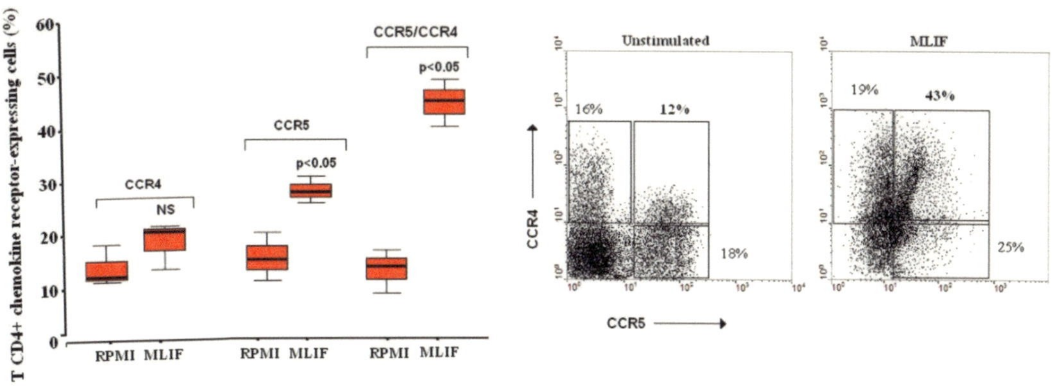

Fig. 6. Expression profiles of CCR4, CCR5, and CCR4/CCR5 on isolated CD4+ T cells. 5×10^5 CD4+ T lymphocytes were cultured for 24 h with RPMI or MLIF (50 μg/mL). Cells were stained with PE or FITC anti- human CCR4, anti-human CCR5, or anti-human CCR4/CCR5 mAbs. Box plots represent range, 25th and 75th percentiles, and vertical lines represent the 10th and 90th percentiles of data. Horizontal bars show significant statistical differences among the different groups. NS = no significant difference. Values (p) were calculated using a Mann-Whitney Test. Dot plots show the co-expression of CCR4/CCR5, and bold numbers are the mean of three independent experiments

5. Intracellular cytokines

The effect of MLIF upon the production of intracellular cytokines was evaluated using a quantitative method of flow cytometry. This was used to assess the production of IL-1β, IL-2, IFN-γ, IL-4, and IL-10. CD4+ T cells were cultured in 24-well plates in RPMI-1640 medium (supplemented with fetal calf serum (FCS), L-glutamine, streptomycin, gentamicin, and sodium pyruvate) with PMA alone or in conjunction with MLIF for 24 h at 37 °C with 5% CO_2. Cell viability was ≥ 90% determined by trypan blue dye (Sigma) exclusion. Once CD4+ T lymphocytes were activated, we determined if the effect of MLIF on cytokine production was related to a Th1 or Th2 cytokine pattern. To stain for intracellular cytokine expression, lymphocytes are labeled with anti-CD antibodies to identify cells by their subset, such as helper lymphocytes, B lymphocytes and cytotoxic lymphocytes. The cells are then stabilized by fixation with formaldehyde. Holes are punched in the cell membrane by detergent to enable the passage of anti-cytokine antibodies to the interior of the cells. By three-color flow cytometry analysis, activated T- lymphocytes can be subdivided into several different populations according to their staining characteristics. CD4 and CD3 positive and negative cells populations are identified using a FITC or PE-labeled anti-CD4 or CD3 antibody, which labels the cell surface. Following the permeabilization step, intracellular cytokines are stained with anti-human mAbs directed against IL-1β, IL-2, IFN-γ, IL-4, and IL-10, and Th1 and Th2-associated cytokine-producing lymphocytes can be counted on a flow cytometer. This procedure helps to differentiate between Th1 (IFN-γ producing) and Th2 (IL-4 producing) cells in specific cell populations. MLIF increased the expression of IL-Iβ, IL-2, IFN-γ, IL-4, and IL-10. Following PMA+MLIF treatment, the production of IFN-γ and IL-1β was inhibited compared to treatment with PMA alone. MLIF possessed the ability to nonspecifically activate CD4+ T cells, and it induced an increase in pro- and anti-inflammatory cytokine production (IL-1β, IL-2, IFN-γ, IL-4, and IL-10) (Rojas-Dotor et al., 2006). In contrast, in PMA +MLIF-incubated cells, we found that IFN-γ and IL-1β production was inhibited and production of IL-10, the prototypical anti-inflammatory cytokine, was increased (Figure 7) (Rojas-Dotor et al., 2009). It is probable that MILF induces a signaling cascade, which results in the activation of transcription factors, such as nuclear factor kB (NF-kB) (Kretschmer et al., 2004). After its translocation into the nucleus, NF-kB binds to genomic sites that regulate a large number of genes implicated in cytokine production. In this way, *E. histolytica* could potentially first establish an acute transitory reaction involving pro-inflammatory cytokines, followed by an increase and dominant pattern of anti-inflammatory signals mainly through increased IL-10. IL-10 could cause the decreased inflammatory reaction observed in the advanced states of invasive amoebiasis (Kretschmer et al., 1985).

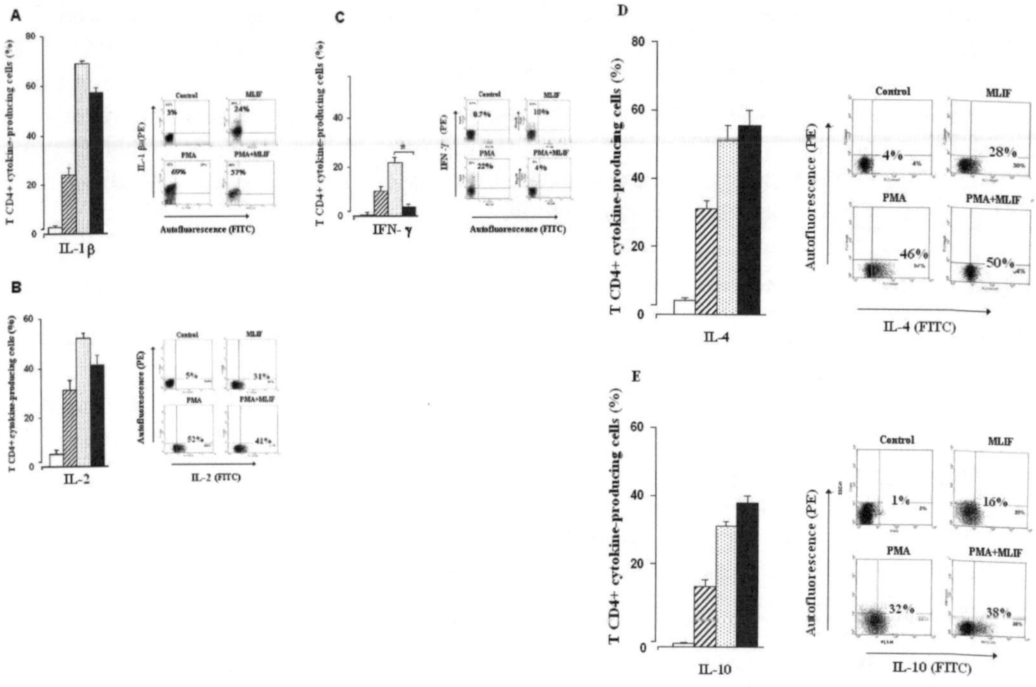

Fig. 7. Intracellular cytokine production

5 × 10^5 CD4+ T lymphocytes were cultured for 24 h in the presence of RPMI, MLIF, PMA, or PMA+MLIF. Brefeldin A, a cellular transport inhibitor was added during the last 6 h of culture . Cells were permeabilized and stained with anti-human cytokine mAbs (IL-1β, IL-2, IFNγ, IL-4, and IL-10) or mouse anti-IgG as an isotype control. FACScan dot plots are representative of control and treated cells. The numbers in each quadrant indicate the mean of the 6 independent experiments. In A, B, C, D, and E, the histograms represent control

(white), MLIF (diagonals), PMA (dotted), and PMAM+ MLIF (black) treated cells and untreated cells represent mean values ± SEM. Asterisk shows comparison among groups, *p <0.05 (Mann-Whitney Test). Bold numbers (dot plots) represent the mean.

6. Cytokines and chemokine receptors

The presence and regulation of cytokines and chemokines receptors were studied with MLIF. The cells were also stained to detect chemokine receptors and cytokine with the following combinations of mAb: anti-IL-1βPE/anti-CCR5FITC, anti-IL2FITC/anti-CCR5PE, anti-IFNγ PE/anti-CCR5FITC, anti-IL-4PE/anti-CCR4FITC and anti-IL-10FITC/anti-CCR4PE (PharMingen). 5 X10^5 $CD4^+$ T cells from each group were incubated in 24-well plates for 24 h; 10 μg/ml brefeldin A were added and incubated for the last 6 hours. After incubation, cells were centrifuged for 5 min at 400g and supernatants were aspirated without disturbing pellets. Cells were washed with PBS/0.5% albumin/2mM EDTA then they were marked with mAb, and incubated for 20 min at 4°C in the dark, and fixed with 1% p-formaldehyde according to the manufacturer's instructions (PharMingen). Acquisition of 10,000 events was conducted in flow cytometry FACScan (BD Biosciences, Sa Jose, USA). For analysis, Facs Diva and Win MDI 2.8 software were used. The results showed that $CD4^+$ T cells control 2% co-expressed IL-lβ/CCR5, IL-2/CCR5, and IFN-γ/CCR5, while 3% co-expressed IL-4/CCR4, and 1% co-expressed IL-10/CCR4. After stimulating $CD4^+$ T cells with MLIF, 15% cells co-expressed IL-1β/CCR5, 21% IL-2/CCR5, and 16% IFN-γ/CCR5, while 18% co-expressed IL-4/CCR4 and 16% IL-10/CCR4. PMA increased the expression of all of them (24%, 28%, 23%, 32%, and 31% respectively) and the combination PMA+MLIF showed that MLIF inhibited significant IL-1β/CCR5 (p<0.05) and IFN-γ/CCR5 (p< 0.002) induced by PMA (figure 8).

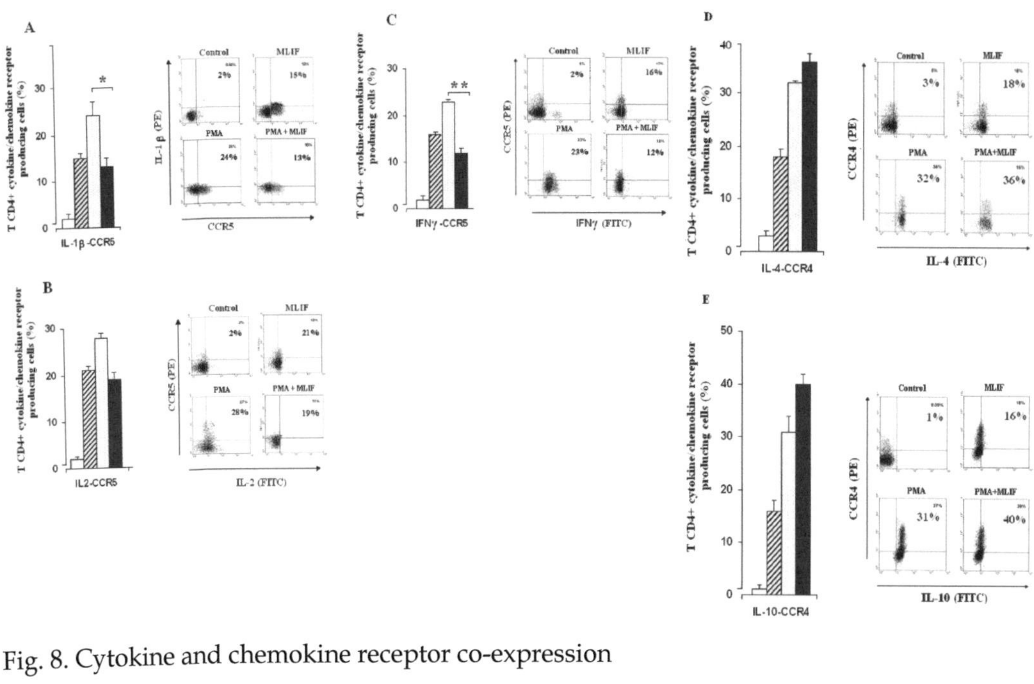

Fig. 8. Cytokine and chemokine receptor co-expression

Cells were cultured with RPMI, MLIF, PMA, or PMA+MLIF for 24 h at the previously mentioned concentrations. Brefeldin A was added during the last 6 h of culture. The cells were first stained to detect the surface cell molecules with anti- human CCR5 or CCR4 mAbs. They were then permeabilized and stained with mAbs directed against IL-1β and CCR5, IL-2 and CCR5, IFNγ and CCR5, IL-4 and CCR4, or IL-10 and CCR4 and were analyzed on a flow cytometer. A, B, C, D, and E. FACScan dot plots are representative staining of the control and the treated cells, bold numbers represent the mean of the 6 additional experiments. The histograms represent control (white), MLIF (diagonals), PMA (dotted), and PMAM+ MLIF (black) treated cells and untreated cells represent mean values ± SEM. Asterisks indicate significant differences between the groups, $^{*}p < 0.05$, $^{**}p < 0.002$ (Mann-Whitney Test).

The precise mechanisms through which MLIF causes these biological effects are unknown, but it is known that MLIF interacts with human leukocytes by means of a mannose-containing receptor (Kretschmer et al., 1991), and that it causes an increase in the number of pericentriolar microtubules and cytoplasmic AMPc concentration without concomitant GMPc diminution (Rico et al., 1995). Recent studies show that the MLIF does not interfere with programmed cell death or necrosis (Rojas-Dotor et al., 2011).

Given the level of activity of the studied cytokines, we observed that MLIF acted to promote cell populations that express IL-2/IL-10 or IFN-γ/IL-10 and CCR4/CCR5 chemokine receptor. These effects have been previously reported and are associated with pro- and anti-inflammatory functions (Katsikis et al., 1995). In previous work, MLIF was found to inhibit the induction of CC, MIP-1α, MIP-1β, and I-309 chemokines, the CCR1 receptor (Utrera-Barrillas et al., 2003), and the IL-1β, IL-5, and IL-6 cytokines (Rojas-Dotor et al., 2006). This behavior may be associated with the atypical inflammation observed in invasive amoebiasis in which there is a decrease in chemotaxis and disequilibrium in cytokine production. This conclusion is supported by observations *in vivo* in which MLIF notably decreased cellular infiltration and inflammatory cytokine expression.

7. Conclusion

Entamoeba *histolytica* produces Monocyte Locomotion Inhibitory Factor (MLIF), a pentapeptide with proven anti-inflammatory properties both *in vitro* and *in vivo*. MLIF may contribute to the exiguous inflammation observed in late amebic liver abscess, through effects exerted directly on monocytes, such as decreased locomotion and respiratory burst, or indirectly by modulating the production and expression of cytokines involved in mononuclear cell recruitment to the inflammatory focus. We evaluated the effect of MLIF on the expression of pro and anti-inflammatory $CD4^{+}$ T cells after 24 h of incubation with RPMI, MLIF, PMA or PMA + MLIF. MLIF treatment increased expression of CD69 by these cells, from which we can infer that MLIF acts as an inducer or activator of $CD4^{+}$ cells under these experimental conditions. The expression of the cytokines IL-1β, IFN-γ, IL-2, IL-4 and IL-10 and co-localization with the chemokine receptors IL-1 β/CCR5, IFN-γ/CCR5, IL-2/CCR5, IL-4/CCR4 and IL-10/CCR4 are induced by MLIF. While PMA-induced production of IL-1 β and IFN- γ was inhibited by MLIF, IL-2 production was not affected, in contrast to the expression of IL-10, which was increased by MLIF. The inhibitory effect of MLIF could be explained by two different and independent mechanisms: inhibition of pro-inflammatory cytokines such as IL-1 β and IFN-γ or increased expression of IL-10, with the concomitant increase in the suppressive effects attributed to IL-10.

MLIF acts at the beginning of the inflammatory process as a nonspecific activator, inducing the production of both pro and anti-inflammatory cytokines. As inflammation progresses, Th2 cytokine production prevails, which may inhibit Th1 cytokines. The observed effect of MLIF in this study could be explained by Th1 inhibition, as decreases in IFN-γ, IL-1β, cytokine and IL-1β/CCR5, IFN-γ/CCR5 cytokine and chemokine receptor co-expression were observed along with increases in the Th2 factors IL-4/CCR4 and IL-10/CCR4, resulting in a predominantly anti-inflammatory Th1<Th2 pattern.

The effects of MLIF on the expression of cell surface molecules and intracellular cytokine expression was made possible by the availability of a range of monoclonal anti- antibodies coupled to fluorochromes, such as FITC or PE, and analysis by flow cytometry.

8. Acknowledgements

The research was supported by the Consejo Nacional de Ciencia y Tecnología (CONACYT), México (No. 38104-M). We also wish to acknowledge American Journal Experts (AJE) for the critical review of the manuscript in English (EE.UU).

9. References

Abbas, A. & Lichtman, A. Ed. Saunders. (2004). *Cellular and molecular immunology*. ISBN 978848174710-2, Elsevier, EEUU.

Aley, SB.; Scott, WA. & Cohn, ZA. (1980). Plasma membrane of Entamoeba histolytica. *J Exp Med*, Vol. 152, No. 2, (Aug 1), pp. 391-404. ISSN: 0022-1007

Campanelli, AP., Brodskyn, CI., Boaventura, V., Silva, C., Roselino, AM., Costa, J., Saldanha, AC., de Freitas, LA., De Oliveira, CI., Barral-Netto, M., Silva, JS. & Barral, A. (2010). Chemokines and chemokine receptors coordinate the inflammatory immune response in human cutaneous leishmaniasis. *Hum Immunol*, Vol. 71, No. 12, (Dec), pp. 1220-7, ISSN:0198-8859

Chadee, K. & Meerovitch, E. (1984). The pathogenesis of experimentally induced amebic liver abscess in the gerbil (Meriones unguiculatus). *Am J Pathol*, Vol. 117, No. 1, (Oct), pp.71-80.

Clark, S., Page, E., Ford, T., Metcalf, R., Pozniak, A., Nelson, M., Henderson, DC., Asboe, D., Gotch, F., Gazzard, BG. & Kelleher, P. (2011). Reduced T(H)1/T(H)17 CD4 T-cell numbers are associated with impaired purified protein derivative-specific cytokine responses in patients with HIV-1 infection. *Allergy Clin Immunol*. Vol. 128, No. 4, (Oct), pp. 838-846.

Collins, DP., Luebering, BJ. & Shaut, DM. (1998). T-lymphocyte functionality assessed by analysis of cytokine receptor expression, intracellular cytokine expression, and femtomolar detection of cytokine secretion by quantitative flow cytometry. *Cytometry*, Vol. 33, No. 2, (Oct), pp.249-55.

D´Ambrosio, D. (2002). Role of chemokine receptors in allergic inflammation and new potential of treatment of bronchial asthma. *Recenti Prog Med*, Vol. 93 No. 6, (Jun), pp. 346-350

D'Ambrosio, D., Panina-Bordignon, P. & Sinigaglia, F. (2003). Chemokine receptors in inflammation: an overview. *J Immunol Methods*, Vol. 273 No.1-2, (Feb), pp.3-13, ISSN:0022-1759

Edman, P. & Begg, G. (1967). A protein sequenator. *Eur J Biochem*, Vol.1, No.1, (Mar), pp. 80-91, ISSN: 0014-2956

García, R. (1999). Mixed Signals Bioergonomics´ MultiFlow Multiple Cytokine Immunoassay Kits. *The Scientist*, Vol. 3, No. 23, (Nov), pp. 1-2

Giménez-Scherer, JA., Pacheco-Cano, MG., Cruz, DE., Lavín, E., Hernández-Jauregui, P., Merchant, MT. & Kretschmer, R. (1987). Ultrastructural changes associated with the inhibition of monocyte chemotaxis caused by products of axenically grown Entamoeba histolytica. *Lab Invest*, Vol. 57, No.1, (Jul), pp. 45-51

Giménez-Scherer, JA., Rico, G., Fernandez-Diez, J. & Kretschmer, RR. (1997). Inhibition of contact cutaneous delayed hypersensitivity reactions to DNBC in guinea pigs by the monocyte locomotion inhibitory factor (MLIF) produced by axenically grown Entamoeba histolytica. *Arch Med Res*, 28 Spec No:237-238

Gimenez-Scherer, JA., Arenas, E., Diaz, L., Rico, G., Fernandez, J. & Kretschmer, R. (2000). Effect of the monocyte locomotion inhibitory factor (MLIF) produced by Entamoeba histolytica on the expression of cell adhesion molecules (CAMs) in the skin of guinea pigs. *Arch Med Res*, Vol. 31, 4 Suppl, (Jul-Aug), S92-S93

Giménez-Scherer, JA., Cárdenas, G., López-Osuna, M., Velázquez, JR., Rico, G., Isibasi, A., Maldonado, M del C., Morales, ME., Fernández-Diez, J., & Kretschmer RR. (2004). Immunization with a tetramer derivative of an anti-inflammatory pentapeptide produced by Entamoeba histolytica protects gerbils (Meriones unguiculatus) against experimental amoebic abscess of the liver. *Parasite Immunol*, Vol. 26, No. 8-9, (Aug-Sep), pp. 343-9, ISSN:0141-9838

Ivashkiv, LB. (2003). Type I interferon modulation of cellular responses to cytokines and infectious pathogens: potential role in SLE pathogenesis. *Autoimmunity*, Vol.36, No. 8, (Dec), pp. 473-479, ISSN:0891-6934

Katakai, T., Hara, T., Sugai, M., Gonda, H., Nambu, Y., Matsuda, E., Agata, Y. & Shimizu, A. (2002). Chemokine-independent preference for T-helper-1 cells in transendothelial migration. *J Biol Chem*, Vol. 277, No. 52, (Dec 27), pp. 50948-50958. ISSN: 0021-9258

Katsikis, PD., Cohen, SB., Londei, M. & Feldmann, M. (1995). Are $CD4^+$ Th1 cells pro-inflammatory or anti-inflammatory? The ratio of IL-10 to IFN-γ or IL-2 determines their function. *Int Immunol*, Vol. 7, No. 8, (Aug), pp. 1287-1294. ISSN: 0953-8178

Katzman, SD. & Fowell, DJ. (2008). Pathogen-imposed skewing of mouse chemokine and cytokine expression at the infected tissue site. *J Clin Invest*, Vol. 118 No2, (Feb), pp. 801-811. ISSN: 0021-9738

Kawakami, K. (2002). Interleukin-18 and host defense against infectious pathogens. *J Immunother*, Vol. 25 Suppl 1, (March-April), S12-S19, ISSN:1053-8550

Kretschmer, R., Collado, ML., Pacheco, MG., Salinas, MC., Lopez Osuna, M., Lecuona, M., Castro, EM. & Arellano, J. (1985). Inhibition of human monocyte locomotion by products of axenically grown E. histolytica. *Parasite Immunol*, Vol. 7, No.5, (Sep), pp. 527-543, ISSN:0141-9838

Kretschmer, R., Castro, EM., Pacheco, G., Rico, G., Diaz-Guerra, O. & Arellano, J. (1991) The role of mannose in the receptor of the monocyte locomotion inhibitory factor produced by Entamoeba histolytica. *Parasitol Res*, Vol. 77, No. 5, pp. 374-378

Kretschmer, RR., Rico, G. & Giménez, JA. (2001). A novel anti-inflammatory oligopeptide produced by Entamoeba histolytica. *Mol Biochem Parasitol*, Vol. 112, No. 2 (Feb), pp 201-219.

Kretschmer, R., Velázquez, J., Utrera-Barillas, D. & Zentella, A. (2004). The amibic anti-inflammatory monocyte locomotion (MLIF) inhibits the NF-kB nuclear translocation in human monocytes. *FASEB J*, Vol. 18, No. A1147, pp. ISSN: 0892-6638

Loetscher, P., Uguccioni, M., Bordoli, L., Baggiolini, M., Moser, B., Chizzolini, C. & Dayer, JM. (1998). CCR5 is characteristic of Th1 lymphocytes. *Nature*, Vol. 391 No.6665, (Jan 22), pp. 344-345 ISSN: 0028-0836

Luscinskas, FW. & Gimbrone, MA. Jr. (1996). Endothelial-dependent mechanisms in chronic inflammatory leukocyte recruitment. *Annu Rev Med*, Vol. 47, pp. 413-21. Review.

Mackay, CR. (1993). Homing of naive, memory and effector lymphocytes. *Curr Opin Immunol*, Vol. 5, No.3, (Jun), pp. 423-427. ISSN: 0952-7915

McHugh, TM. (1994). Flow microsphere immunoassay for the quantitative and simultaneous detection of multiple soluble analytes. *Methods Cell Biol*, 42 Pt B: 575-95

Mosmann, TR. & Fong, TA. (1989). Specific assays for cytokine production by T cells. *J Immunol Methods*, Vol.116, No.2, (Jan), pp151-158. ISSN: 0022-1759

Mosmann, TR., Li, L., Hengartner, H., Kagi, D., Fu, W. & Sad, S. (1997). Differentiation and functions of T cell subsets. *Ciba Found Symp*, Vol.204, pp. 148-154, discussion 154-158.

Rico, G., Diaz-Guerra, O., Gimenez-Scherer, JA. & Kretschmer, RR. (1992). Effect of the monocyte locomotion inhibitory factor (MLIF) produced by Entamoeba histolytica upon the respiratory burst of human leukocytes. *Arch Med Res*, Vol.23, No.2, pp:157-159

Rico, G., Díaz-Guerra, O. & Kretschmer, R. (1995). Cyclic nucleotide changes induced in human leukocytes by a product of axenically grown Entamoeba histolytica that inhibits human monocyte locomotion. *Parasitol Res*, Vol. 81, No.2, pp. 158-162.

Rico, G., Ximenez, C., Ramos, F. & Kretschmer RR. (1997). Production of the monocyte locomotion inhibitory factor (MLIF) by axenically grown Entamoeba histolytica: synthesis or degradation? *Arch Med Res*, Suppl 28:235-236

Rico, G., Leandro, E., Rojas, S., Giménez, JA. & Kretschmer, RR. (2003). The monocyte locomotion inhibitory factor produced by Entamoeba histolytica inhibits induced nitric oxide production in human leukocytes. *Parasitol Res*, Vol. 90, No. 4, (Jul), pp. 264-267.

Roitt. (Ed. UK9). (1998) *Immunology*. ISBN 0723429189, Mosby London, EEUU.

Rojas-Dotor, S., Rico, G., Pérez, J., Velázquez, J., & Kretscmer, R. (2006). Cytokine expression in CD4+ cells exposed to the monocyte locomotion inhibitory factor (MLIF) produced by Entamoeba histolytica. *Parasitol Res*, Vol.98, No. 5, (Apr), pp. 493-495.

Rojas-Dotor, S., Pérez-Ramos, J., Giménez-Scherer, JA., Blanco-Favela, F. &, Rico, G. (2009). Effect of the Monocyte Locomotion Inhibitory Factor (MLIF) produced by E. histolityca on cytokines and chemokine receptors in T CD4+ lymphocytes. *Biol Res*, Vol. 42 No.4, (Jan), pp. 415-425.

Rojas-Dotor, S., Vargas-Neri L., & Blanco-Favela, F (2011). Effect of the monocyte locomotion inhibitory factor (MLIF) a natural anti-Inflammatory produced by E. histolytica on apoptosis in human CD4+ T lymphocytes. *Pharmacology and Pharmacy*, Vol. 2, (Oct), pp. 248-255.

Ruschpler, P. & Stiehl, P. (2002). Shift in Th1 (IL-2 and IFN-gamma) and Th2 (IL-10 and IL-4) cytokine mRNA balance within two new histological main-types of rheumatoid-arthritis (RA). *Cell Mol Biol*, Vol. 48, No. 3, (May 2002), pp.285-293, ISSN: 0145-5680

Sallusto, F., Lenig, D., Mackay, CR. & Lanzavecchia, A. (1998). Flexible programs of chemokine receptor expression on human polarized T helper 1 and 2 lymphocytes. *J Exp Med*, Vol. 187, No.6, (Mar), pp. 875-883, ISSN: 0022-1007

Soriano-Correa, C., Sánchez-Ruíz, JF., Rico-Rosillo, G., Giménez-Scherer, JA., Velázquez, JR. & Kretschmer, R. (2006). Electronic structure and physicochemical properties of the anti-inflammatory pentapeptide produced by Entamoeba histolytica: Theoretical study. *J Mol Struct: Theochem*, Vol. 769 (May 22), pp. 91-95.

Spagnoli, GC., Juretic, A., Schultz-Thater, E., Dellabona , P., Filgueira, L., Hörig, H., Zuber, M., Garotta, G. & Heberer, M. (1993). On the relative roles of interleukin-2 and interleukin-10 in the generation of lymphokine-activated killer cell activity. *Cell Immunol,* Vol. 146, No. 2 (Feb), pp. 391-405. ISSN: 0008-8749

Talvani, A., Rocha, MO., Ribeiro, AL., Correa-Oliveira, R. & Teixeira, MM. (2004). Chemokine receptor expression on the surface of peripheral blood mononuclear cells in Chagas disease. *J Infect Dis*, Vol. 189, No. 2, (Jan), pp. 214-20. ISSN: 0022-1899

Trask, BJ., Van den Engh, GJ. & Elgershuizen, JH. (1982). Analysis of phytoplankton by flow cytometry. *Cytometry*, Vol.2 No. 4, (Jan), pp. 258-64.

Utrera-Barrillas, D., Velázquez, JR., Enciso, A., Cruz, SM., Rico. G., Curiel-Quezada, E., Terán, LM. & Kretschmer, R. (2003). An anti-inflammatory oligopeptide produced by Entamoeba histolytica down-regulates the expression of pro-inflammatory chemokines. *Parasite Immunol*, Vol.25, No.10, (Oct), pp. 475-482. ISSN:0141-9838

Zingoni, A., Soto, H., Hedrick, JA., Stoppacciaro, A., Storlazzi, CT., Sinigaglia, F., D'Ambrosio, D., O'Garra, A., Robinson, D., Rocchi, M., Santoni, A., Zlotnik, A. & Napolitano, M. (1998). The chemokine receptor CCR8 is preferentially expressed in Th2 but not Th1 cells. *J Immunol*, Vol. 161, No.2, (Jul), pp. 547-551. ISSN: 0022-1767

2

Applications of Flow Cytometry to Clinical Microbiology

Barbara Pieretti, Annamaria Masucci and Marco Moretti
Laboratorio di Patologia Clinica, Ospedale S. Croce Fano
A.O.R.M.N. Azienda Ospedali Riuniti Marche Nord
Fano (PU),
Italy

1. Introduction

Microbiology in general and clinical microbiology in particular have witnessed important changes during the last few years. Traditional methods of bacteriology and mycology require the isolation of the organism prior to identification and other possible testing. In most cases, culture results are available in 48 to 72 h. Virus isolation in cell cultures and detection of specific antibodies have been widely used for the diagnosis of viral infections (*Weinstein, 2007*). These methods are sensitive and specific, but, the time required for virus isolation is quite long and is governed by viral replication times. Additionally, serological assays on serum from infected patients have often most limits in specificity and sensitivity. Life-threatening infections require prompt antimicrobial therapy and therefore need rapid and accurate diagnostic tests. Procedures which do not require culture and which detect the presence of antigens or the host's specific immune response have shortened the diagnostic time. More recently, the emergence of molecular biology techniques, particularly those based on nucleic acid probes combined with amplification techniques, has provided speediness and specificity to microbiological diagnosis. These techniques have led to a revolutionary change in many of the traditional routine tests used in clinical microbiology laboratories.

The current organization of clinical microbiology laboratories is now subject to increased use of automation exemplified by systems used for detecting bacteremia, screening of urinary tract infections, antimicrobial susceptibility testing and antibody detection. To obtain better sensitivity and speed, manufacturers continuously modify all these systems. Nevertheless, the equipment needed for all these approaches is different, and therefore the initial costs, both in equipment and materials, are high.

Indeed, in recent years microbiological techniques have been increasingly complemented by technologies such as those provided by flow cytometry.

We have gotten used to consider the flow cytometry applicable only in the field of hematology, then associate it with clinical microbiology makes it even more mysterious.

Over the past forty years we have witnessed several attempts of application of the flow cytometry to microbiology, with good results but also with many difficulties.

In particular, the problems encountered relate the difficulty of measuring microbes by flow due to their small size and point towards the development of instrumentation that has managed to overcome this limitation of standard instrumentation used for routine flow cytometry in different fields from microbiology.

The aim of this chapter is to provide a complete overview of the applications of flow cytometry in microbiology, referring mainly to what is published in the literature. Will be presented innovative methods and practical examples of applications of flow cytometry in different areas of microbiology following the scheme outlined in paragraphs listed below.

The authors report in paragraph "References" articles that offer important points of discussion to make useful chapter to the various professionals in the targeted book.

2. Flow cytometry and microbiology

Flow cytometry is a powerful fluorescence based diagnostic tool that enables the rapid analysis of entire cell populations on the basis of single-cell characteristics (*Brehm-Stecher, 2004*). Flow cytometry (FCM) could be successfully applied in bacteremia and bacteriuria, for rapidly microorganism's detection on the basis of its cytometric characteristics. Although FCM offers a broad range of potential applications for susceptibility testing, a major contribution would be in testing for slow-growing microorganisms, such as mycobacteria and fungi.

This technique could also be applied to study the immune response in patients, in detection of specific antibodies and monitor clinical status after antimicrobial treatments.

In the last years of the 1990s, the applications of FCM in microbiology have significantly increased (*Fouchet, 1993*).

Earlier works had demonstrated the applicability of dual-parameter analysis (light scattered vs fluorescence coupled to cellular components as protein and DNA or auto-fluorescence) to discriminate among different bacteria in the same sample.

FCM has also been used in metabolic studies of microorganisms (es. autofluorescence due to NADPH and flavins as metabolic status markers), in DNA's analysis, protein, peroxide production, and intracellular pH, for count of live and dead bacteria and/or yeasts, and for the discrimination of gram-positive from gram-negative bacteria on the basis of the fluorescence emitted when the organisms are stained with two fluorochromes.

Also it offers the possibility to investigate in yeasts and bacteria the respective gene expression (*Alvarez-Barrientos, 2000*).

3. Applications of flow cytometry to clinical microbiology

FCM is an analytical method that allows the rapid measurement of light scattered (intrinsic parameters: cell size and complexity) and fluorescence emission produced by suitably illuminated cells (fluorochromes). The cells, or particles, are suspended in liquid and produce signals when they flow individually through a beam of light, and the results represent cumulative individual cytometric characteristics. An important analytical feature of flow cytometers is their ability to measure multiple cellular parameters (analytical flow cytometers). Some flow cytometers are able to physically separate cell subsets (sorting) based on their cytometric characteristics (cell sorters).

Fluorochromes can be classified according to their mechanism of action: those whose fluorescence increases with binding to specific cell compounds such as proteins (fluorescein isothiocyanate [FITC]), nucleic acids (propidium iodide [PI]), and lipids (Nile Red); those whose fluorescence depends on cellular physiological parameters (pH, membrane potential, etc.); and those whose fluorescence depends on enzymatic activity (fluorogenic substrates) such as esterases, peroxidases, and peptidases. Fluorochromes can also be conjugated to antibodies or nucleotide probes to directly detect microbial antigens or DNA and RNA sequences (*see Table 1*).

Several articles of literature propose flow cytometry as rapid diagnostic tool in the fight against infection (*Alvarez-Barrientos, 2000*). In fact this methodology can be used in the isolation of microbes and their identification, in the determination of antibodies to a particular pathogen in different stages of the disease and in direct detection of essential microbial components such as nucleic acids and proteins directly in clinical specimens (tissues, body fluids, etc.) and for evaluation of effectiveness of antimicrobial therapy in general.

Recently, the Sysmex UF-100 flow cytometer has been developed to automate urinalysis. *Penders et al.* have valuated this instrument to explore the possibilities of flow cytometry in the analysis of peritoneal dialysis fluid and have compared the obtained data with those of counting chamber techniques, biochemical analysis and bacterial culture (*Penders, 2004*); while *Pieretti et al.* have applied this technology at diagnosis of bacteriuria, for example (*Pieretti, 2010*).

3.1 Direct detection of bacteria, fungi, parasites, viruses

Several studies are reported in the literature concerning the use of flow cytometry to determine the presence of bacteria, viruses, parasites, etc, in a biological sample. In this section we describe the techniques used for this purpose.

Microorganisms are small and they are very different in structure and function, and both these factors lead to technological and methodological problems in studying them.

Conventionally, microorganisms are studied at the population scale because cultures of microbes are considered to be uniform populations which can be adequately described by average values. However, the availability of tools such as flow cytometry and image analysis which allow measurements to be made on individual cells has changed our perception of microbes within both the laboratory and the natural environment. Only a small proportion of the diversity of microorganisms has been identified and a smaller proportion still has been characterized through laboratory studies.

Microbes cannot be investigated without technological assistance, meaning that methods such as microscopy and flow cytometry with appropriate fluorochomes are essential for the acquisition of both qualitative and quantitative information. Although these methods have become conventional tools in microbial cell biology and in the analysis of environmental samples, their use in investigations of bacteria is limited by the physical constraint of optical resolution. Application of cell markers is also a challenge, simply because the cells have only

Applications	Substrate	Dye	Excitation/ Emission Wavelength (λmax)nm
Viability [a] **DNA quantification** [b] **RNA quantification** [c] **Cell cycle studies** [d]	DNA-RNA	*SYTOX Green* [a,b]	504-525
		Propidium Iodide (PI) [a,b,d]	536-625
		Ethidium bromide [b,d]	510-595
		SYTO 13 [a,b,d]	488-509
	DNA (GC pairs)	*Hoechst 33258/33342* [d]	340-450
	DNA	*Mithramycin* [d]	425-550
	RNA	*Pyronine Y* [c]	497-563
Microbe detection	Proteins	*Fluorescein isothiocyanate (FITC)*	495-525
		Texas Red	580-620
		Oregon Green Isothiocyanate	496-526
	Antigens	*Antibodies labeled with flurochromes*	*Depends on fluorochrome conjugated*
	Nucleotide sequences	*Fluorescently labeled oligonucleotides*	
Ca2+ mobilization	Ca2+	*Indo-1*	340-(398–485)
		Fura-2	340-549
		Fluor-3	469-545
Metabolic variations	pH	*BCECF*	(460–510)-(520–610)
		SNARF-1	510-(587–635)
Antibiotic susceptibility Metabolic variations	Membrane potential	*DiOC$_6$(3)*	484-501
		Oxonol [DiBAC$_4$(3)]	488-525
		Rhodamine 123	507-529
Cell wall composition Microbe detection	Membrane oligosaccharides	*Lectins*	*Depends on fluorochrome conjugated*
Metabolic activity	Enzyme activities	*Substrates linked to fluorochromes*	
Yeast metabolic state [e] **Fungal detection** [f]	Lipids	*Nile Red* [e]	(490–550)-(540–630)
	Vacuolar enzyme activity	*Fun-1* [e]	508-(525–590)
	Chitin and other carbohydrate polymers	*Calcofluor white* [f]	347-436

Table 1. Features of same fluorescent molecules used in flow cytometry (*modified from Alvarez-Barrientos 2000*)

a thousandth of the volume of a normal blood cell and correspondingly small amounts of cellular constituents. This is the reason why multicolor approaches in bacteria with small cell volumes will not work, as the close spatial interaction of the dyes prevents quantitative analysis (*Muller, 2009*).

Mueller and Davey (*2009*) have proposed a bibliometric analysis of flow cytometric studies in last forty-years in which appear that the role of flow cytometry in microbiology is steadily increasing.

A survey was made of the Web of Science database of the Institute for Scientific Information counting all papers whose topic database field contained the words flow and cytometr* (es. citometry, citometric, etc) plus one or more of the following words: bacteri*, microorganism, procaryot* or yeast. The percentage of flow cytometry papers in general shows a steady growth after the 1990s, and in particular 8% of flow cytometry articles includes studies of microbes.

Earlier works had demonstrated the applicability of dual-parameter analysis to discriminate among different bacteria in the same sample. One parameter was light scattered (size), and the other was either fluorescence emission from fluorochromes coupled to cellular components (protein and DNA) or autofluorescence, or light scattered acquired from another angle. For example dual-parameter analysis of forward light scatter and red fluorescence signals (FSC-H vs FL3-H) allowed the discrimination between two species of *Candida,* as *Candida lusitaniae* and *Candida maltosa,* based on different fluorochrome staining backgrounds. These yeast species are indistinguishable by monoparametric analysis of forward light scatter or red autofluorescence.

In addition it is possible the quantification of different protein amounts (measured as FITC fluorescence) to distinguish different microorganisms (bacteria and/or yeasts) present in mixed cultures by histogram representation (FITC fluorescence vs number of events); or use dual-fluorescence to discrimination of specific fungal spores. For example, *Alvarez-Barrientos* et al. (2000) have proposed Calcofluor fluorescence vs PI fuorescence for detection of *Aspergillus, Mucor, Cladosporium,* and *Fusarium.* In particular, Calcofluor binds chitin in the spore wall, while PI stains nucleic acids. However, the use of several fluorochromes for direct staining or through antibody or oligonucleotide conjugates plus size detection is the simplest way to visualize or identify microorganisms by FCM.

The simple and rapid assessment of the viability of a microorganism is another important aspect of FCM. The effect of environmental stress or starvation on the membrane potential of bacteria has been studied by several groups using fluorochromes that distinguish among nonviable, viable, and dormant cells.

FCM has also been used in metabolic studies of microorganisms using autofluorescence due to NADPH and flavins as metabolic status markers. Other authors studied DNA, proteins, peroxide production, and intracellular pH, detection of live and dead bacteria and fungi, detection of gram-positive and gram-negative on the basis of the fluorescence emitted when the organisms are stained with two fluorochromes, and gene expression.

FCM has been extensively used for studying virus-cell interactions for cytomegalovirus (CMV), herpes simplex virus (HSV), adenovirus, human immunodeficiency virus (HIV), and hepatitis B virus (HBV).

3.1.1 Bacteria

Pianetti et al. (*2005*) compared traditional methods (spectrophotometric and plate count) used in bacteria counting cells with FCM for the determination of the viability of *Aeromonas hydrophila* in different types of water. They studied the presence of a strain of *Aeromonas hydrophila* in river water, spring water, brackish water and mineral water.

Flow cytometric determination of viability was carried out using a dual-staining technique that enabled us to distinguish viable bacteria from damaged and membrane-compromised bacteria. The traditional methods showed that the bacterial content was variable and dependent on the type of water. The plate count method is a widely used technique for determining the bacterial charge, but it supplies information related only to viability and growth capacity; while the absorbance method have a sensitivity who appears to be correlated with microbiological culture density.

The flow cytometric nucleic acid double-staining protocol is based on simultaneous use of permeable fluorescent probes (SYBR Green dyes) and an impermeable fluorescent probe (PI) and can distinguish viable, membrane-damaged, and membrane-compromised cells.

The results obtained from the plate count analysis correlated with the absorbance data. In contrast, the flow cytometric analysis results did not correlate with the results obtained by traditional methods; in fact, this technique showed that there were viable cells even when the optical density was low or no longer detectable and there was no plate count value. According to their results, flow cytometry is a suitable method for assessing the viability of bacteria in water samples. Furthermore, it permits fast detection of bacteria that are in a viable but nonculturable state, which are not detectable by conventional methods.

Similar study was proposed to *McHugh et al.* (*2007*) who investigated FCM for the detection of bacteria in cell culture production medium, using a nucleic acid stain, thiazole orange, which binds to nucleic acids of viable and nonviable organisms. They analyzed different bacteria: Gram positive (*Microbacterium species*) and Gram negative (*Acinetobacter species, Burkholderia cepacia, Enterobacter cloacae, Stenotrophomonas maltophilia*) vegetative bacteria, and Gram positive spore former (*Bacillus cereus*).

Loehfelm T.W. (*2008*) proposed a new application of FCM: identification and characterization of protein associated to biofilm in *Acinetobacter baumannii*, an opportunistic pathogen that is particularly successful at colonizing and persisting in the hospital environment, able to resist desiccation and survive on inanimate surfaces for months (*Kramer, 2006*). The authors have identified a new *A. baumannii* protein, Bap, expressed on the surface of these bacteria that is involved in biofilm formation in static culture, and that is detectable with FCM applied the following settings: forward scatter voltage, E02 (log); side scatter voltage, 582 (log); FL1 voltage, 665 (log); event threshold, forward scatter 434 and side scatter 380.

Weiss Nielsen and collaborators (*2011*) proposed an interesting video-protocol for detection of *Pseudomonas aeruginosa* and *Saccharomyces cerevisiae* present in biofilm by flow cell system.

Tracy et al. (*2008)* described the development and application of flow-cytometric and fluorescence assisted cell-sorting (FACS) techniques for study endospore-forming bacteria. In particular, they showed that by combining flow-cytometry light scattering with nucleic acid staining it's possible discriminate, quantify, and enrich all sporulation associated morphologies exhibited by the endospore-forming anaerobe *Clostridium acetobutylicum*. By light scattering discrimination they detect the temporal aspects of sporulation, accurately quantify the proportion of the population participating in sporulation, and sort cultures into enriched populations for subsequent analysis. By coupling with nucleic acid staining (SYTO-9 plus PI), they effectively discriminated between different sporulation-associated phenotypes, and by using FACS they were able to enrich for the various sporulation phenotypes.

3.1.1.1 Bacterial detection and live/dead discrimination by flow cytometry

Flow cytometry is a sensitive analytical technique that can rapidly monitor physiological states of bacteria (reproductively viable, metabolically active, intact, permeabilized) and can be readily applied to the enumeration of viable bacteria in a biological sample (*Khan, 2010*).

Accurate determination of live, dead, and total bacteria is important in many microbiology applications.

Traditionally, viability in bacteria is synonymous with the ability to form colonies on solid growth medium and to proliferate in liquid nutrient broths.

FCM makes specificity of different fluorochrome-labeled antibodies to binding at specific antigens present in the surface of microorganisms for their identification in short period of time (less than 2 h), but with the extent of availability of specific antibodies.

The first fluorochome used to detect bacteria was ethidium bromide in association with light-scatter signal, and the second was propidium iodide (PI).

Live cells have intact membranes and are impermeable to dyes such as PI which only leaks into cells with compromised membranes, while thiazole orange (TO) is a permeant dye and enters all cells, live and dead, to varying degrees. With gram-negative organisms, depletion of the lipopolysaccharide layer with EDTA greatly facilitates TO uptake. Thus a combination of these two dyes provides a rapid and reliable method for discriminating live and dead bacteria. An intermediate or "injured" population can often be observed between the live and dead populations.

It is possible to create a gating strategy for bacterial populations (es. *Escherichia coli*) staining the sample with thiazole orange (TO) and propidium iodide (PI), and analyze FSC vs SSC dot plot. You can set liberally a region (R1) around the target population and another (R2) around the beads. Then you can analyze FL2 vs SSC dot plot setting another region (R3) around the stained bacteria. At this point you can observed FL1 vs FL3 dot plot gated on (R1 or R2) and R3, with regions set around the live, "injured" and dead bacterial populations.

Very interesting is the work that *Khan et al.* have proposed in 2010 on enumeration of viable but non-culturable and viable-culturable Gram-Negative Bacteria using flow cytometry.

The traditional culture methods for detecting indicator and pathogenic bacteria in food and water may underestimate numbers due to sub-lethal environmental injury, inability of target bacteria to take up nutrient components in the medium, and other physiological factors which reduce culturability; however, these methods are also time-consuming and cannot detect non-culturable (VBNC) cells. An issue of critical about microbiology is the ability to detect viable but non-culturable (VBNC) and viable-culturable (VC) cells by methods other than existing approaches. Culture methods are selective and underestimate the real population, and other options (direct viable count and the double-staining method using epifluorescence microscopy and inhibitory substance-influenced molecular methods) are also biased and time-consuming. A rapid approach that reduces selectivity, decreases bias from sample storage and incubation, and reduces assay time is needed (*Davey, 1996*).

Flow cytometry is a sensitive analytical technique that can rapidly monitor physiological states of bacteria. This report outlines a method to optimize staining protocols and the flow cytometer instrument settings for the enumeration of VBNC and VC bacterial cells within 70 min (*Khan 2010*), using SYTO dyes with different fluorescent probes (SYTO 9, SYTO 13, SYTO 17, SYTO 40) for detection of total cells and PI for detection of dead cells.

Khan et al. (*2010*) reported a study using FCM methods to detect cells with intact and damaged membranes. They assumed that cells having intact membranes are live (VC) and those with damaged membranes are dead or theoretically dead (VBNC).

The main objective of this study was to establish the quickest, most accurate, and easiest ways to estimate the proportions of VBNC and VC states and dead cells, as indicated by membrane integrity of these four Gram-negative bacteria: *Escherichia coli* O157:H7, *Pseudomonas aeruginosa, Pseudomonas syringae,* and *Salmonella enterica* serovar *Typhimurium* (*Khan, 2010*).

The FCM data were compared with those for specific standard nutrient agar to enumerate the number of cells in different states. By comparing results from cultures at late log phase, 1 to 64% of cells were nonculturable, 40 to 98% were culturable, and 0.7 to 4.5% had damaged cell membranes and were therefore theoretically dead. Data obtained using four different Gram-negative bacteria exposed to heat and stained with PI also illustrate the usefulness of the approach for the rapid and unbiased detection of dead versus live organisms.

Similar analysis was proposed by McHugh (2007) for detection of Gram positive and Gram negative vegetative bacteria (*Acinetobacter species, Burkholderia cepacia, Enterobacter cloacae, Stenotrophomonas maltophilia, Mycobacterium species, and Bacillus cereus*).

Another way in which FCM can achieve direct diagnosis is by use of different-sized fluorescent microspheres coated with antibodies against microbes. In this case is possible determine the absolute count of bacteria per unit of volume present in the sample analyses using following equation:

$$\frac{\#\ of\ events\ in\ region\ containing\ cell\ population}{\#\ of\ events\ in\ bead\ population} \times \frac{\#\ of\ beads\ per\ test}{test\ volume} \times dilution\ factor = \begin{matrix} Concentration\ of \\ bacterial\ population \end{matrix}$$

Flow cytometry (FCM) has potential as an alternative method for the quantification of fluorescently labeled bacterial cells in drinking water; it is fast, accurate, and quantitative.

Füchslin et al. (*2010*) have proposed an interesting method for the rapid and quantitative detection of *Legionella pneumophila* in water samples in according to ISO 11371. The method comprised concentrating by filtration and resuspension, immunostaining followed by immunomagnetic separation using labeling with paramagnetic MicroBeads (size 50 nm), separation on a high-gradient column, and finally flow cytometric detection. The individual steps of the procedure were separately validated under laboratory conditions, and the results were compared with established standard methods such as cell enumeration with fluorescence microscopy and colony-forming units on selective agar plates. Furthermore, the whole method was tested with spiked tap water, and the detection limit was determined.

Use of fluorescent stains or fluorogenic substrates in combination with FCM allows the detection and discrimination of viable culturable, viable nonculturable, and nonviable organisms, can be used to microbial analysis of milk. *Gunasekera et al.* (*2000*) have demonstrated the potential application of flow cytometers in milk analyses developing a rapid method (less than 60 minutes) for detecting of total bacteria (*Gunasekera, 2000*). The authors have considered as potential contaminants of milk for represent gram-negative rods *Escherichia coli* and for gram-positive cocci *Staphylococcus aureus*.

Pure populations of *E. coli* and *S. aureus* were easily detected by FCM when they were suspended in phosphate-buffered saline (PBS), but when they were inoculated into ultra-heat-treated (UHT) milk, no distinct separation appeared. This is due to the presence of proteins and lipid globules that can bind nonspecifically to fluorescent stains and interfere with staining and detection of bacteria. Treatment of milk by centrifugation to remove lipids without also treating samples with proteases was insufficient to allow definition of bacteria. For these reason the authors have applied enzymatic treatment with protease K or savinase to remove or modify proteins and thereby enable distinction of bacteria by flow cytometry. The FCM procedure described estimates numbers of total bacteria in the processed sample, since SYTO BC binds to live culturable, live non-culturable, and dead cells.

This study demonstrates the ability of FCM to determine total bacterial numbers after clearing of milk and staining of bacteria with a reaily available fluorescent stain (SSC vs green fluorescence). The sensitivity of the FCM procedure was $\leq 10^4$ total bacteria ml of milk^{-1}.

Pianetti et al. (*2005*) proposed a protocol for the determination of the viability of *Aeromonas hydrophila* in different types of water by flow cytometry and compared this results with classical methods as spectrophotometric and plate count techniques. Flow cytometric determination of viability was carried out using a dual-staining technique that enabled us to distinguish viable bacteria from damaged and membrane-compromised bacteria, using simultaneous permeable (SYBR Green dyes) and impermeable fluorescent probe (PI). The traditional methods showed that the bacterial content was variable and dependent on the type of water. The results obtained from the plate count analysis correlated with the absorbance data. In contrast, the flow cytometric analysis results did not correlate with the results obtained by traditional methods; in fact, this technique showed that there were viable cells even when the optical density was low or no longer detectable and there was no plate count value. Furthermore, it permits fast detection of bacteria that are in a viable but nonculturable state, which are not detectable by conventional methods.

FCM can be used to demonstrate multiplexed detection of bacteria and toxins using fluorescent coded microspheres.

Antibodies specific for selected bacteria and toxins were conjugated to the coded microspheres to achieve sensitive and selective binding and detection. The respective limits of detection for bacteria and toxin are different (*Kim, 2009*). The microflow cytometer can detect for *Escherichia coli, Listeria*, and *Salmonella* 10^3, 10^5, and 10^4 cfu/mL, respectively, while the limits of detection for the toxins as cholera toxin, staphylococcal enterotoxin B, and ricin were 1.6, 0.064, and 1.6 ng/mL respectively (*Kim, 2009*).

3.1.2 Fungi

The use of FCM to detect fungal pathogens was first described by *Libertin et al.* in 1984 for *Pneumocystis carinii* (now *Pneumocystis jirovecii*) and following was evaluated by *Lapinsky* in 1991.

Pneumocystis jirovecii is an opportunistic pathogen responsible for severe pneumonia in immune-compromised patients. Its diagnosis has been based upon direct microscopy either by classic staining or by epifluorescence microscopy (immunofluorescence staining, IFS), both of which are time-consuming and low on sensitivity. Its aim was to develop a flow cytometric (FC) protocol for the detection of *P. jirovecii* on respiratory samples. *Barbosa et al. (2010)* analyzed in parallel by IFS and FC, 420 respiratory samples and compared the results with clinical diagnosis to its resolution upon specific anti-Pneumocystis therapy. The optimum specific antibody concentration for FC analysis was determined to be 10 μg/ml, without any cross-reactions to bacteria or fungi. All positive cases detected by IFS were positive by FC; however, FC classified eight samples to be positive which were classified as negative by routine technique. These samples were obtained from patients with respiratory symptoms who responded favourably to Pneumocystis-specific therapy and were subsequently considered to be true-positives. Using clinical diagnosis as a reference method, FC showed 100% sensitivity and specificity, whereas IFS showed 90.9% sensitivity and 100% specificity. According to their results, a new diagnostic approach is now available to detect *P. jirovecii* in respiratory samples.

Prigione et al. (2004) proposed an alternative study to traditional methods for the enumeration of airborne fungi: the possibility to evaluate by FCM the assessment of exposure to the fungus aerosol. They compared FCM with epifluorescence microscopy direct counting (gold standard). Setting up of the method was achieved with pure suspensions of *Aspergillus fumigatus* and *Penicillium brevicompactum* conidia at different concentrations, and then analyses were extended to field samples collected by an impinger device. Detection and quantification of airborne fungi by FCM was obtained combining light scatter and propidium iodide red fluorescence parameters. Since inorganic debris are unstainable with propidium iodide, the biotic component could be recognized, whereas the preanalysis of pure conidia suspensions of some species allowed us to select the area corresponding to the expected fungal population. Moreover, data processing showed that FCM can be considered more precise and reliable at any of the tested concentrations, and suggest that FCM could also be used to detect and quantify airborne fungi in environments different, including agricultural environments (*Prigione, 2004*).

Page et al. (2005) have developed two assays utilizing two different methods capable of identifying clinically important ascomycetous yeast species in a single-well test. They identified different species of *Candida* (*C. albicans, C. krusei, C. parapsilosis, C. glabrata, C. tropicalis*) using a direct hybridization method and allele-specific primer extension method. The amplicons are analyzed by FCM.

3.1.3 Parasites

FCM may also be applied to study parasites included analysis of the cell cycle, DNA quantification and analysis of membrane antigens. Specific clinical applications came later, when used associations of monoclonal antibodies, FCM, and immunofluorescence microscopy for the direct identification of parasites, as *Naegleria fowleri* and *Acanthamoeba spp.*, in clinical specimens (*Flores, 1990*).

Other applications of FCM regarding malaria's detection. The diagnosis of malaria is primarily cell-based and involves visual detection of intraerythrocytic parasites by transmitted light microscopy in a peripheral blood smear stained with Giemsa's stain, a mixture of eosin and methylene azure dyes first described over a century ago. Identification of the various stages of parasites depends heavily on morphologic information, requiring observation at high power. Although it has been known for many years that methods based on fluorescence microscopy, using acridine orange and other dyes, compare in accuracy with light microscopy and may require less time and a less skilled observer, the required fluorescent microscope has, until recently, been too expensive for most laboratories in areas where malaria is most prevalent. If malaria were more common in affluent countries, we might expect that cytometry would, by now, have supplanted microscopy of Giemsa stained smears for malaria diagnosis, just as it has for differential leukocyte counting and reticulocyte counting.

In clinical diagnosis, it is important to distinguish between malaria caused by *Plasmodium falciparum* and malaria due to the other species (*Shapiro, 2007*), because microscopy is an imperfect "Gold Standard" diagnostic device (*Makler, 1998*).

Many recent publications on cytometry in malaria (*Li, 2007*) have used asymmetric cyanine nucleic acid dyes of the SYTO and YOYO series. These dyes, structurally related to thiazole orange (*Makler, 1987*), can be excited with blue or blue-green (488 nm) light and emit in the green or yellow spectral region. Unlike acridine orange, which quenches on binding to nucleic acids, the cyanines are not DNA-selective and enhance fluorescence substantially on binding, typically by a factor of 1,000 or more; this results in lower background fluorescence, which makes it easier to detect smaller (haploid) forms of the malaria parasite (*Shapiro, 2007; Shapiro, 2010*).

Several approaches have been developed in the last few years to detect intracellular parasites, such as *Plasmodium;* but these all rely on clinical suspicion and, consequently, an explicit clinical request. Such work took adventage of the absence of DNA in erythrocytes. Thus, if the parasite is inside the cell, its DNA can be stained with specific fluorochromes and detected by FCM. The multiparameter analysis permitted by FCM can be used to study other characteristics, such as parasite antigens expressed by the erythrocyte (which can be detected by antibodies conjugated with fluorochromes) or the viability state of the parasitised cell using fresh or fixed cells (*Janse, 1994; Jouin, 1995*).

Although some methods lend themselves to automation (e.g. flow cytometry), no technique can yet be used for routine clinical automated screening. *Li et al.* (*2007*) have recently proposed a new methodology to measure a parasitemia of *Plasmodium falciparum* using flow cytometry analysis, because the microscopic analysis of patient blood smears represent an imperfect "Gold Standard" diagnostic device (*Makler, 1987*). In fact, there was reported significant misdiagnosis with regard to false positives (7–36%), false negatives (5–18%), and false species (13–15%) and an high frequency of technical errors (e.g. wrong pH or a poor quality film).

Different dyes, such as Hoechst 33258 (*Brown, 1980*), acridine orange (*Whaun, 1983*), thiazole orange (*Makler, 1987*), or hydroethidine (*Wyatt, 1991*), have been considered for the determination of parasitemia in cultures of *P. falciparum* by FCM.

Jacobberger et al. (*1984*) used DiOC1, a membrane potential responsive dye and Hoechst 33342 to evaluate parasitemia levels in mice (*Makler, 1987*). YOYO-1, a dimeric cyanine nucleic acid dye, is among the highest sensitivity fluorescent probes available for nucleic acid staining and has been added to this list (*Rye 1992; Barkan 2000*). YOYO-1 has an extremely high affinity for DNA, and it can be excited at 488 nm, which is the excitation wavelength available from most lasers employed in FCM. Its bright fluorescence signal and low background make it ideal for flow cytometric analysis of stained malaria nucleic acids (*Barkan, 2000; Jimenez-Diaz, 2005; Xie, 2007*). The FCM analysis in cultured *P. falciparum* models of malaria is impeded by significant reduction of reticulocytes and normocytes containing detectable amounts of nucleic acids after blood treated. Therefore, the absence of reticulocytes and normocytes may reduce the interference in measurement of parasitemia (*Hirons, 1994*). *Li et al.* (*2007*) compared FCM method to traditional microscopic analysis of blood smears and the microdilution radioisotope method for the evaluation of parasitemia in parasite culture with *P. falciparum*. They report a dual-parameter procedure using autofluorescence to make a distinction of infected erythrocytes from uninfected erythrocytes and normocytes. This method is particularly well suited for measuring low and high parasitemias and significantly increased the sensitivity.

Several reports show YOYO-1 is better than Hoechst 33258 to easily differentiate between uninfected and infected RBC when parasitemia is low. The parasites in the reticulocytes population should exhibit the same YOYO-1 associated fluorescence intensity as the parasites in the normal RBC. Compensation of YOYO-1 emission in FL-2 is an essential step whose only objective is to set up accurately the region of infected cell events. The region must be empirically determined by comparison of blood samples from uninfected and malaria infected rats by increasing compensation of YOYO-1 emission in FL-2 until a defined region for infected cell events is obtained (*Li, 2007*).

Other important parasite for malaria is *Plasmodium vivax* which preferentially invades reticulocytes. It is therefore relevant for vaccine development purposes to identify and characterize *P. vivax* proteins that bind specifically to the surface of reticulocytes. *Tran et al.* (*2005*) have developed a two-color flow cytometric erythrocyte binding assay (F-EBA) using the *P. vivax* Duffy binding protein region II (PvDBP-RII) recombinant protein as a model. This protein binds to all erythrocytes that express the Duffy receptor (Fy) and discriminates binding between normocytes and reticulocytes. This technique have several advantages over traditional erythrocyte binding assays (T-EBAs) used in malaria research. Interesting is the Malaria's detection with haematology analysers, as diagnostic tool in the work-up of febrile patients. For more than a decade, flow cytometry-based automated haematology analysers have been studied for malaria diagnosis, and recently work for incorporate into modern analysers different "malaria alert" especially in scenarios with low pre-test probability for the disease. Ideally, a flag for malaria could be incorporated and used to guide microscopic evaluation of the patient's blood to establish the diagnosis and start treatment promptly. Automation of a "malaria alarm" is currently possible for some analysers as Cell-Dyn®, Coulter® GEN S and LH 750, and the Sysmex XE-2100®.

The Cell-Dyn instruments use a multiple-angle polarized scatter separation for WBC analysis to distinguish eosinophils from neutrophils based on the light depolarizing properties of their granules, but has also been found to detect haemozoin-containing monocytes and granulocytes. The malaria-related events are shown in a scatter-plot with 90°

side-scatter on the x-axis and 90° depolarized side-scatter on the y-axis. Coulter GEN S and LH 750 haematology analysers use Volume-Conductance-Scatter (VCS) technology to obtain positional parameters of all WBC by measuring impedance for cell volume; radiofrequency conductivity for internal structure and nuclear characteristics; and flow cytometry-based helium-neon laser light scatter analysis for cellular granularity, nuclear lobularity and cell surface structure.

The Sysmex XE-2100 automated haematology analyser uses combined impedance and radiofrequency conductance detection, semiconductor diode laser light 90° side-scatter (SSC) and 0° frontal-scatter (FSC) detection, and polymethyne fluorescence nucleic acid staining 90° side-fluorescence (SFL) detection (*Campuzano-Zuluaga, 2010*).

Other applications of FCM regarding the use of FCM in combination with immunofluorescence, conventional or immunofluorescence microscopy for detection of samples containing small number of cysts as *Giardia lamblia* (*Dixon, 1997*).

In recent years, flow cytometry has been gaining in popularity as a novel method of detecting and enumerating different parasites as *Giardia* cysts and *Cryptosporidium* oocysts present in environmental and fecal samples (*Ferrari, 2003; Moss, 2001; Power, 2003*). Many papers reported flow cytometry as a method more sensitive than either conventional or immunofluorescence microscopy for the detection of *Giardia sp.* cysts in fecal samples (*Dixon, 1997; Dixon, 2002; Ferrari, 2003*), in detection of *Cryptosporidium* in SCID mice (*Arrowood, 1995*), seeded horse feces (*Cole, 1999*), and seeded human stool specimens (*Valdez, 1997*). In addition to detection and enumeration, large-scale sorting could also be used in conjunction with flow cytometry to yield partially purified oocysts for research purposes, such as food-spiking and recovery experiments, viability determination, or molecular characterization (*Dixon, 2005*).

All *Cryptosporidium* and *Giardia* surface monoclonal antibodies (mAbs) isolated thus far are directed against the same immunodominant epitope, therefore independent noncompeting mAbs are not available. Multiparameter FCM analysis largely depends on the use of noncompeting mAbs to quantify phenotype percentages or cellular activation.

Ferrari et al. (*2003*) proposed an analysis for detection of *Giardia* who combining Immunomagnetic Separation (IMS) and Two-Color flow cytometry (Green fluorescence vs Orange fluorescence). In particular a two-color assay using competing surface mAbs has been developed for the detection of *Cryptosporidium* oocysts. Regions were defined around mAb-PE–stained cysts (R1), FITC-stained cysts (R2), and dual-stained cysts (R3); a gate was defined whereby any particle present within R1, R2, and R3 was positive and was sorted on membranes for microscopic confirmation.

In this assay the immunoglobulin G1 (IgG1) oocyst wall-specific mAb CRY104 was conjugated to phycoerythrin (PE) and fluorescein isothiocyanate (FITC). The greatest specificity in water was obtained with this combination over other *Giardia* cysts were spiked into a backwash water sample with and without prior hybridization to peptide nucleic acid (PNA) probes. Immunomagnetic separation (IMS) as a pre-enrichment step was compared with filtration of the water sample. Cysts were recovered with two-color FCM. Those cysts hybridized with PNA and fluorescein isothiocyanate (FITC) were dual stained with monoclonal antibody (mAb) conjugated to phycoerythrin (PE); those not hybridized to PNA were dual stained with mAb-FITC and mAb-PE. A fourfold increase in fluorescent signal intensity was obtained when combining the mAb-PE and PNA probe compared with two-colors antibody staining. When combined with IMS, *Giardia* was successfully identified by FCM, with no false positives detected. Analysis-only FCM detection of *Giardia* in water is feasible. Further method development incorporating PNA probe hybridization after IMS is necessary.

Moreover, the authors developed PNA probes directed to *Cryptosporidium* oocysts, so a dual *Cryptosporidium* and *Giardia* detection method is possible. This method described can be used in small cytometers with no cell sorting capabilities. Such a system would provide a rapid, online method for screening water samples. This method using PNA probes also was species specific; therefore, water utilities would gain important information on the potential public health risks of a contamination event. This research demonstrated that analysis-only FCM detection of *Giardia* is feasible. To achieve the sensitivity required, a combination of IMS and two-color immunofluorescence staining with independent probes (mAb and PNA probe) was necessary, followed by two-color FCM analysis. Although we could detect the cysts, the cyst seed used was hybridized to the PNA probes before spiking in water. Further method development is required for the hybridization of cysts to be carried out after IMS and before FCM.

Cryptosporidium parvum is transmitted through water and can cause severe diarrhea. The diagnosis is usually based upon observer-dependent microscopic detection of oocysts, with rather low sensitivity and specificity. *Barbosa et al.* (*2008*) recently proposed a study with an objective to optimize a FCM protocol to detect *Criptosporidium parvum* oocysts in spiked human stools, using specific monoclonal antibodies. In particular, a specific monoclonal antibody conjugated with R-phycoerythrin was incubated with dead oocysts to determine the optimal antibody concentration, who was calculated in 3.0 mg/ml. Staining procedure was specific, as no cross-reactions were observed. This reliable and easy FC protocol allow the specific detection of *Cryptosporidium* oocysts, even at very low concentrations, which is important for public health and further studies of treatment efficacy.

Comparison of fluorescence signal intensities of *Cryptosporidium parvum* oocysts analyzed at FL2 showing autofluorescence of $2x10^5$ oocysts/ml and different concentrations of labeled oocysts with specific antibody (R-Phycoerythrin vs Counts) (*Barbosa, 2008*).

Dixon et al. (*2005*) involves an evaluation of the effectiveness of flow cytometry for the detection and enumeration of *Cyclospora cayetanensis* oocysts in human fecal specimens. Using flow cytometry, oocysts could be separated according to their autofluorescence, size, and complexity, and a cluster representing *Cyclospora* oocysts could be clearly observed on the dot plots of positive samples (autofluorescence vs SSC, with gate region R1 for *Cyclospora* oocysts). *Dixon et al.* concluded that while the sample preparation time for flow cytometry may be similar to or even longer than that for microscopy, depending upon the concentration and staining procedures used, the time it takes to analyze a sample by flow cytometry is considerably shorter than the time it takes to analyze a sample by microscopy. Sample analysis took only minutes, whereas microscopic examination is often a very time-consuming procedure. As a result, a larger number of samples could be analyzed by flow cytometry in a relatively short period of time. More importantly, as the method is largely automated, the results are not influenced by an analyst's levels of fatigue and expertise, as they may be with microscopy. While stool specimens are generally not examined for *Cyclospora* oocysts unless specifically requested, the results of the present study suggest that flow cytometry may be a useful alternative to microscopy in the screening of large numbers of fecal specimens for the presence of *Cyclospora* oocysts.

3.1.4 Virus

With FCM is possible to detect and quantify virus-infected cells present simultaneously (directly) in clinical samples, using antibodies that specifically recognize surface or internal antigens. We can investigate particular components of virus, as proteins or nucleic acids.

For example FCM could be applied to the detection of animal or human viruses in different clinical sample, such as the simultaneous detection of CMV, HSV, and HBV in organs destined for transplantation as well as in transplanted patients and co-infections in HIV-infected individuals.

It's possible discriminate stages of virus antigen expression (es. immediate-early, early, late) using monoclonal antibodies, detect viremia or FCM can be applied in a single device for the detection of HIV-1 viral load in association with other parameters to monitoring in the blood the success of antiretroviral therapy (HAART), as: CD4 Tcell count, CD4 percentage of lymphocytes (CD4%), and viral load (*Greeve, 2009*).

Greeve et al. (*2009*) proposed a new viral load test based on flow cytometric to detect HIV-1 viral load. They performed a FCS/SSC plot, and set a gate on each population, using PE-specific fluorescence and measure the sample in fluorescence 2 (FL2 with a 590 nm bandpass filter). In particular ten thousand events were collected, and the mean fluorescence intensity was calculated by setting a range over the whole measuring scale (0–1,000) in FL2 (log 4) separately for each microbead population.

Different methods have been routinely used to detect specific antibodies to viral antigens (ELISA, complement fixation, indirect immune-fluorescence microscopy, Western blotting), but the detection and quantification of antibodies to viral antigens can be carried out by FCM.

This technique has been used to detect and quantify antibodies to CMV, herpesvirus (HSV-1 and HSV-2), hepatitis C virus (HCV) and HIV-1 virus.

3.1.4.1 Detection and quantification of viral antigens

FCM can detect viral antigens other on the surface and/or within infected cells. It can rapidly detect and quantify virus-infected cells using antibodies that specifically recognize surface or internal antigens; in the latter case, permeabilization of the cells is required.

Direct and indirect fluorescent-antibody methods are used. Direct detection involves the use of fluorescently labeled antibody (labeled with FITC or phycoerythrin). In the indirect fluorescent-antibody method, unlabeled antibody is bound to infected cells, which are then incubated with fluorescence-labeled anti-Ig that binds to the first viral antibody.

Based on the potential of FCM for multiparametric analysis, there are two key advantages to its use in studying viral infection: its ability to analyze several parameters in single infected cells at the same time and its ability not only to detect but also to quantify infected cells. These parameters may be related to particular components or events of the infected cell or components (proteins or nucleic acids) of the virus. For this reason, FCM has been a powerful tool to characterize the mechanisms of viral pathogenesis. Furthermore, FCM allows simultaneous detection of several viruses in a sample by using antibodies to different viral antigens conjugated to different fluorochromes, or specific viral antibodies conjugated to latex particles of different sizes. As stated above, the presence of different viral antigens is detected by differences in the forward-scattered light as a consequence of the different sized particle used for each antibody. Different plant, animal or human viruses in any clinical sample is possible simultaneously detected.

3.1.4.2 Detection and quantification of viral nucleic acids

The emergence of PCR and RT-PCR techniques has allowed the highly sensitive detection of specific viral nucleic acids (DNA or RNA) in virus-infected cells. These methods are indeed the most sensitive for the detection and characterization of viral genomes, especially in rare target viral sequences. However, the association between the viral nucleic acid and an individual cell is lost, and therefore no information about productively infected cell populations is obtained by this method. FCM analysis of fluorescent in situ hybridization in cell suspension overcomes this problem, since this assay can be coupled with simultaneous cell phenotyping (by using specific antibodies to different cell markers).

With FCM is possible to monitor EBV-infected cells in blood sample using in situ hybridization combined use with two or more fluorochromes.

3.2 Serological diagnosis

The diagnosis of acute hepatitis C virus (HCV) infection is based on the detection in serum or plasma of HCV RNA, anti-HCV IgG, and elevation of alanine aminotransferase levels. However, none of these markers alone or in combination can be used to identify acute infection, since they may also be detectable during the chronic phase of infection.

Araujo et al. (*2011*) developed a multiplexed, flow-cytometric microsphere immunoassay, to measure simultaneously anti-HCV-IgG responses to multiple structural (E1, E2, core) and nonstructural (NS3, NS4, NS5) HCV recombinant proteins. Furthermore this assay has the potential to discriminate between the acute and chronic phases by testing of single specimens (*Araujo, 2011*).

The detection of specific antibody to HCV is an important assay in the identification of individuals infected with HCV. Routinely screening (enzyme immunoassay or EIA) and confirmation analysis (recombinant immunoblot assay or RIBA) of blood sample is well addressed using the commercially available assays. *McHugh et al.* (*2005*) considered that the increased rate of false-positive antibody test results coupled with the data indicating that the concentration of HCV specific antibody can help to indicate the likelihood of antibody positivity proposed a semi-quantitative assay to improvement the resolution of low levels of specific HCV antibody using microsphere assay.

Bhaduri-McIntosh et al. (*2007*) propose flow cytometry–based assay to investigated IgA antibodies are a marker for primary Epstein-Barr virus (EBV) infection, and compared this assay to presence of IgM antibodies to viral capsid antigen and the absence of antibodies to EB nuclear antigen (EBNAs). The authors compare the occurrence of IgA serologic responses to EBV total antigens and early antigen (EAs) during primary EBV infection and in healthy individuals persistently infected with EBV, for differentiation between individuals with primary EBV infection and healthy EBV-seropositive individuals, using flow cytometry–based assay.

The use of flow cytometry to measure the number of infected cells has been demonstrated previously for other types of viruses (*McSharry, 2000*). These methods were aimed at the measurement to quantify virus infectivity in a sample previously infected with a virus suspension and relied on the assumption that only one round of infection had occurred and that virus adhesion is quantitative and synchronous. These has been described for various enveloped and non-enveloped viruses.

These studies are based on direct enumeration of infected cells in the flow cytometer and discrimination from noninfected cells by immunostaining using monoclonal antibodies specific for viral antigens.

Recently *Gates et al.* (*2009*) introduced a semi-automated flow cytometry protocol to quantitative measurement of Varicella-Zoster Virus Infection. They describe an alternate infectivity assay for the attenuated VZV strain, based on the enumeration of infected cells 24 to 72 h post-infection by semi-automated capillary flow cytometry. The discrimination of infected cells from non infected cells is performed by indirect immunofluorescence to detect the expression of viral glycoproteins on the surface of infected cells. The new assay provides a rapid, higher-throughput alternative to the classical plaque assay. It was used a semi permeable vitality dye (7-AAD) to identify and quantify live-infected cells.

Measurement of VZV infection using flow cytometry was made considering FSC (x axis) and red fluorescence intensity channel (RED; y axis) correlation dot plot showing selective gating on 7-AAD-negative events (live cells and non nucleated debris) and tested monoclonal antibodies which are directed at both immediate early/early genes (IE62) and late, structural proteins (VZV gE, gI, gB, and gH and MCP) and were titrated to measure mean fluorescence intensities at saturation (*Gates, 2009*).

Lemos et al. (*2007*) developed a flow cytometry-based methodology to detect anti-*Leishmania* (*Leishmania*) *chagasi* immunoglobulin G as a reliable serological approach to monitor post-therapeutical cure in patients affected by Visceral Leishmaniasis. They have demonstrated that although conventional serology (indirect immunofluorescence and enzyme-linked immunosorbent assay) remained positive after treatment, the antimembrane-specific antibodies detected by flow cytometry were present only during active disease and not detected after successful chemotherapy.

Similar work was proposed by *Rocha et al.* (*2006*) for clinical value of anti-live *Leishmania* (Viannia) *braziliensis* immunoglobulin G subclasses for diagnosing active localized cutaneous leishmaniasis.

3.3 Antimicrobial effects and susceptibility testing by flow cytometry

In the 1990s, there were interesting advances in this field from microbiology laboratories, and the number of scientific articles addressing the antimicrobial responses of bacteria (including mycobacteria), fungi, and parasites to antimicrobial agents increased considerably (*Gant, 1993*).

FCM has proved to be very useful for studying the physiological effects of antimicrobial agents (bactericidal or bacteriostatic effect) on bacterial cells due to their effect on particular metabolic parameters (membrane potential, cell size, and amount of DNA).

Pina-Vaz et al. (*2005*) described a flow cytometric assay, simple, fast, safe and accurate, to assess the susceptibility of *Mycobacterium tuberculosis* to the antimicrobial susceptibility (streptomycin, isoniazid, rifampicin, ethambutol) and compared it with standard laboratory procedure (BACTEC MGIT 960). The described assay is a quick, safe and accurate method, as heatinactivated mycobacteria cells are analysed following staining with SYTO 16, a nucleic acid stain, which distinguishes them from debris. The time needed to obtain susceptibility results of *Mycobacterium tuberculosis* using classical methodologies is still too long (two months), and flow cytometry is a promising technique in the setting of the clinical laboratory, giving fast results. A safe, reliable and rapid method to study susceptibility to streptomycin, isoniazide, rifampicin and ethambutol is described. Isolates of mycobacteria, grown for 72 h in the absence or presence of antimycobacterial drugs in the mycobacteria growth indicator tube (MGIT), were heat-killed, stained with SYTO 16 (a nucleic acid fluorescent stain that only penetrates cells with severe lesion of the membrane) and then analysed by flow cytometry. Comparing the intensity of fluorescence of *Mycobacterium* cells incubated with antimycobacterial drugs with that of drug-free cells, after staining with SYTO 16, it was possible to distinguish between sensitive, intermediate and resistant phenotypes. Bacterial cells respond to different antimicrobial agents by decreasing or increasing their membrane potential. Antimicrobial susceptibility show a decrease in green fluorescence (live cells) and an increase in red fluorescence (dead cells).

Piuri et al. (*2009*) describe a virus-based assay in which fluoro-mycobacteriophages are used to deliver a GFP or ZsYellow fluorescent marker gene to *M. tuberculosis*, which can then be monitored by fluorescent detection approaches including fluorescent microscopy and flow cytometry. Pre-clinical evaluations show that addition of either Rifampicin or Streptomycin at the time of phage addition obliterates fluorescence in susceptible cells but not in isogenic resistant bacteria enabling drug sensitivity determination in less than 24 hours. Detection requires no substrate addition, fewer than 100 cells can be identified, and resistant bacteria can be detected within mixed populations. Fluorescence withstands fixation by paraformaldehyde providing enhanced biosafety for testing MDR-TB and XDR-TB infections (*Piuri, 2009*).

3.4 Monitoring of infections and antimicrobial therapy

FCM can be used to monitoring patient's responses to antimicrobial treatments during the infections' treatment with antimicrobial therapy.

Rudensky et al. (*2005*) develop a rapid flow-cytometric antifungal susceptibility test for determining susceptibility of different species of *Candida* to fluconazole and echinocandin, and compare results with the standard methods (MIC determined by macrodilution and/or Etest according to National Committee for Clinical Laboratory Standard, now Clinical laboratory and Standard Institute).

They used reference and laboratory strains of *Candida* (*C. albicans, C. tropicalis, C. parapsilosis, C. glabrata, C. krusei*) who tested for susceptibility to fluconazole and echinocandin by fluorescent flow cytometry using Acridine Orange (AO) as indicator of viability (AO fluorescence versus SSC). The flow method produced results in 5 h or less, and give excellent sensitivity and specificity to distinguish between sensitive, susceptible dose-dependent and resistant strains. The advantages of this method is to produce daily results and assist clinicians in the selection of appropriate antifungal therapy. The method is easy, reproducible, permit to measure the percentage of damaged yeasts in relation with drug concentration, and can be implemented in any laboratory with access to a flow cytometer.

In the same period, *Ramani et al.* (*2003*) test with FCM antifungal susceptibility of *Aspergillus fumigates* against three important antifungal (voriconazole, amphotericin B and itraconazole) used in therapy of aspergillosis. The results obtained within 3 to 4 h proved to be a reliable indicator of a drug's antifungal activity against *A. fumigatus* isolates, and indicate a good correlation with the drug MICs obtained by the CLSI broth microdilution method.

Flow cytometry can be used to monitoring anti-leishmanial drugs susceptibility (pentavalent antimonial, pentamidine, amphotericin B, sodium stibogluconate). In particular, *Singh and Dube* (*2004*) proposed a flow citometry assay based on green fluorescent protein a marker for *Leishmania* causing kala-azar (visceral leishmaniasis) and for transgenic *L. donovani* promastigotes that constitutively express GFP in their cytoplasm.

3.5 Other application of flow cytometry

Several strategies to optimize the detection of bacterial contamination in platelet preparations (PLTs) have been examined in the past. In fact, bacterial contamination is the major infectious hazard associated with transfusion of PLTs.

Screening of PLTs for bacterial contamination by prospective culture testing has been implemented as part of the quality assurance program in several blood services. Despite screening of PLTs for bacterial contamination by culture, it has been demonstrated that there is still a substantial infection risk associated with transfusing PLTs, and septic complications have been observed in recipients (*Dreier, 2009*).

Routine testing for bacterial contamination in PLTs has become common, but transfusion-transmitted bacterial sepsis has not been eliminated. *Dreier et al.* (*2009*) describe a new flow cytometry-based method for point-of-issue screening of PLTs for bacterial contamination. They used flow cytometry to detect and count bacteria based on esterase activity in viable cells, and compared the flow-cytometric assay to incubation culture system and rapid nucleic acid-based or immunoassay (reverse transcription PCR) methods.

Flow cytometry is rapidly becoming an essential tool in the field of aquatic microbiology. *Wang et al.* (2010) proposed an interesting application of FCM in aquatic microbiology, in the development range from straightforward total cell counts to community structure analysis, and further extend to physiological analysis at a single-cell level (*Wang, 2010*).

Hammes and Egli (2010) describe as the rapid detection of microbial cells is a challenge in microbiology, particularly when complex indigenous communities or subpopulations varying in viability, activity and physiological state are investigated. Numerous FCM applications have emerged in industrial biotechnology, food and pharmaceutical quality control, routine monitoring of drinking water and wastewater systems, and microbial ecological research in soils and natural aquatic habitats. They focused the information that can be gained from the analysis of bacteria in water, highlighting some of the main advantages, pitfalls and applications (*Hammes, 2010)*.

In fact *Comas-Riu and Rius* (2009) proposed a mini-review to gives an overview of the principles of flow cytometry and examples of the application of this technique in the food industry. By analysing large numbers of cells individually using light-scattering and fluorescence measurements, this technique reveals both cellular characteristics and the levels of cellular components. Flow cytometry has been developed to rapidly enumerate microorganisms; to distinguish between viable, metabolically active and dead cells, which is of great importance in food development and food spoilage; and to detect specific pathogenic microorganisms by conjugating antibodies with fluorochromes, which is of great use in the food industry. In addition, high-speed multiparametric data acquisition, analysis and cell sorting, which allow other characteristics of individual cells to be studied, have increased the interest of food microbiologists in this technique (*Comas-Riu and Rius, 2009*).

Penders et al. (*2004*) proposed an automated flow cytometry analysis of peritoneal dialysis fluid. Peritonitis is the major frequent complication of peritoneal dialysis fluid. The diagnosis and effective treatment of peritonitis depends on clinical evaluation and correlation with laboratory examination of the dialysate. Various techniques have been used to facilitate the recovery of microorganisms from dialysate, among them the use of selected broth media, processing of large volumes of dialysis effluent by concentration techniques or total volume culture. Nevertheless, microorganisms are not always recovered from dialysate during peritonitis. The authors have evaluated the possibilities to applied flow cytometry in the analysis of peritoneal dialysis fluid. In particular they have analyzed 135 samples with automated instrument Sysmex UF-100 and compared the obtained data with those of counting chamber techniques, biochemical analysis and bacterial culture (*Penders, 2004*). They concluded that flow cytometric analysis can be an useful additional tool for peritoneal dialysis fluid examination, especially in the emergency setting for detect leukocytes, bacteria and/or yeast cells.

Another application of flow cytometry regards screening of urine sample (*Jolkkonen, 2010; Pieretti, 2011*).

Urinary tract infection (UTI) is a widespread disease, and thus, the most common samples tested in diagnostic microbiology laboratories are urine samples. The "gold standard" for diagnosis is still bacterial culture, but a large proportion of samples are negative. Unnecessary culture can be reduced by an effective screening test. *Pieretti et al.* (*2011*) have evaluated the performance of a new urine cytometer, the Sysmex UF-1000i (Dasit), on 703 urine samples submitted to our laboratory for culture. They have compared bacteria and leukocyte (WBC) counts performed with the Sysmex UF-1000i to CFU-per-milliliter quantification on CPS agar to assess the best cutoff values. Different cutoff values of bacteria/ml and WBC/ml were compared to give the best discrimination. On the basis of the results obtained in this study, we suggest that when the Sysmex UF-1000i analyzer is used as a screening test for UTI the cutoff values should be 65 bacteria/ml and 100 WBC/ml. Diagnostic performance in terms of sensitivity (98.2%), specificity (62.1%), negative predictive value (98.7%), positive predictive value (53.7%), and diagnostic accuracy (73.3%) were satisfactory. The authors concluded that the screening with the Sysmex UF-1000i is acceptable and applicable for routine use because have reduced the number of bacterial cultures by 43% and decreased the inappropriate use of antibiotics.

Similar study was proposed by *Jolkkonen et al.* (*2010*).

Li et al. (*2010*) have demonstrated as FCM represent a rapid and quantitative method to detect infectious Adenoviruses in environmental water and clearly distinguish them from inactivated viruses. This method has the potential for application in detection of infectious Adenoviruses in environments and evaluation of viral stability and inactivation during the water treatment and disinfection's process.

Cantera et al. (*2010*) described an alternative approach at classical serological and viral nucleic acid detection, that utilizes engineered cells expressing fluorescent proteins undergoing fluorescence resonance energy transfer (FRET) upon cleavage by the viral 2A protease (2Apro) as an indication of infection. Quantification of the infectious-virus titers was resolved by using flow cytometry, and utility was demonstrated for the detection of poliovirus 1 (PV1) infection.

Those methods, however, are time-consuming and labor-intensive, as the procedures included cell fixation, permeabilization, labeling, and washing steps prior to flow cytometry. Viral titers determined by FC were comparable to titers obtained by the plaque assay.

4. Concluding remarks and future perspectives

In this chapter we remark the different applications of flow cytometry in clinical microbiology.

It's a wide field for many aspects still to be explored, and for future we think that it's very important introduce automation in routine of clinical microbiology laboratories the flow cytometric assay, but is necessary optimize the cost-benefit ratio of FCM.

5. Acknowledgments

We would like to thank you all referenced Authors since, due to their works, we were able to finalize this chapter.

6. References

Alvarez-Barrientos, A., Arroyo, J., Cantòn, R., Nombela, C., & Sànchez-Pérez, M. (2000). Applications of Flow Cytometry to Clinical Microbiology. *Clinical Microbiology Reviews*. Vol. 13, No. 2, pp. 167–195, ISSN: 0893-8512.

Araujo, A.C., Astrakhantseva, IV., Fields, H.A., & Kamili S. (2011). Distinguishing Acute from Chronic Hepatitis C Virus (HCV) Infection Based on Antibody Reactivities to Specific HCV Structural and Nonstructural Proteins. *Journal of Clinical Microbiology*. Vol. 49, No. 1, pp. 54–57, ISSN: 0095-1137.

Arrowood, M.J., Hurd, M.R., & Mead, J.R. (1995). A new method for evaluating experimental cryptosporidial parasite loads using immunofluorescent flow cytometry. *The Journal of Parasitology*. Vol. 81, pp. 404–409, ISSN: 0022-3395.

Barbosa, J., Bragada, C., Costa-de-Oliveira, S., Ricardo, E., Rodrigues, A.G., & Pina-Vaz, C. (2010). A new method for the detection of *Pneumocystis jirovecii* using flow cytometry. *European Journal of Clinical Microbiology and Infection Diseases*. Vol. 29, No. 9, pp. 1147-1152, ISSN: 0934-9723.

Barbosa, J.M., Costa-de-Oliveira, S., Rodrigues, A.G., Hanscheid, T., Shapiro, H., & Pina-Vaz, C. (2008). A Flow Cytometric Protocol for Detection of *Cryptosporidium spp*. *Cytometry Part A*. Vol. 73, pp. 44-47, ISSN: 1552-4922.

Barkan, D., Ginsburg, H., & Golenser, J. (2000). Optimisation of flow cytometric measurement of parasitaemia in plasmodium-infected mice. *International Journal for Parasitology*. Vol. 30, pp. 649–653, ISSN: 0020-7519.

Bhaduri-McIntosh, S., Landry, M.L., Nikiforow, S., Rotenberg, M., El-Guindy, A., & Miller, G. (2007). Serum IgA Antibodies to Epstein-Barr Virus (EBV) Early Lytic Antigens Are Present in Primary EBV Infection. *The Journal of Infectious Diseases*. Vol. 195, pp. 483-492, ISSN: 0022-1899.

Brehm-Stecher, B.F., & Johnson, E.A. (2004). Single-Cell Microbiology: Tools, Technologies, and Applications. *Microbiology And Molecular Biology Reviews*. Vol. 68, No. 3, pp. 538–559, ISSN: 1092-2172.

Brown, G.V., Battye, F.L., & Howard, R.J. (1980). Separation of stages of *P. falciparum*-infected cells by means of fluorescence activated cell sorter. *The American Journal of Tropical Medicine and Hygiene*. Vol. 29, pp. 1147–1149, ISSN: 0002-9637.

Campuzano-Zuluaga, G., Hänscheid, T., & Grobusch, M.P. (2010). Automated haematology analysis to diagnose malaria. Review. *Malaria Journal*. Vol. 9, pp. 346-361, ISSN: 1475-2875.

Cantera, J.L., Chen, W., & Yates, M.V. (2010). Detection of Infective Poliovirus by a Simple, Rapid, and Sensitive Flow Cytometry Method Based on Fluorescence Resonance Energy Transfer Technology. *Applied and Environmental Microbiology*. Vol. 76, No. 2, pp. 584–588, ISSN: 0099-2240.

Cole, D.J., Snowden, K., Cohen, N.D., & Smith, R. (1999). Detection of *Cryptosporidium parvum* in horses: thresholds of acid-fast stain, immunofluorescence assay, and flow cytometry. *Journal of Clinical Microbiology*. Vol. 37, pp. 457–460, ISSN: 0095-1137.

Comas-Riu, J., & Rius, N. (2009). Flow cytometry applications in the food industry. *Journal of Industrial Microbiology & Biotechnology*. Vol. 36, No. 8, pp. 999-1011, ISSN: 1637-5435.

Davey, H.M., & Kell, D.B. (1996). Bacterial Detection and Live/Dead Discrimination by Flow Cytometry. Flow cytometry and cell sorting of heterogeneous microbial populations: the importance of single cell analyses. *Microbiological Reviews*. Vol. 60, pp. 641-696, ISSN: 0146-0749.

Dixon, B.R., Parenteau, M., Martineau, C., & Fournier, J. (1997). A comparison of conventional microscopy, immunofluorescence microscopy and flow cytometry in the detection of *Giardia lamblia* cysts in beaver fecal samples. *Journal of Immunological Methods*. Vol. 202, pp. 27–33, ISSN: 0022-1759.

Dixon, B.R., Bussey J., Parrington, L., Parenteau, M., Moore, R., Jacob, J., Parenteau, M.P., & Fournier., J. (2002). A preliminary estimate of the prevalence of *Giardia sp.* in beavers in Gatineau Park, Quebec, using flow cytometry. In: B. E. Olson, M. E. Olson, and P. M. Wallis (ed.), Giardia: the cosmopolitan parasite. CAB International, Wallingford, United Kingdom, pp. 71–79, ISBN: 9780851996127.

Dixon, B.R., Bussey, J.M., Parrington, L.J., & Parenteau, M. (2005). Detection of *Cyclospora cayetanensis* Oocysts in Human Fecal Specimens by Flow Cytometry. *Journal of Clinical Microbiology*. Vol. 43, No. 5, pp. 2375–2379, ISSN: 0095-1137.

Dreier, J., Vollmer, T., & Kleesiek, K. (2009). Novel Flow Cytometry–Based Screening for Bacterial Contamination of Donor Platelet Preparations Compared with Other

Rapid Screening Methods. *Clinical Chemistry*. Vol. 55, No. 8, pp. 1492–1502, ISSN: 0009-9147.

Ferrari, B.C., & Veal, D. (2003). Analysis-only detection of *Giardia* by combining immunomagnetic separation and two-color flow cytometry. *Cytometry Part A*. Vol. 51, pp. 79–86, ISSN: 1552-4922.

Flores, B.M., Garcia, C.A., Stamm, W.E., & Torian, B.E. (1990). Differentiation of *Naegleria fowleri* from *Acanthamoeba* species by using monoclonal antibodies and flow cytometry. *Journal of Clinical Microbiology*. Vol. 28, pp. 1999–2005, ISSN: 0095-1137.

Fouchet, P., Jayat, C., Héchard, Y., Ratinaud, M.H., & Frelat, G. (1993). Recent advances of flow cytometry in fundamental and applied microbiology. *Biology of the Cell*. Vol. 78, No. 1-2, pp. 95-109, ISSN: 0248-4900.

Füchslin, H.P., Kötzsch, S., Keserue, H.A., & Egli, T. (2010). Rapid and Quantitative Detection of *Legionella pneumophila* Applying Immunomagnetic Separation and Flow Cytometry. *Cytometry Part A*. Vol. 77A, pp. 264-274, ISSN: 1552-4922.

Gant, V.A., Warnes, G., Phillips, I., & Savidge, G.F. (1993). The application of flow cytometry to the study of bacterial responses to antibiotics. *Journal of Medical Microbiology*. Vol. 39, pp. 147-154, ISSN: 0022-2615.

Gates, I.V., Zhang, Y., Shambaugh, C., Bauman, M.A., Tan, C., & Bodmer, J.L. (2009). Quantitative Measurement of Varicella-Zoster Virus Infection by Semi-automated Flow Cytometry. *Applied and Environmental Microbiology*. Vol. 75, No. 7, pp. 2027–2036, ISSN: 0099-2240.

Greve, B., Weidner, J., Cassens, U., Odaibo, G., Olaleye, D., Sibrowski, W., Reichelt, D., Nasdala, I., & Göhde, W. (2009). A New Affordable Flow Cytometry Based Method to Measure HIV-1 Viral Load. *Cytometry Part A*. Vol. 75, pp. 199-206, ISSN: 1552-4922.

Gunasekera, T.S., Attfield, P.V., & Veal, D.A. (2000). A Flow Cytometry Method for Rapid Detection and Enumeration of Total Bacteria in Milk. *Applied and Environmental Microbiology*. Vol. 66, No. 3, pp. 1228–1232, ISSN: 0099-2240.

Hammes, F., & Egli, T. (2010). Cytometric methods for measuring bacteria in water: advantages, pitfalls and applications. *Analytical and Bioanalytical Chemistry*. Vol. 397, No. 3, pp.1083-1095, ISSN: 1618-2642.

Hirons, G.T., Fawcett, J.J., & Crissman, HA. (1994). TOTO and YOYO: New very bright fluorochromes for DNA content analysis by flow cytometry. *Cytometry*. Vol. 15, pp. 129–140, ISSN: 0196-4763.

Jacobberger, J.W., Horan, P.K., & Hare, J,D. (1984). Flow cytometric analysis of blood cells stained with the cyanine dye DiOC1[3]: reticulocyte quantification. *Cytometry*. Vol. 5, pp. 589–600, ISSN: 0196-4763.

Janse, C.J., & Van Vianen, P.H. (1994). Flow cytometry in malaria detection. *Methods in Cell Biology*. Vol. 42 (B), pp. 295–318, ISSN: 0091-679X.

Jimenez-Diaz, M.B., Rullas, J., Mulet, T., Fernández, L., Bravo, C., Gargallo-Viola, D., & Angulo-Barturen, I. (2005). Improvement of detection specificity of Plasmodium-infected murine erythrocytes by flow cytometry using autofluorescence and YOYO-1. *Cytometry Part A*. Vol. 67, pp. 27–36, ISSN: 1552-4922.

Jolkkonen, S., Paattiniemi, E.L., Kärpänoja, P., & Sarkkinen, H. (2010). Screening of Urine Samples by Flow Cytometry Reduces the Need for Culture. *Journal of Clinical Microbiology*. Vol. 48, No. 9, pp. 3117–3121, ISSN: 0095-1137.

Jouin, H., Goguet de la Salmonière, Y.O., Behr, C., Huyin Qan Dat, M., Michel, J.C., Sarthou, J.L., Pereira da Silva, L., & Dubois, P. (1995). Flow cytometry detection of surface antigens on fresh, unfixed red blood cells infected by *Plasmodium falciparum*. *Journal of Immunology Methods*. Vol. 179, pp. 1–12, ISSN: 0022-1759.

Khan, M.M., Pyle, B.H., & Camper, A.K. (2010). Specific and Rapid Enumeration of Viable but Nonculturable and Viable-Culturable Gram-Negative Bacteria by Using Flow Cytometry. *Applied and Environmental Microbiology*. Vol. 76, No. 15, pp. 5088–5096, ISSN: 0099-2240.

Kim, J.S., Anderson, G.P., Erickson, J.S., Golden, J.P., Nasir, M., & Ligler, F.S. (2009). Multiplexed Detection of Bacteria and Toxins Using a Microflow Cytometer. *Analytical Chemestry*. Vol. 81, No. 13, pp. 5426–5432, ISSN: 0003-2700.

Kramer, A., Schwebke, I., & Kampf, G. (2006). How long do nosocomial pathogens persist on inanimate surfaces? A systematic review. *BMC Infectious Diseases*. Vol. 6, page 130, ISSN: 1471-2334.

Lapinsky, S.E., Glencross, D., Car, N.G., Kallenbach, J.M., & Zwi, Set. (1991). Quantification and Assessment of Viability of *Pneumocystis carinii* Organisms by Flow Cytometry. *Journal of Clinical Microbiology*. Vol. 29, No. 5, pp. 911-915, ISSN: 0095-1137.

Lemos, E.M., Gomes, I.T., Carvalho, S.F., Rocha, R.D., Pissinate, J.F., Martins-Filho, O.A., & Dietze, R. (2007). Detection of Anti-*Leishmania* (*Leishmania*) *chagasi* Immunoglobulin G by Flow Cytometry for Cure Assessment following Chemotherapeutic Treatment of American Visceral Leishmaniasis. *Clinical and Vaccine Immunology*. Vol. 14, No. 5, pp. 569–576, ISSN: 1556-6811.

Li, Q., Gerena, L., Xie, L., Zhang, J., Kyle, D., & Milhous, W. (2007). Development and Validation of Flow Cytometric Measurement for Parasitemia in Cultures of *P. falciparum* Vitally Stained with YOYO-1. *Cytometry Part A*. Vol. 71, pp. 297-307, ISSN: 1552-4922.

Li., D., He, M., & Jiang, S.C. (2010). Detection of Infectious Adenoviruses in Environmental Waters by Fluorescence-Activated Cell Sorting Assay. *Applied And Environmental Microbiology*. Vol. 76, No. 5, pp. 1442–1448, ISSN: 0099-2240.

Libertin, C.R., Woloschak, G.E., Wilson, W.R., & Smith, T.F. (1984). Analysis of *Pneumocystis carinii* cysts with a fluorescence-activated cell sorter. *Journal of Clinical Microbiology*. Vol. 20, pp. 877–880, ISSN: 0095-1137.

Loehfelm, T.W., Luke, N.R., & Campagnari, A.A. (2008). Identification and Characterization of an *Acinetobacter baumannii* Biofilm-Associated Protein. *Journal of Bacteriology*. Vol. 190, No. 3, pp. 1036–1044, ISSN: 0021-9193.

Makler, M.T., Lee, L.G., & Recktenwald, D. (1987). Thiazole orange: A new dye for Plasmodium species analysis. *Cytometry*. Vol. 8, pp. 568–570, ISSN: 0196-4763.

Makler, M.T., Palmer, C.J., & Ager, A.L. (1998). A review of practical techniques for the diagnosis of malaria. *Annals of Tropical Medicine and Parasitology*. Vol. 92, pp. 419–433, ISSN: 0003-4983.

McHugh T.M. (2005). Performance Characteristics of a Microsphere Immunoassay Using Recombinant HCV Proteins as a Confirmatory Assay for the Detection of Antibodies to the Hepatitis C Virus. *Cytometry Part A*. Vol. 67, pp. 97-103, ISSN: 1552-4922.

McHugh, I.O., & Tucker, A.L. (2007). Flow Cytometry for the Rapid Detection of Bacteria in Cell Culture Production Medium. *Cytometry Part A*. Vol. 71, pp. 1019-1026, ISSN: 1552-4922.

McSharry J.J. (2000). Analysis of virus-infected cells by flow cytometry. *Methods*. Vol. 21, pp. 249–257, ISSN: 1046-2023.

Moss, D.M., & Arrowood, M.J. (2001). Quantification of *Cryptosporidium parvum* oocysts in mouse fecal specimens using immunomagnetic particles and two-color flow cytometry. *The Journal of Parasitology*. Vol. 87, pp. 406–412, ISSN: 0022-3395.

Mueller, S., & Davey, H. (2009). Recent Advances in the Analysis of Individual Microbial Cells. *Cytometry Part A*. Vol. 75A, pp. 83-85, ISSN: 1552-4922.

Page, B.T., & Kurtzman, C.P. (2005). Rapid Identification of *Candida* species and Other Clinically Important Yeast Species by Flow Cytometry. *Journal of Clinical Microbiology*. Vol. 43, No. 9, pp. 4507–4514, ISSN: 0095-1137.

Penders, J., Fiers, T., Dhondt, A.M., Claeys, G., & Delanghe, J.R. (2004). Automated flow cytometry analysis of peritoneal dialysis fluid. *Nephrology, dialysis, transplantation : official publication of the European Dialysis and Transplant Association - European Renal Association*. Vol. 19, pp. 463–468, ISSN: 0931-0509.

Pianetti, A., Falcioni, T., Bruscolini, F., Sabatini, L., Sisti, E., & Papa, S. (2005). Determination of the Viability of *Aeromonas hydrophila* in Different Types of Water by Flow Cytometry, and Comparison with Classical Methods. *Applied and Environmental Microbiology*. Vol. 71, No. 12, pp. 7948–7954, ISSN: 0099-2240.

Pieretti, B., Brunati, P., Pini, B., Colzani, C., Congedo, P., Rocchi, M., & Terramocci, R. (2010). Diagnosis of Bacteriuria and Leukocyturia by Automated Flow Cytometry Compared with Urine Culture. *Journal of Clinical Microbiology*. Vol. 48, No. 11, pp. 3990-3996, ISSN: 0095-1137.

Pina-Vaz, C., Costa-de-Oliveira, S., & Rodrigues, AG. (2005). Safe susceptibility testing of *Mycobacterium tuberculosis* by flow cytometry with the fluorescent nucleic acid stain SYTO 16. *Journal of Medical Microbiology*. Vol. 54, pp. 77–81, ISSN: 0095-1137.

Piuri, M., Jacobs, W.R. Jr., & Hatfull, G.F. (2009). Fluoromycobacteriophages for Rapid, Specific, and Sensitive Antibiotic Susceptibility Testing of *Mycobacterium tuberculosis*. *PLoS One*. Vol. 4, No. 3, pp. 1-12, ISSN: 1932-6203.

Power, M.L., Shanker, S.R., Sangster, N.C., & Veal, DA. (2003). Evaluation of a combined immunomagnetic separation/flow cytometry technique for epidemiological investigations of *Cryptosporidium* in domestic and Australian native animals. *Veterinary Parasitology*. Vol. 112, pp. 21–31, ISSN: 0304-4017.

Prigione, V., Lingua, G., & Filipello Marchisio, V. (2004). Development and Use of Flow Cytometry for Detection of Airborne Fungi. *Applied and Environmental Microbiology*. Vol. 70, No. 3, pp. 1360–1365, ISSN: 0099-2240.

Ramani, R., Gangwar, M., & Chaturvedi, V. (2003). Flow Cytometry Antifungal Susceptibility Testing of *Aspergillus fumigatus* and Comparison of Mode of Action of Voriconazole vis-a`-vis Amphotericin B and Itraconazole. *Antimicrobial Agents And Chemotherapy*. Vol. 47, No. 11, pp. 3627–3629, ISSN: 0066-4804.

Rocha, R.D., Gontijo, C.M., Elói-Santos, S.M., Teixeira-Carvalho, A., Corrêa-Oliveira, R., Ferrari, T.C., Marques, M.J., Mayrink, W., & Martins-Filho, O.A. (2006), Clinical value of anti-live *Leishmania* (Viannia) *braziliensis* immunoglobulin G subclasses, detected by flow cytometry, for diagnosing active localized cutaneous leishmaniasis. *Tropical Medicine & International Health.* Vol. 11, No. 2, pp 156–166, ISSN: 1360-2276 .

Rudensky, B., Broidie, E., Yinnon, A.M., Weitzman, T., Paz, E., Keller, N., & Raveh, D. (2005). Rapid flow-cytometric susceptibility testing of *Candida* species. *The Journal of Antimicrobial Chemotherapy.* Vol. 55, pp. 106–109, ISSN: 0305-7453.

Rye, H.S., Yue, S., Wemmer, D.E., Quesada, M.A., Haugland, R.P., Mathies, R.A., & Glazer, A.N. (1992). Stable fluorescent complexes of double-stranded DNA with bis-intercalating asymmetric cyanine dyes: Properties and applications. *Nucleic Acids Research.* Vol. 20, pp. 2803–2812, ISSN: 0305-1048.

Shapiro, H.M., & Mandy, F. (2007). Cytometry in Malaria: Moving Beyond Giemsa. *Cytometry Part A.* Vol. 71A, pp. 643-645, ISSN: 1552-4922.

Shapiro, H.M., & Ulrich, H. (2010). Cytometry in Malaria: From Research Tool to Practical Diagnostic Approach? *Cytometry Part A.* Vol. 77A, pp. 500-501, ISSN: 1552-4922.

Singh, N., & Dube, A. (2004). Short report: fluorescent *Leishmania*: application to anti-leishmanial drug testing. *American Journal of Tropical Medicine Hygiene.* Vol. 71, No. 4, pp. 400–402, ISSN: 0002-9637.

Tracy, B.P., Gaida, S.M., & Papoutsakis, E.T. (2008). Development and Application of Flow-Cytometric Techniques for Analyzing and Sorting Endospore-Forming Clostridia. *Applied and Environmental Microbiology.* Vol. 74, No. 24, pp. 7497–7506, ISSN: 0099-2240.

Tran, T.M., Moreno, A., Yazdani, S.S., Chitnis, C.E., Barnwell, J.W., & Galinski, M.R. (2005). Detection of a *Plasmodium vivax* Erythrocyte Binding Protein by Flow Cytometry. *Cytometry Part A.* Vol. 63, pp. 59-66, ISSN: 1552-4922.

Valdez, L.M., Dang, H., Okhuysen, P.C., & Chappell, C.L. (1997). Flow cytometric detection of *Cryptosporidium* oocysts in human stool samples. *Journal of Clinical Microbiology.* Vol. 35, No. 8, pp. 2013–2017, ISSN: 0095-1137.

Wang, Y., Hammes, F., De Roy, K., Verstraete, W., & Boon, N. (2010). Past, present and future applications of flow cytometry in aquatic microbiology. *Trends in Biotechnology.* Vol. 28, No. 8, pp. 416-24, ISSN: 0167-7799.

Weinstein, M.P. (2007). Diagnostic technologies in clinical microbiology, In: Murray, P.R., Baron, E.J., Jorgensen, J.H., Landry, M.L., & Pfaller, M.A. Manual of clinical microbiology, 9th ed. ASM Press, Washington, D.C., Vol. 1, pp. 173-270, ISBN: 9781555813710.

Weiss Nielsen, M., Sternberg, C., Molin, S., & Regenberg B. (2011). *Pseudomonas aeruginosa* and *Saccharomyces cerevisiae* Biofilm in Flow Cells. *Video* Article Journal of Visualized Experiments. Vol. 47, www.jove.com, ISSN: 1940-087X.

Whaun, J.M., Rittershaus, C., & Ip, S.H. (1983). Rapid identification and detection of parasitized human red cells by automated flow cytometry. *Cytometry.* Vol. 4, No. 2, pp. 117–122, ISSN: 0196-4763.

Wyatt, C.R., Goff, W., & Davis, WC. (1991). A flow cytometric method for assessing viability of intraerythrocytic hemoparasites. *Journal of Immunology Methods.* Vol. 140, pp. 23–30, ISSN: 0022-1759.

Xie, L.H., Li, Q., Johnson, J., Zhang, J., Milhous, W., & Kyle, D. (2007). Development and validation of flow cytometric measurement for parasitemia using autofluorescence and YOYO-1 in rodent malaria. *Parasitology.* Vol. 134, Pt 9, 1151-1162, ISSN: 031-1820.

3

High-Throughput Flow Cytometry for Predicting Drug-Induced Hepatotoxicity

Marion Zanese[1], Laura Suter[2], Adrian Roth[2],
Francesca De Giorgi[1] and François Ichas[1]
[1]*Fluofarma,*
[2]*F. Hoffmann-La Roche,*
[1]*France*
[2]*Switzerland*

1. Introduction

The development of a new drug is a long, expensive and complex process which aims to identify a pharmacologically-active low toxicity drug candidate. Large amount of resources and time are wasted if a drug fails in late stages of development or is withdrawn from the market because of toxicity. Hepatotoxicity in particular is a frequent cause for the failure of a drug to get approved, or for the withdrawal of already marketed medicines (Stevens & Baker, 2009). Current preclinical testing systems lack predictivity and need to be significantly improved in order to allow the identification of potentially hepatotoxic drug candidates, and the safety-based prioritization of compounds early in the development process. A cost-effective identification of compounds with potential liver liabilities in the initial preclinical phase of drug development would undoubtedly reduce the number of drug nonapprovals and withdrawals.

We present here the development of an optimized methodology for predicting drug-induced hepatotoxicity, which could be used early in the drug development process (e.g. during lead optimization), relying on the assessment of multiple cellular readouts by high-throughput flow cytometry.

This methodology is based on the measurement of key intracellular events reflecting the main cellular and metabolic changes occurring in hepatocytes in response to hepatotoxicant exposition (i.e. cytolysis, mitochondrial membrane depolarization, NAD(P)H depletion, ROS production, glutathione (GSH) depletion, and variations in lipid content). Each measurement was optimized in terms of robustness (reproducibility), sensitivity and dynamic range, and when possible multiplexed, in 3 hepatic cellular models: the HepG2 cell line, fresh rat hepatocytes and cryopreserved human hepatocytes.

The HepG2 cell line, derived from a human hepatoma, is probably the most utilized cell line in hepatotoxicological studies. HepG2 cells are attractive because they are cheap, easy to handle and generate reproducible results. However, they are known to have a reduced drug metabolizing activity compared to primary hepatocytes. Fresh primary rat hepatocytes provide a model of fully functional hepatocytes, well suited to flow cytometry experiments, although the results obtained are not always relevant to human, due to species differences in metabolism and cell biology between rat and man. Primary human hepatocytes are considered the "gold standard" but the reduced viability of frozen human hepatocytes and the significant donor-to-donor variability both in terms of quality and metabolic activity, as well as their restricted availability constitute important limiting factors for their extensive use. Nevertheless, these biological systems with their inherent advantages and flaws are the methods of choice for *in vitro* assessment of hepatotoxicity. The high-throughput flow cytometry approach presented here is applicable to all these biological test systems.

2. Drug testing process

The entire drug testing process (from the seeding of the cells until the flow cytometry analysis) was performed in 96-well plates. Each step of this process was optimized. First the cell density and the medium composition were adjusted for each cell type in order to obtain a confluent monolayer of hepatocytes with high viability.

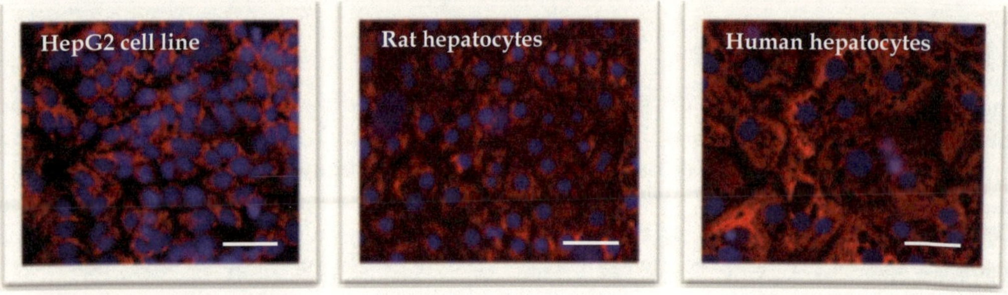

Fig. 1. Hepatic cellular models

HepG2 cells (*left*), freshly isolated primary rat hepatocytes (*middle*), and cryopreserved human hepatocytes (*right*) were observed 72 h post-seeding in 96-well plates. Nuclei (in blue) were stained with Hoechst 33342 and mitochondria (in red) of viable cells were stained with the potentiometric probe TMRM (scale bar = 50µm).

The cell detachment process was adapted to each cellular model and its innocuousness was checked by comparing flow cytometry results on suspended cells with imaging results on adherent cells.

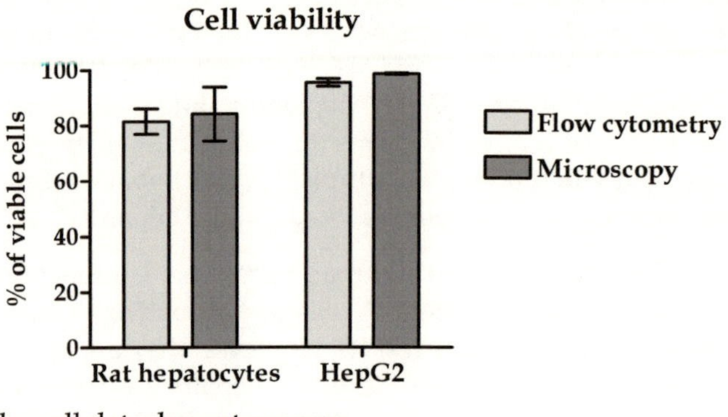

Fig. 2. Innocuousness of the cell detachment process

The cell viability of rat hepatocytes and HepG2 cells after 48 h in culture was assessed on adherent cells in microscopy and after cell detachment in flow cytometry (on suspended cells). Viable cells were identified by staining polarized mitochondria with a potentiometric probe. Results are expressed as the mean ± SD of 3 replicates.

In addition, several probes and staining protocols were tested for each functional assay in order to maximize the dynamic range (signal/noise ratio) of the measurement, and to ensure sufficient signal stability over time (compatible with flow cytometry analysis).

Flow cytometry experiments were performed using a special order BD LSRFortessa™ cell analyzer equipped with 3 excitation sources (355 nm, 488 nm, and 561 nm) and a high-throughput injection module capable of handling 96-well plates. In our customized configuration, the instrument allows the simultaneous detection of up to 10 colors. As the optical filters are removable and interchangeable, this flow cytometer has the flexibility to support a large variety of multicolor flow cytometry assays, which allowed us to multiplex most of the assays we developed. Analysis of flow cytometry outputs was performed using BD FACSDiva software. Typically a few thousands cells per well were analyzed, and the wells in which less than 100 cells could be analyzed were rejected.

Thanks to the extensive optimization of the entire drug testing process, we were able to develop robust and sensitive assays with low variability, in all 3 cellular models. This allowed us to generate accurate data by performing experiments in duplicate (2 replicates per experimental condition). Both the multiplexing of assays and the use of a reduced number of experimental replicates contribute to the high throughput of the assay, required for the rapid testing of numerous compounds in the early stage of drug development.

Although the functional assays we developed were multiplexed, they are presented separately for easier understanding.

3. Cell death measurements

Cytolysis is a conventional cytotoxicity indicator. Indeed, loss of plasma membrane integrity is a measure of cell death and quantitates a general cytotoxicity that is not necessarily unique to liver. In our experiments, cytolysis is assessed with a fluorescent high affinity nucleic acid stain that easily penetrates cells with compromised plasma membranes but do not cross healthy cell membranes. It is thus very easy to distinguish fluorescent cytolytic cells from non-fluorescent viable cells in flow cytometry.

The loss of the mitochondrial inner transmembrane potential ($\Delta\psi$) maintained by the respiratory chain can be triggered by many different drug-induced toxic mechanisms, leading to cell death either by apoptosis or by necrosis.

Mitochondrial potential can be readily measured with fluorescent cationic dyes (rhodamines, carbocyanines, etc.). The accumulation of these amphiphilic cationic probes is dependent on the mitochondrial potential value, and thus cells with active mitochondria (high $\Delta\psi$) will brightly fluoresce whereas cells in which mitochondria are depolarized (low $\Delta\psi$) will be barely fluorescent.

Cytolysis and mitochondrial transmembrane potential measurements were optimized in the 3 cellular models using acetaminophen (APAP) as a model compound for drug-induced hepatotoxicity. APAP is widely used for the treatment of pain and fever. Although it is safe and effective at therapeutic levels, the drug causes severe liver injury following overdosing (whether on purpose or by accident) with the potential to progress to liver failure (Tang, 2007). Partly because of its widespread use, APAP hepatotoxicity accounts for more than a third of drug-related acute liver failure cases in the US.

The results obtained in the mitochondrial depolarization assay after 24 h of treatment with acetaminophen are very similar to those obtained in the cytolysis assay. In rat hepatocytes, the EC_{50} is slightly lower in the mitochondrial assay compared to the cytolysis assay, and there is no significant difference between EC_{50} for mitochondrial depolarization and cytolysis in HepG2 cells or human hepatocytes.

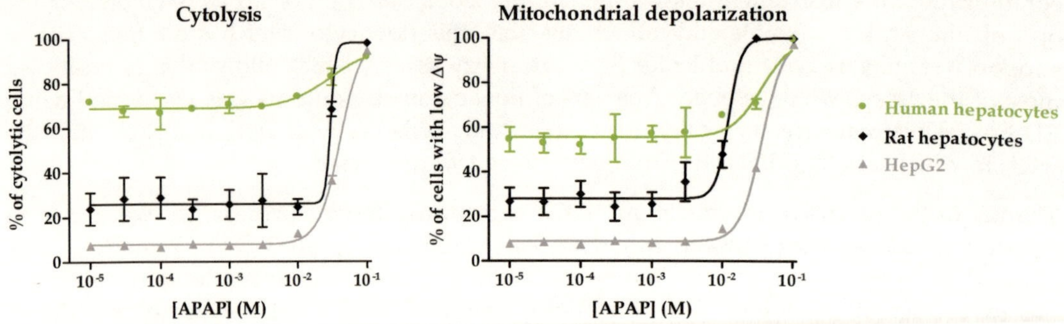

Fig. 3. Acetaminophen-induced cell death in hepatocytes

Primary human hepatocytes, primary rat hepatocytes and HepG2 cells were incubated for 24 h with increasing concentrations of acetaminophen. Cytolysis and mitochondrial membrane depolarization were measured in high-throughput flow cytometry with SYTOX Green and TMRM respectively. Results are expressed as the mean ± SD of 2 replicates. Sigmoidal curve fitting was performed with GraphPad Prism software.

The EC_{50} of the curves representing the percentage of non-viable cells after 24 h of treatment with acetaminophen are very similar from one cell type to another. The 3 cellular models are thus equally sensitive to acetaminophen cytotoxicity. In contrast the signal/noise ratio differs greatly between cellular models. This is the direct consequence of the differences in the cytolysis rate in basal (vehicle-treated) conditions: less than 10% in HepG2 cells, around 25% in primary rat hepatocytes and more than 60% in cryopreserved human hepatocytes. Note that the basal percentage of non viable cells after 48 h in culture (which determines the dynamic range of the cell death assays) varies substantially (from 30% to 80% in our tests) from one batch of cryopreserved human hepatocytes to another (not shown).

More than 80 other drugs were tested and gave similar results in the cytolysis assay and in the mitochondrial depolarization assay, confirming that both are direct indicators of cell death.

Regarding the relationship between *in vitro* cell death induction and clinically observed drug-induced hepatotoxicity, we show here the results obtained with two drugs which are considered non-hepatotoxic, namely metformin and entacapone (Fig. 4).

Metformin, an orally available biguanine derivative, is a cornerstone for the treatment of type 2 diabetes, in particular in overweight and obese people. Metformin is safe, cost effective and remains the first line of diabetes therapy with diet and exercise (Andujar-Plata et al., 2011). The drug may also be used in polycystic ovary syndrome (PCOS), non-alcoholic fatty liver disease (NAFLD) and premature puberty, three other conditions that feature insulin resistance. Although metformin mechanism of action is not well understood, it includes a decrease of hepatic insulin resistance and a change in bile acids metabolism. As expected for a safe drug, no toxicity of metformin was evidenced in our cell death assays (cytolysis and mitochondrial depolarization) after 24 h of treatment, in all three cellular models.

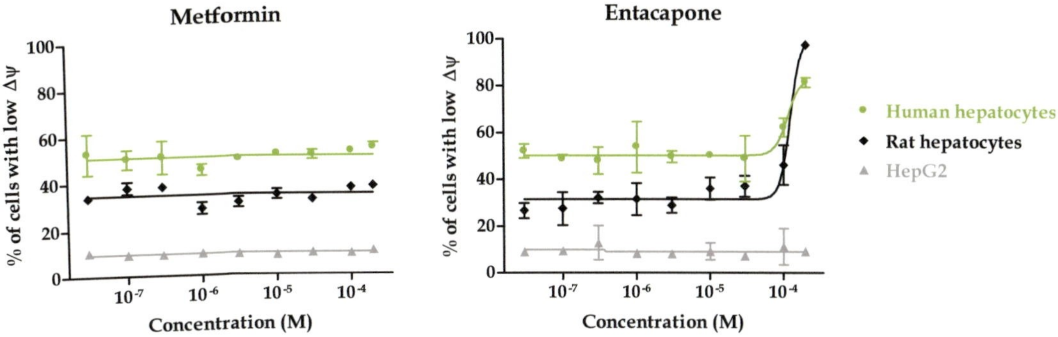

Fig. 4. Assessment of cell death induced by non-hepatotoxic drugs

Primary human hepatocytes, primary rat hepatocytes and HepG2 cells were incubated for 24 h with increasing concentrations of metformin or entacapone. Cell death was quantified in high-throughput flow cytometry by measuring mitochondrial membrane depolarization. Results are expressed as the mean ± SD of 2 replicates. Sigmoidal curve fitting was performed with GraphPad Prism software.

Entacapone is a catechol-O-methyl transferase (COMT) inhibitor used in the treatment of Parkinson's disease. It is usually administered in conjunction with the dopaminergic agent L-DOPA in order to increase its bioavailability by preventing COMT from metabolizing L-DOPA into 3-methoxy-4-hydroxy-L-phenylalanine (3-OMD). Entacapone is often used in hepatotoxicological studies in parallel with tolcapone, another COMT inhibitor with liver liabilities, to form a model drug pair: "non-liver toxic drug" (entacapone) versus "hepatotoxic drug" (tolcapone). In our assays, entacapone elicited mitochondrial depolarization in primary hepatocytes after 24 h of treatment at the highest tested concentration of 200 µM (Fig. 4). However, no effect was observed in HepG2 cells in the same experimental conditions evidencing differences in susceptibility to entacapone-induced toxicity between the primary cells and the HepG2 cell line. The fact that entacapone induces cell death in primary hepatocytes is not incompatible with the fact that it is a safe drug. Indeed as Paracelsus pointed out 500 years ago, the *dose* makes the *poison,* and all drugs can be toxic at high enough concentrations. What determines whether a drug is safe or not is the difference between the therapeutically active dose and the toxic dose, in other words, the safety margin of the drug.

By measuring mitochondrial depolarization or cytolysis, we could determine the exposure levels that lead to cell death *in vitro*. Using lower doses, we could explore earlier indicators of toxicity which are more hepato-specific and reflect the initial cellular processes that may lead to cell death.

4. Energetic metabolism and oxidative stress measurements

To improve sensitivity of the assay, we chose to measure NAD(P)H depletion, ROS production and glutathione depletion as earlier indicators of toxicity.

Nicotinamide adenine dinucleotide (NAD^+) and nicotinamide adenine dinucleotide phosphate ($NADP^+$) are two of the most used coenzymes in cellular metabolism. They can exist in two different redox states (reduced and oxidized) that change into each other by accepting or donating electrons. The balance between the oxidized and reduced forms of these coenzymes is an important component of what is called the *redox state* of a cell, a measurement that reflects both the metabolic activity and the health of cells.

Hundreds of enzymes use $NAD(P)^+$ to catalyze reduction-oxidation reactions reversibly. Some of these are among the most abundant and well-studied enzymes participating in energetic metabolism (glycolysis, Krebs cycle, Lynen helix), biosynthesis, degradation, defense against oxidative damage, etc.

The reduced and oxidized forms of these coenzymes have distinct fluorescence characteristics: NADH and NADPH are fluorescent, while their oxidized forms (NAD^+ and $NADP^+$ respectively) are not. Fluorescence signals consistent with NAD(P)H can be measured to monitor cellular activity through redox status. As a cell changes its metabolic activity, the balance between NAD(P)H and $NAD(P)^+$ shifts correspondingly as the reduction-oxidation (redox) state of the cell fluctuates.

In our experiments, cells are measured in suspension and thus there are little effects of absorption and morphology on fluorescence emission. The sole contributors are intracellular fluorophores (in this case, endogenous fluorescence). Autofluorescence signals consistent with NAD(P)H are measured to monitor energetic metabolism through redox status. The use of flow cytometry is of real advantage because NADH has a very short fluorescence lifetime (0.4 nanoseconds) and cannot be easily quantified by fluorescence microscopy.

The NADH quantitation assay is attractive because, as it relies on cell autofluorescence and no staining step is required, it is cheap and quickly performed. In particular we used this assay to characterize batches of cryopreserved human hepatocytes (Fig. 5).

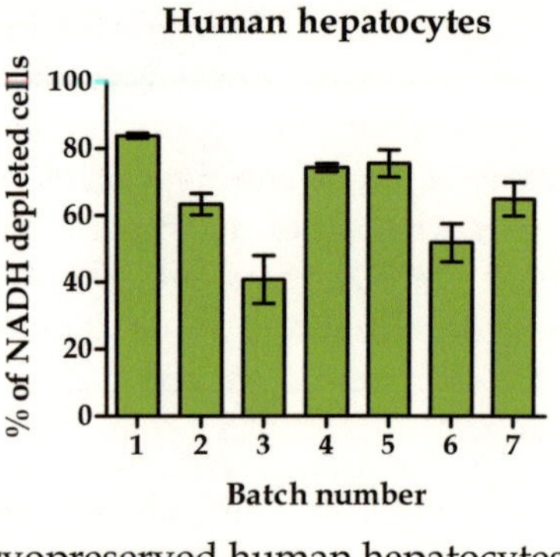

Fig. 5. Characterization of cryopreserved human hepatocytes batches

The quality of 7 different batches (i.e. donors) of human hepatocytes was assessed by measuring NADH depletion in high-throughput flow cytometry (excitation 355 nm - emission 450±20 nm) after 3 days in culture. Results are expressed as the mean ± SD of 2 replicates.

We generated dose-response curves for 25 chemicals, which all showed almost identical NADH depletion and mitochondrial depolarization results. However, a stronger NADH depletion than mitochondrial depolarization was evident for a few chemicals, including Alpha-naphtylisotiocianate (ANIT) (Fig. 6).

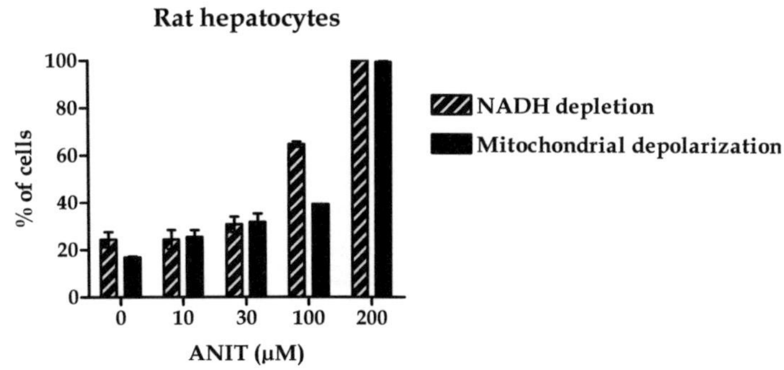

Fig. 6. NADH depletion "precedes" mitochondrial depolarization

Primary rat hepatocytes were incubated for 48 h with the indicated concentrations of ANIT. NADH depletion and mitochondrial membrane depolarization were measured in high-throughput flow cytometry as mentioned above. Results are expressed as the mean ± SD of 2 replicates.

ANIT is a known hepatotoxicant used in rodents to model human intrahepatic cholestasis. Cholestasis is the disruption of bile flow from the liver to the duodenum which leads to the accumulation of bile acids and other bile components in the liver and, ultimately, hepatobiliary toxicity. Cholestasis is often divided into two categories, extrahepatic and intrahepatic, based upon etiology. Extrahepatic cholestasis is the consequence of a mechanical blockage in the duct system (typically observed in patients with gallstones or tumors of the common biliary tract) whereas intrahepatic cholestasis is caused by physiological and pathological factors including genetic defects and chemicals. In rats, a single administration of ANIT induces intrahepatic cholestasis through damage to biliary epithelium cells (Orsler et al., 1999).

Measuring NADH depletion results in only a small improvement in sensitivity compared to cytolysis and mitochondrial depolarization. Perhaps the high correlation between the 3 assays is in part due to the fact that measurements are performed after 24 hours of treatment. Shorter exposures may be needed to increase the differences between these readouts.

Oxidative stress is an important mechanism of drug-induced toxicity. Oxidative stress is characterized by both increased production of oxidants or free radicals, and intracellular macromolecular change due to oxidative injury such as decreased glutathione.

Oxidative stress was first assessed by measuring intracellular levels of reactive oxygen species (ROS). ROS are molecules or ions (e.g. singlet oxygen, superoxides, peroxides, hydroxyl radical, and hydroperoxides) formed by the incomplete one-electron reduction of oxygen. ROS form as a natural byproduct of the normal metabolism of oxygen and have important roles in cell signaling and homeostasis. However ROS levels can increase dramatically under different conditions of cell stress. The accumulation of these strong oxidants can result in significant damage to cell structures. Among the most important of these are the actions of free radicals on the fatty acid side chains of lipids in the various membranes of the cell, especially mitochondrial membranes (which are directly exposed to the superoxide anions produced during cellular respiration).

Most of the commercially available probes to monitor ROS production by flow cytometry in living cells are cell-permeant chemicals that undergo changes in their fluorescence spectral properties once oxidized by ROS. Two different probes were used in our assay: dihydroethidium (DHE, also called hydroethidine) and CM-H_2DCFDA (chloromethyl-dichlorodihydrofluorescein diacetate). DHE exhibits blue fluorescence in the cytosol until oxidized by superoxide to 2-hydroxyethidium which intercalates within the DNA staining the cell nucleus a bright fluorescent red. In contrast the nonfluorescent CM-H_2DCFDA is first hydrolyzed to DCFH in the cell by intracellular esterases and DCFH is oxidized to form the highly fluorescent DCF in the presence of ROS such as hydrogen peroxide.

We applied the ROS production assay to many drugs including troglitazone, a thiazolidinedione which was approved in 1997 for the treatment of type 2 diabetes. Troglitazone was an effective antidiabetic drug with a fundamentally new mechanism of action but several cases of liver injury and failure were reported in troglitazone-treated patients. The drug was eventually withdrawn from the market in 2000, after the approval of a newer generation of thiazolidinediones (i.e. rosiglitazone and pioglitazone) with diminished incidence of toxicity. Since then, a significant effort has been made to elucidate the mechanisms underlying troglitazone-induced hepatotoxicity. Possible mechanisms of troglitazone-induced cell injury include the formation and accumulation of toxic metabolites, mitochondrial dysfunction and oxidant stress, ATP depletion and subsequent cell death (Tang, 2007).

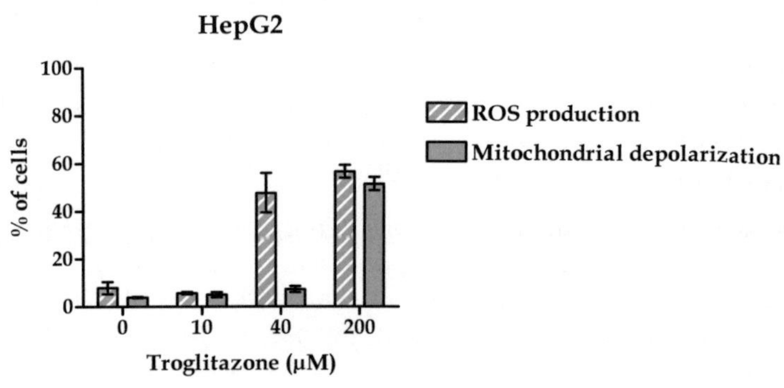

Fig. 7. ROS production "precedes" mitochondrial depolarization

HepG2 cells were incubated for 72 h with the indicated concentrations of troglitazone. ROS production and mitochondrial membrane depolarization were measured in high-throughput flow cytometry as mentioned above. Results are expressed as the mean ± SD of 2 replicates.

As shown in Fig. 7, after 72 h of treatment with troglitazone in HepG2 cells, a significant mitochondrial depolarization could be evidenced but only at the highest tested concentration of 200 µM. In contrast a significant ROS production was detected at a concentration of 40 µM. This pre-lethal assay is thus sensitive enough to detect ROS production at lower troglitazone concentrations than those needed for cytotoxicity.

Oxidative stress was also assessed by quantifying intracellular glutathione (GSH) levels. Glutathione (a tripeptide composed of three amino acids: cysteine, glutamic acid, and glycine) is the most abundant and important nonprotein thiol in mammalian cells. Glutathione plays a major role in the protection of the liver against several hepatotoxicants. Indeed, in addition to its central role in protecting cells of all organs against damage produced by free radicals, glutathione is involved in drug detoxification.

Xenobiotics including drugs are subject to metabolism which most likely acts as a self-defense mechanism of the body. Drugs are metabolized through a complex series of biochemical reactions which are categorized into two major pathways, referred to as Phase I (oxidative reactions) and Phase II (conjugation reactions). This can result in toxification or detoxification (the activation or deactivation respectively) of the chemical. While both toxification and detoxification occur, the major metabolites of most drugs are detoxification products.

During phase I and phase II, drugs are converted into more polar products that can be excreted in the urine or the bile depending on the particular characteristics of the end product. In phase I a variety of enzymes acts to introduce reactive and polar groups into their substrate. These reactions are mainly catalyzed by cytochrome P450 enzymes (often abbreviated as CYPs), amine oxidase, peroxidases, and flavin-containing monooxygenase. The cytochrome P450 superfamily is a large and diverse group of enzymes which catalyze the oxidation of organic substances. CYPs are the major enzymes involved in drug metabolism accounting for about 75% of the total number of different metabolic reactions. A significant side effect of phase I oxidative metabolism is the formation of potentially harmful reactive electrophiles which are mostly neutralized by glutathione that is in turn oxidized to glutathione disulfide (GSSG). Phase 2 reactions, also known as conjugation reactions, are usually detoxificating in nature and consist in the conjugation of phase I metabolites with charged species such as glutathione, sulfate, glycine or glucuronic acid. The conjugates formed are highly hydrophilic, which promotes their excretion. In this process, reduced glutathione levels decrease at the expense of the formation of glutathione conjugates. Thus GSH plays a key role in drug metabolism and depletion of reduced form of glutathione was reported to be a marker of hepatotoxicity (Xu et al., 2004).

In our experiments, reduced glutathione content was assessed with monochlorobimane. This non fluorescent bimane derivative reacts with GSH (but do not react with GSSG) to form a highly fluorescent conjugated product readily quantified in viable cells by flow cytometry.

The measurement of GSH in the 3 cellular models was first optimized using buthionine sulfoximine (BSO) which inhibits GSH neosynthesis thus reducing cellular GSH levels. The quantitation of GSH levels was restricted to non cytolytic cells (Fig. 8) based on cell morphology using the forward and side scatter channels (FSC and SSC) which are related to the cell size and the internal complexity respectively.

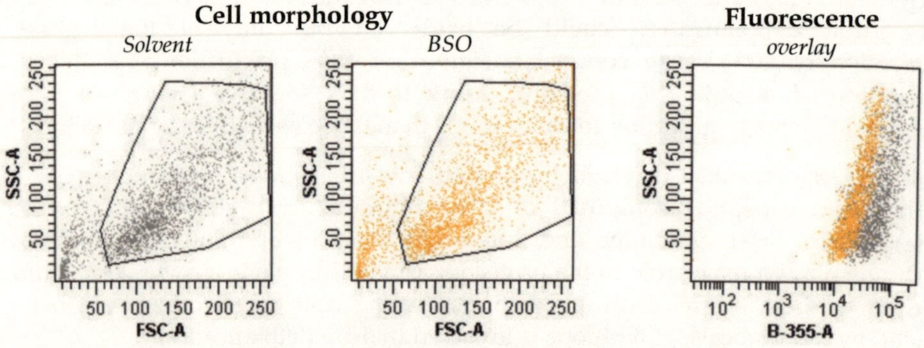

Fig. 8. Analysis of flow cytometry outputs for the GSH depletion assay

Biparametric cell morphology plots show the selection of non-cytolytic HepG2 cells incubated with solvent (*left plot*) or 300 μM BSO (*middle plot*) for 72 h. The decrease in the fluorescence intensity of monochlorobimane staining after treatment with BSO is clearly visible in the overlay of the fluorescence outputs from both conditions (*right plot*): the fluorescence of the non-cytolytic solvent-treated cells (in grey) is more intense than the fluorescence of the non-cytolytic BSO-treated cells (in orange).

As only viable cells are analyzed, the obtained dynamic range is high in all tested cell types (Fig. 9), even in cryopreserved human hepatocytes. After 24 hours of treatment with 300 μM BSO, a complete depletion in GSH is observed in all cellular models. However the EC_{50} of glutathione depletion is lower in HepG2 cells than in primary hepatocytes revealing differences in kinetics of GSH depletion between the cell line and the primary cells.

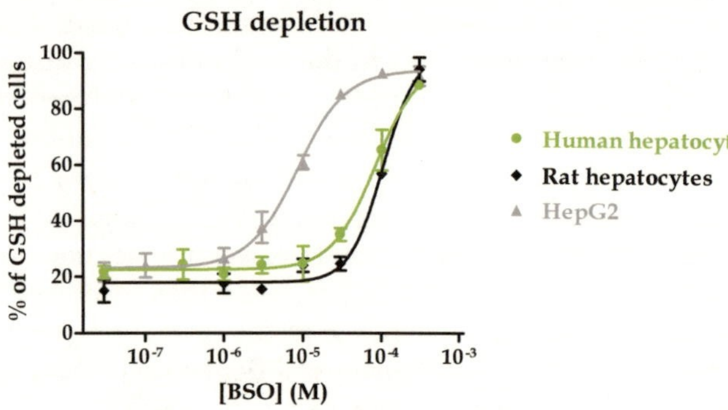

Fig. 9. Optimization of the GSH depletion assay with BSO

Primary human hepatocytes, primary rat hepatocytes and HepG2 cells were incubated for 24 h with increasing concentrations of BSO. GSH depletion was measured in high-throughput flow cytometry as mentioned above. Results are expressed as the mean ± SD of 2 replicates. Sigmoidal curve fitting was performed with GraphPad Prism software.

Acetaminophen hepatotoxicity is mediated by the formation of NAPQI (N-acetyl-p-benzoquinone imine), a reactive metabolite produced by a minor APAP clearance pathway mainly catalyzed by CYP2E1. Because of its chemical reactivity, NAPQI undergoes a conjugation with GSH. When large quantities of APAP are metabolized, the amount of hepatic GSH is not sufficient to detoxify NAPQI. Glutathione pools are depleted and the reactive metabolite accumulates and binds to critical mitochondrial proteins ultimately causing cell death. Intracellular events resulting in hepatocyte death may include: disturbance of cellular calcium homeostasis, mitochondrial oxidative stress, collapse of mitochondrial membrane potential, decreased ATP synthesis, DNA fragmentation, and cytolysis (Tang, 2007).

After 24 hours of treatment with 10 mM acetaminophen, a significant proportion of GSH-depleted cells is observed in primary hepatocytes (from rat and human). However no GSH depletion is detected in the HepG2 cell line (Fig. 10).

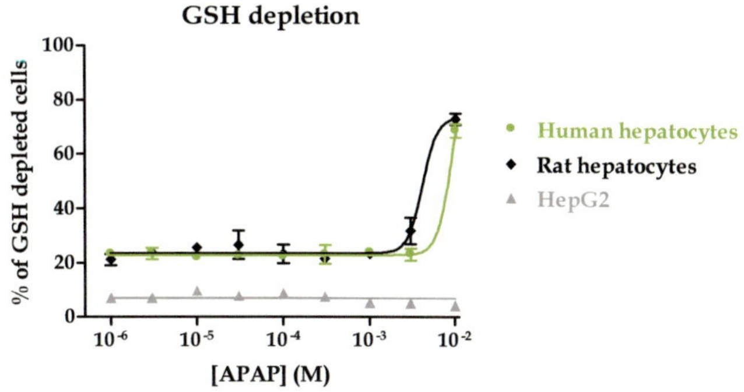

Fig. 10. Acetaminophen-induced GSH depletion in hepatocytes

Primary human hepatocytes, primary rat hepatocytes and HepG2 cells were incubated for 24 h with increasing concentrations of APAP. GSH depletion was measured in high-throughput flow cytometry as mentioned above. Results are expressed as the mean ± SD of 2 replicates. Sigmoidal curve fitting was performed with GraphPad Prism software.

Acetaminophen-induced glutathione depletion is a CYP-dependent mechanism and HepG2 cells are known to have a reduced metabolic activity. The absence of glutathione depletion in the cell line is thus probably due to a reduced or inexistent formation of NAPQI. But interestingly acetaminophen is as toxic in HepG2 cells as it is in primary cells, as far as cell death is concerned (Fig. 3). Therefore the intracellular events leading to cell death in response to acetaminophen exposure appear to be different in HepG2 cells and primary hepatocytes, suggesting that a "non canonical" mechanism of action is involved in APAP-induced cell death in the cell line.

5. Lipid content measurement

Drug-induced liver injury encompasses a large spectrum of lesions, some of which are the consequence of steatosis and phospholipidosis.

Drugs are known to be able to induce steatosis, an abnormal accumulation of neutral lipids which can lead to liver failure. When fat accumulates, lipids are primarily stored as triglycerides. Steatosis is believed to result from an imbalance between hepatic free fatty acids inflow and triglyceride synthesis and excretion. Steatosis most often occurs in the liver which is the primary organ of lipid metabolism, although it may occur in any organ, such as the kidneys, heart, and muscles. The risk factors associated with steatosis are varied, and include diabetes mellitus, hypertension and obesity. Macrovesicular steatosis, characterized by the presence of large lipid vesicles that displace the nucleus of hepatocytes, is the most common form of fatty degeneration, and may be caused by oversupply of lipids due to obesity, insulin resistance, or alcoholism. Microvesicular steatosis, the accumulation of multiple small lipid droplets, can be caused by several diseases including Reye's syndrome and hepatitis D. Fat accumulation is not necessarily a pathological condition and drug-induced steatosis is often reversible.

Prolonged exposure to certain drugs can cause macrovesicular steatosis, a benign hepatic lesion. Nevertheless chronic macrovesicular steatosis can evolve in certain cases into steatohepatitis (a liver inflammation resulting from steatosis) and ultimately into cirrhosis. Moreover, in a few patients, some drugs induce microvesicular steatosis which can potentially lead to liver failure with fatal consequences.

One of the major mechanisms involved in drug-induced liver steatosis is the inhibition of beta-oxidation (degradation of long chain fatty acids) either by direct inhibition of mitochondrial beta-oxidation enzymes or by sequestration of the cofactors involved in this metabolic pathway. Other drugs eventually reduce beta-oxidation as a result of mitochondrial dysfunction (because the oxidized cofactors NAD+ and FAD which are produced by mitochondrial respiration are needed for beta-oxidation).

Mitochondrial dysfunction plays a key role in the pathophysiology of steatohepatitis. Indeed, respiratory chain deficiency results in decreased ATP formation and increased ROS generation. The combination of decreased beta-oxidation (resulting in lipid accumulation) and increased ROS generation (resulting in lipid peroxidation and release of aldehydic derivatives with detrimental effects on hepatocytes) is an important mechanism of drug-induced steatohepatitis.

Phospholipidosis is a lysosomal storage disorder characterized by the excess accumulation of phospholipids in cells. The mechanisms of drug-induced phospholipidosis involve trapping or selective uptake of the phospholipidosis-inducing drugs within the lysosomes and acidic vesicles of affected cells. Drug trapping is followed by a gradual accumulation of drug-phospholipid complexes within the internal lysosomal membranes. The increase in undigested materials results in the abnormal accumulation of multi-lammellar bodies (myeloid bodies) in tissues. Many cationic amphiphilic drugs, including anti-depressants and cholesterol-lowering agents, are reported to cause drug-induced phospholipidosis in animals and humans.

Phospholipidosis is often accompanied with various associated toxicities in the liver. It does not *per se* constitute frank toxicity but is reportedly predictive of drug or metabolite accumulation in affected tissues (Xu et al., 2004).

Thus, the variations in both neutral lipids content and polar lipids (phospholipids) content may be early indicators of drug-induced hepatotoxicity. Various probes are available for use in intact cells that either titrate the lipid pool of interest or get accumulated as a lipid mimetic. We developed a proprietary probe formulation and detection methodology (lipotracker) that allows the simultaneous quantitation of neutral lipids and polar lipids (quantitation service available at www.fluofarma.com). The ratio of neutral lipids content upon polar lipids content at the single cell level is directly generated by the flow cytometry platform. This lipid ratio can be used to normalize cell size and dye uptake and provides a reliable and precise measurement. As it has a very low variability it allows the detection of slight variations in lipid content. By using FSC and SSC outputs, lipid content is only measured in intact (non-cytolytic) cells, as it is the case for the glutathione depletion assay.

The lipid content assay was first optimized with valproic acid (2-n-propylpentanoic acid), a drug commonly prescribed worldwide in the treatment of epilepsy and in the control of several types of seizures affecting both children and adults. The mechanism of the antiepileptic action of VPA involves the regional changes in the concentration of the neurotransmitter gamma-aminobutyric acid (GABA). VPA is well tolerated by the vast majority of patients but it can induce severe and sometimes fatal hepatotoxicity that is characterized by microvesicular steatosis and most likely results from beta-oxidation inhibition.

A prerequisite to beta-oxidation is the uptake of fatty acids by mitochondria. Short- and medium-chain fatty acids may pass through the mitochondrial membrane directly, whereas long-chain fatty acids are transported across the mitochondrial membrane by a CoA/carnitine-dependent carrier system. Through several mechanisms, valproic acid inhibits the CoA/carnitine-dependent transport of fatty acids resulting in their accumulation in the cytoplasm. Besides a few valproic acid metabolites are suspected to directly inhibit specific enzyme(s) in the beta-oxidation pathway (Tang, 2007).

Consistent with its known steatotic potential, VPA induces an increase in the lipid ratio, and this increase is identical in the 3 studied cell types after 24 h of treatment (Fig. 11).

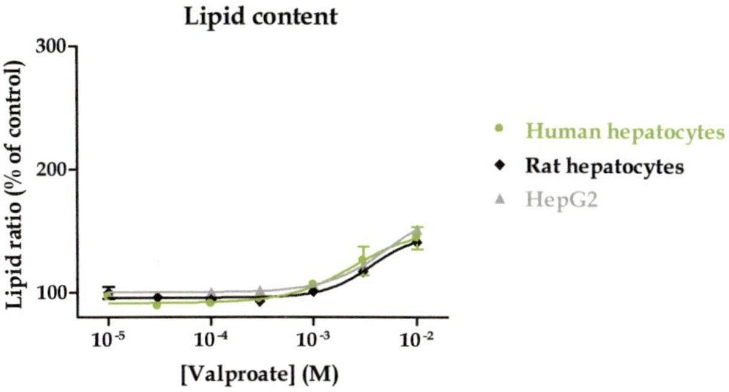

Fig. 11. Valproate-induced variations in lipid content after short exposure

Primary human hepatocytes, primary rat hepatocytes and HepG2 cells were incubated for 24 h with increasing concentrations of VPA. Variations in lipid content were assessed by measuring the single cell lipid ratio (neutral lipids / polar lipids) in high-throughput flow cytometry as mentioned above. Results are expressed as a percentage of the control value (solvent-treated cells) and correspond to the mean ± SD of 2 replicates. Sigmoidal curve fitting was performed with GraphPad Prism software.

In contrast, with a longer exposure to VPA, the observed effects are significantly different from one cellular model to another (Fig. 12).

Primary hepatocytes (from human and rat) and HepG2 cells were incubated with increasing concentrations of VPA for 48 h or 72 h respectively. Variations in lipid content were assessed by measuring the single cell lipid ratio (neutral lipids / polar lipids) in high-throughput

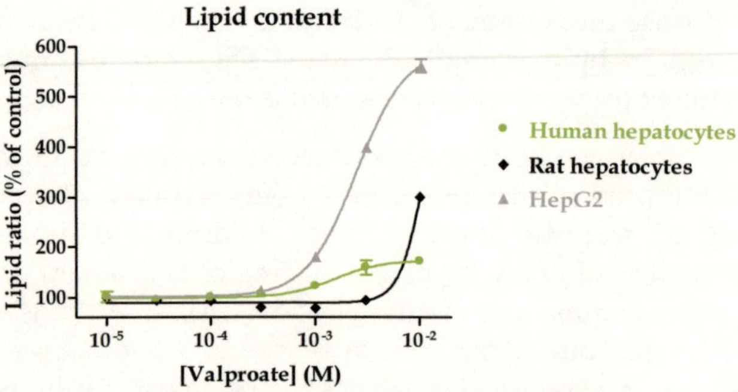

Fig. 12. Valproate-induced variations in lipid content after long exposure

flow cytometry as mentioned above. Results are expressed as a percentage of the control value (solvent-treated cells) and correspond to the mean ± SD of 2 replicates. Sigmoidal curve fitting was performed with GraphPad Prism software.

The accumulation of neutral lipids (evidenced by an increase in lipid ratio) is much more pronounced in HepG2 cells than in primary hepatocytes, with human hepatocytes exhibiting the smallest amplitude of variation. This is probably due to the fact that the basal content in neutral lipids (in vehicle-treated condition) varies considerably between cell types (i.e. the lipid ratio is higher in primary hepatocytes than in HepG2 cells).

Variations in neutral lipid content and polar lipid content were also examined separately to corroborate that the observed VPA-induced augmentation in lipid ratio corresponds to an increase in neutral lipids (and not a decrease in phospholipids content). The same experiment was performed using amiodarone, an antiarrhythmic drug which induces both phospholipidosis and steatosis (Fig. 13).

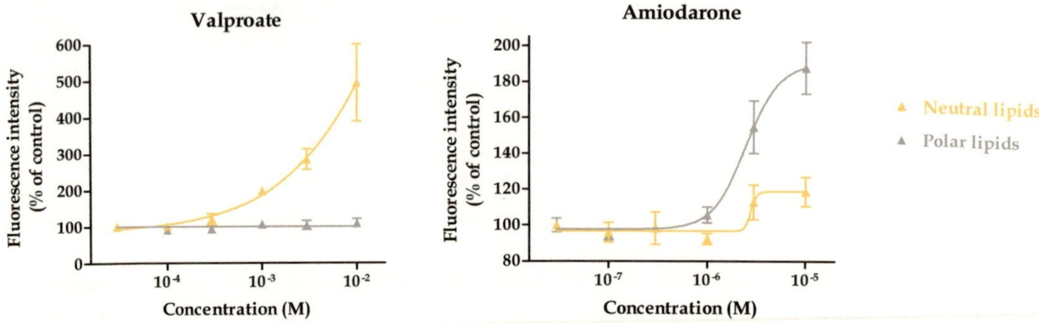

Fig. 13. Steatosis and phospholipidosis in HepG2 cells

HepG2 cells were incubated for 72 h with increasing concentrations of valproate or amiodarone. The fluorescence intensities of the neutral lipids and the polar lipids stainings were quantified in high-throughput flow cytometry as mentioned above. Fluorescence intensity is expressed as a percentage of the control value (solvent-treated cells). Data are given as mean ± SD of 2 replicates. Sigmoidal curve fitting was performed with GraphPad Prism software.

As expected, VPA caused an increase in neutral lipid content with no effect on polar lipid content whereas amiodarone elicited an increase in phospholipids and a smaller rise in neutral lipid content. These results are in accordance with published data reporting that although amiodarone induces both phospholipidosis and steatosis, the accumulation of phospholipids appears after a shorter exposure than those required to provoke an accumulation of neutral lipids (Antherieu et al., 2011).

The lipid assay was subsequently applied to tetracycline, a broad-spectrum antibiotic which inhibits protein synthesis by binding to the 30S subunit of microbial ribosomes. Tetracycline hepatotoxicity seems related to the use of large doses and unlike most other antibiotics, is predictable and reproducible in animal models. With normal low oral doses, tetracycline only rarely causes liver injury. Intravenous or large oral doses of tetracycline induce microvesicular steatosis most likely by direct inhibition of mitochondrial beta-oxidation enzyme(s) (Donato et al, 2009). In our assay, variations in lipid content are detected in cells incubated with sub-cytotoxic concentrations of tetracycline (Fig. 14).

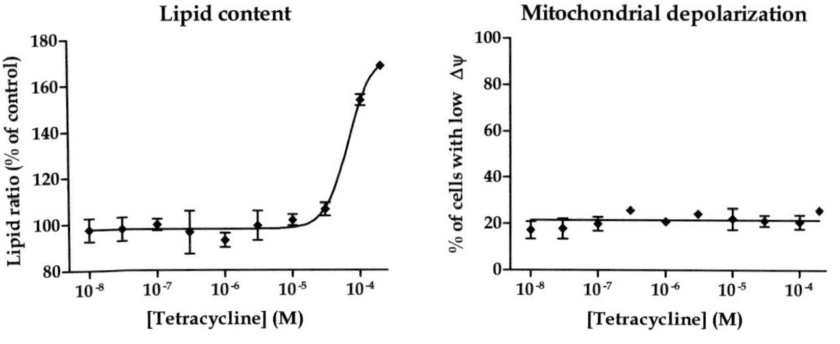

Fig. 14. Variations in lipid content "precede" mitochondrial depolarization

Primary rat hepatocytes were incubated for 48 h with increasing concentrations of tetracycline. Variations in lipid content were assessed by measuring the single cell lipid ratio and results are expressed as a percentage of the control value (solvent-treated cells). Both lipid content and mitochondrial membrane depolarization assays were performed in high-throughput flow cytometry as mentioned above. Results are expressed as the mean ± SD of 2 replicates. Sigmoidal curve fitting was performed with GraphPad Prism software.

Our optimized lipid assay can thus be useful for detecting variations in lipid content with a high sensitivity (thanks to the use of a lipid ratio), and for determining drugs mechanism of action (steatosis and/or phospholipidosis).

6. Idiosyncratic DILI prediction

Although most of the toxic candidate compounds are screened out during preclinical safety studies, each year several new drugs do not get approval or are withdrawn from the market because their toxicity is detected only in late clinical phases or in postmarketing evaluation. Idiosyncratic drug-induced liver injury (DILI) refers to severe (and potentially fatal) hepatic reactions with a low frequency of occurrence (<0.1%), that do not occur in most patients at any dose of the drug, and typically have a delayed onset of weeks or months after initial exposure. Examples of drugs withdrawn from the market because of idiosyncratic DILI include troglitazone and alpidem. In order to assess whether the assays we developed could prove useful for the identification of drugs with an idiosyncratic hepatotoxic potential, we tested pairs of compounds which are related in chemical structure and mechanism of action but show marked differences in hepatotoxic potential.

First we tested troglitazone and rosiglitazone, two antidiabetic drugs that belong to the thiazolidinedione family. As mentioned above, troglitazone was withdrawn from the market because of idiosyncratic DILI and was replaced by newer thiazolidinediones (including rosiglitazone) with diminished incidence of hepatotoxicity. In HepG2 cells, both drugs produced ROS although a marked effect was obtained with 40 μM of troglitazone whereas 200 μM of rosiglitazone were required to induce an equivalent ROS production (Fig. 15). These results are consistent with published data reporting that 50 μM troglitazone induced ROS production in another human hepatocytes cell line (Shishido et al., 2003). Cell death was only evidenced at the highest tested dose of troglitazone, and a similar GSH depletion was observed with both drugs. In addition, alterations in lipid content were much more pronounced with troglitazone than with rosiglitazone.

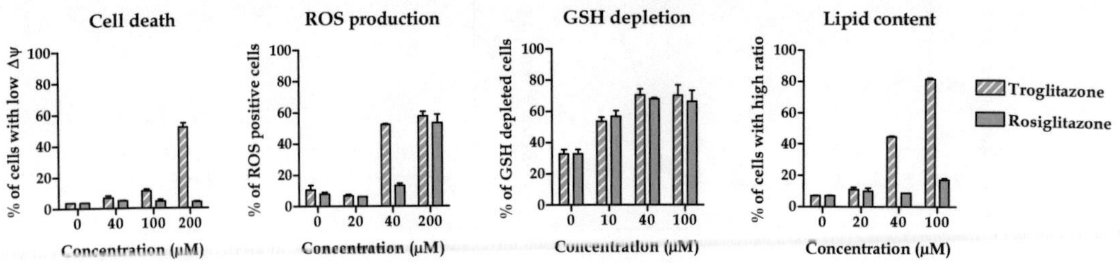

Fig. 15. Multiparametric assessment of troglitazone and rosiglitazone effects in HepG2 cells

HepG2 cells were incubated for 72 h with the indicated concentrations of troglitazone and rosiglitazone. Cell death, ROS production, GSH depletion and lipid content were assessed in high-throughput flow cytometry as mentioned above. Results are expressed as the mean ± SD of 2 replicates.

Our assays were also applied to one pair of drugs from the imidazopyridine class, namely alpidem (a "DILI positive" compound) and zolpidem (a "DILI negative" compound). Although alpidem is related to the better known sleeping medication zolpidem, it does not produce sedative effects at normal doses and was thus used specifically for the treatment of anxiety. Alpidem was released in France in 1991 but was withdrawn from the market a few years later because several cases of severe hepatitis had been reported. The test of these drugs in HepG2 cells (Fig. 16) revealed that neither alpidem nor zolpidem induced ROS production, even at high concentrations. In contrast, as previously reported in rat hepatocytes, both drugs reduced GSH content, with alpidem exhibiting more pronounced effects than zolpidem (Berson et al., 2001). Cell death was apparent only after treatment with alpidem, but not zolpidem. Finally, a very significant increase in lipid ratio was measured at low sub-cytotoxic concentrations of alpidem (2 μM) whereas no effect was observed with equimolar concentrations of zolpidem.

HepG2 cells were incubated for 72 h with the indicated concentrations of alpidem and zolpidem. Cell death, ROS production, GSH depletion and lipid content were assessed in high-throughput flow cytometry as mentioned above. Results are expressed as the mean ± SD of 2 replicates.

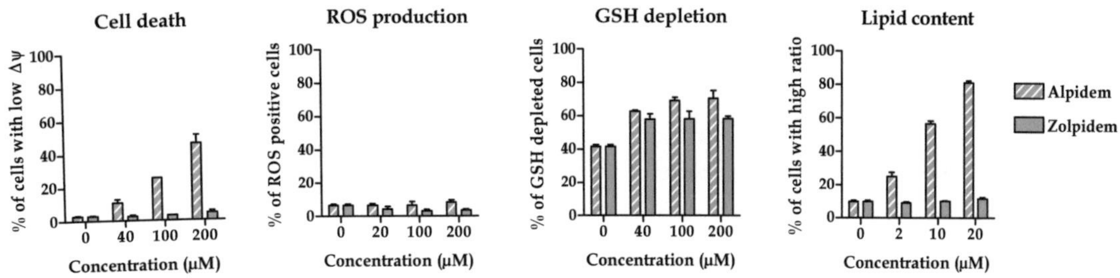

Fig. 16. Multiparametric assessment of alpidem and zolpidem effects in HepG2 cells

All together these data show that the tested drug pairs have very different profiles in our assays. In particular alterations in lipid content seem to be a good indicator of the idiosyncratic hepatotoxic potential of a drug. Our tests could certainly be of great value in preclinical studies, in particular for safety-based prioritization of compounds.

7. Conclusion

Thanks to an extensive optimization, high quality measurement of endpoints could be obtained in all 3 hepatic cellular models: the HepG2 cell line, freshly isolated rat hepatocytes and cryopreserved human hepatocytes. The good quality of these measurements, and in particular the low experimental variability, allowed the detection of small variations in the measured parameters. Combined with the use of early intracellular indicators of hepatotoxicity, we could detect cell alterations at much lower concentrations than those needed for gross cytotoxicity. Moreover these measurements could be performed at high throughput with a flow cytometry platform by multiplexing the assays in 96-well plates and using only 2 replicates per experimental condition.

As expected with a cell line, HepG2 cells generated reproducible results with very low variability. For all the assays we developed, the results obtained with these cells also had an extended dynamic range, indicative of the excellent technical performance of the described assays. However, probably in part due to their reduced drug metabolizing activity, the response of these cells to certain compounds differed from the one obtained in primary hepatocytes. Therefore HepG2 cells are not the most adequate cellular model to elucidate drug toxicity mechanism of action. However, these cells have prove useful for particular studies such as the analysis of drug-induced alterations in lipid content (steatosis and phospholipidosis), and the prioritization of compounds based on their potential to cause liver injury.

Measurements performed with primary cells have a higher variability (in comparison with HepG2 cells) but which is still quite low and compatible with the use of duplicates. In primary hepatocytes, the dynamic range of certain assays is also reduced compared to HepG2 cells, in particular for human hepatocytes. This is largely due to the low basal viability (in untreated conditions) of cryopreserved human hepatocytes, after several days in culture. As a result, although human hepatocytes theoretically represent the best cellular model, the use of frozen hepatocytes with a reduced viability and the lot-to-lot variability constitute limiting factors for their utilization in large scale screening studies. These cells appear to be more suited to mechanistic studies.

As a cellular model for liver toxicity studies, freshly isolated rat hepatocytes represent a good compromise in terms of cell availability and handling, quality of the results (experimental variability, dynamic range and reproducibility), and hepato-specific differentiation and functionality.

In summary, the individual assays we developed can provide insights into the underlying mechanism of action of drug-induced hepatotoxicity and we are currently evaluating whether combinations of these assays could be routinely used early in the drug development process for the prediction of acute hepatotoxicity or the prioritization of compounds based on their potential to cause idiosyncratic liver toxicity.

8. Acknowledgement

The authors would like to thank Lucie Balaguer and Florian Simon for generating experimental data, and Loic Cerf for project management.

9. References

Andújar-Plata, P.; Pi-Sunyer, X. & Laferrère, B. (2011). Metformin effects revisited. *Diabetes research and clinical practice*, DOI:10.1016/j.diabres.2011.09.022

Anthérieu, S.; Rogue, A.; Fromenty, B.; Guillouzo, A. & Robin MA. (2011). Induction of vesicular steatosis by amiodarone and tetracycline is associated with up-regulation of lipogenic genes in HepaRG cells (2011). *Hepatology*, Vol. 53, No. 6, (June 2011), pp. 1895-1905, DOI: 10.1002/hep.24290

Berson, A.; Descatoire, V.; Sutton, A.; Fau, D.; Maulny, B.; Vadrot, N.; Feldmann, G.; Berthon, B.; Tordjmann, T. & Pessayre D. (2001). Toxicity of alpidem, a peripheral benzodiazepine receptor ligand, but not zolpidem, in rat hepatocytes: role of mitochondrial permeability transition and metabolic activation. *The Journal of pharmacology and experimental therapeutics*, Vol. 299, No. 2, pp. 793-800, ISSN: 0022-3565

Donato, MT.; Martínez-Romero, A.; Jiménez, N.; Negro, A.; Herrera, G.; Castell, JV.; O'Connor, JE. & Gómez-Lechón, MJ. (2009). Cytometric analysis for drug-induced steatosis in HepG2 cells. *Chemico-biological interactions*, Vol. 181, No. 3, pp. 417-423

Orsler, DJ.; Ahmed-Choudhury, J.; Chipman, JK.; Hammond, T. & Coleman, R. (1999). ANIT-induced disruption of biliary function in rat hepatocyte couplets. *Toxicological sciences*, Vol. 47, No. 2, pp. 203-210

Shishido, S.; Koga, H.; Harada, M.; Kumemura, H.; Hanada, S.; Taniguchi, E.; Kumashiro, R.; Ohira, H.; Sato, Y.; Namba, M.; Ueno, T. & Sata, M. (2003). Hydrogen peroxide overproduction in megamitochondria of troglitazone-treated human hepatocytes. *Hepatology*, Vol. 37, No. 1, pp. 136-147

Stevens, JL. & Baker TK. (2009). The future of drug safety testing: expanding the view and narrowing the focus. *Drug discovery today*, Vol. 14, No. 3/4, pp. 162-167

Tang, W. (2007). Drug metabolite profiling and elucidation of drug-induced hepatotoxicity. *Expert opinion on drug metabolism and toxicology*, Vol. 3, No. 3, pp. 407-420, ISSN 1742-5255

Xu, JJ.; Diaz, D. & O'Brien, PJ. (2004). Applications of cytotoxicity assays and pre-lethal mechanistic assays for assessment of human hepatotoxicity potential. *Chemico-biological interactions*, Vol. 150, No. 1, pp. 115-128

4

B Cells in Health and Disease – Leveraging Flow Cytometry to Evaluate Disease Phenotype and the Impact of Treatment with Immunomodulatory Therapeutics

Cherie L. Green, John Ferbas and Barbara A. Sullivan
Department of Clinical Immunology, Amgen Inc.
USA

1. Introduction

Flow Cytometers are key devices used to monitor the composition of cells in the blood in the setting of a variety of disease states. Recent advances have produced a range of instruments that range from simple desktop-type devices to multi-laser platforms that allow for high complexity measurements. This variety of instrumentation makes the technology suitable for different budgets, expertise levels and intended uses (research versus diagnostic) with a set of reagents that can effectively be used on any platform so long as the laser line can excite the given fluorochrome and the optics are set up to discriminate emission from the excitation wavelength. Traditional medical applications for flow cytometers include evaluation of CD4 T cell depletion and associated immunophenotypic changes in HIV-infected persons as well as characterization of aberrant cell types used to diagnose hematologic malignancies. More recently, investigators have not only extended immunophenotyping campaigns to other disease settings, but have also taken advantage of fluorescent probes that provide insight into cellular function. For example, it can be inferred that a cell that expresses CD107 on its surface has likely participated in the delivery of cytotoxic granules to a target cell (Michael R.Betts, 2004). Likewise, amine-reactive dyes can be used to track cell division, probes that fluoresce only after enzymatic cleavage can report on caspase activities in apoptosis experiments and intracellular phosphorylation can be measured with specific antibodies and cell permeabilization buffers (phosphoflow) (Maxwell et al., 2009; Krutzik and Nolan, 2006; Wu et al., 2010). The elegance of the flow cytometry platform relies on its simplicity in as much as any combination of fluorescently-conjugated probes can be used to address contemporary hypotheses in cell biology and immunology. It is therefore not surprising that investigators have introduced flow cytometric measurements in biomarker campaigns to study a variety of activities of an immunomodulatory therapeutics), including effects of proximal signaling events as influenced by agonist or antagonistic drugs, or cell immunophenotype as a representative distal pharmacodynamic marker in treated persons.

The breadth of flow cytometric biomarker activities programs by members of our laboratory is quite broad, and we have leveraged our collective expertise to attempt to address contemporary issues in biomarker campaigns that include such assessments. Despite the availability and precision of measurements performed by flow cytometers, it is important to realize that these measurements are made in the absence of accuracy standards; this is true even in the case of established assays. Thus, the strength of clinical flow cytometry is a function of the approach used for assay set-up and validation. One of the goals of this chapter is to share some of our strategies for the use of imunophenotyping data in the setting of disease and to further discuss the potential limitations of immunophenotyping in settings where correlative functional data may not be available. Even though the technology of flow cytometry is over 30 years old, the applications and ideas of using this platform as biomarker tools are in some ways in their infancy. Questions regarding the reliability of a given measurement, specimen and reagent stability, and methods to improve upon assay performance persist. It is our hope to contribute to maturation of this process and to begin to put forth ideas that could ultimately be used to standardize biomarker measurements in the clinic as executed by the flow cytometry laboratory. We have focused on immunophenotyping of blood from Systemic Lupus Erythematosus (SLE) patients in this chapter, but the principles put forth here are applicable to any disease and cell-type setting. This chapter is divided into four sections - an Overview of B cell development, B cell classification by flow cytometry, Technical Considerations, and B cell flow cytometry in contemporary biomarker campaigns.

2. Overview of B cell development

B cells are a central component of the immune system, not only because they produce one of the most important (and abundant) molecules in human serum - the class-switched high affinity antibody - but also by sensing innate stimuli, processing and presenting antigens to T cells and by producing pro- and anti-inflammatory cytokines. Class-switched antibodies (IgG, IgA, IgE) play critical effector roles as well: directing antibody-dependent cellular cytotoxicity (ADCC), phagocytosis and complement fixation to neutralize pathogens. The terminally differentiated plasma cell, residing primarily in the bone marrow, produces high affinity antibodies, sometimes providing high titer antibodies for as long as 75 years, depending on the antigen (Amanna et al., 2007; Crotty et al., 2003; Wrammert et al., 2009).

B cells originate from hematopoietic stem cells, starting their journey in the bone marrow (Figure 1). The B cell receptor (BCR) variable region of the heavy chain locus is rearranged to produce a functional heavy chain and spliced together with the μ constant region to produce IgM. The heavy chain is paired with the surrogate light chain forming the pre-BCR. If a productive signal is transmitted, the light chain undergoes rearrangement. Together, the newly paired heavy and light chain undergo selection in the bone marrow: most immature B cells with a high affinity for self proteins undergo apoptosis or the variable region of either the heavy or light chain can be rearranged anew; those with unproductive BCRs undergo 'death by neglect' and the small fraction that signals optimally proceeds down the developmental pathway. B cells that survive this process are now considered immature and begin to transition out of the bone marrow and to the secondary lymphoid organs. Further deletion of the transitional B cell population can occur (Carsetti et al., 1995), and the variable region of either the heavy or light chain can be rearranged further (Toda et al., 2009; Nemazee, 2006). The transitional B cell traffics to the secondary lymphoid organs and differentiates into a mature naïve B cell, now expressing the variable regions of the heavy chain spliced together with the δ constant region to produce IgD (Monroe et al., 2003). A key difference between the transitional B cell and the mature naïve B cell is the response to antigen – a transitional B cell will undergo apoptosis if the BCR is triggered with a cognate antigen, the naïve B cell will become activated (Monroe et al., 2003). An activated naïve B cell proliferates, internalizes the antigen via the BCR, and processes and presents antigen-derived peptides on MHC class II. With help from a specialized population of CD4+ T follicular helper cells (TFH), the B cell forms a germinal center. Through the course of the germinal center reaction, the B cell proliferates and daughter cells rearrange the BCR locus, resulting in class-switching (from IgM and IgD to either IgG, IgA, or IgE) and introduction of non-germline encoded nucleotides that result in unique BCR specificities. Each new daughter cell tests its BCR for affinity on follicular dendritic cells; those with higher affinity tend to survive. This process is collectively referred to as somatic hypermutation and affinity maturation. A subset of the activated B cells further differentiates into memory B cells and plasma cells. With a higher affinity BCR than those in the naïve pool, memory cells can respond faster and with greater magnitude than their naïve counterparts. Plasma cells are the final stage of B lineage development and travel to the bone marrow (and in some cases the secondary lymphoid organs) where they can produce antibodies for many years.

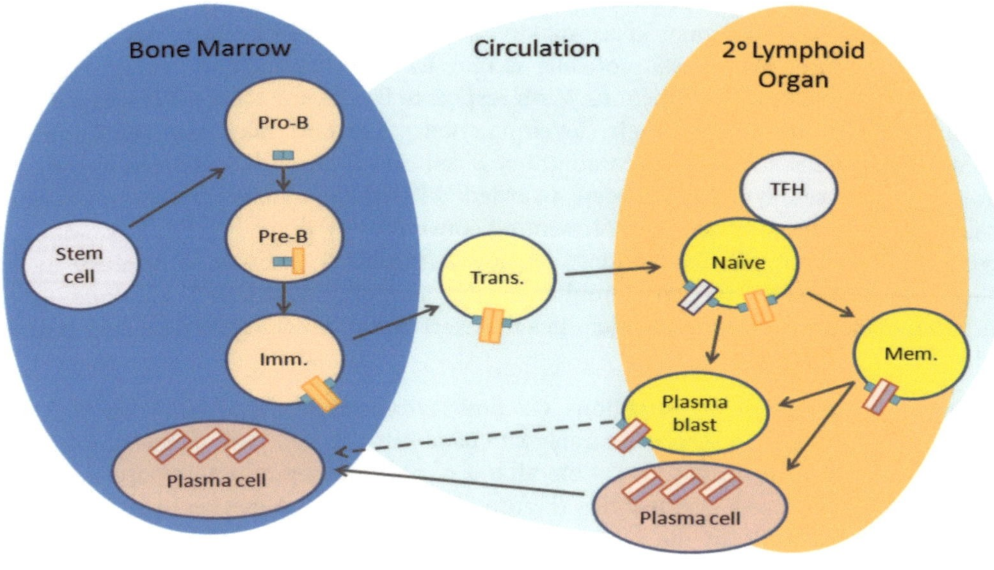

Fig. 1. An overview of B cell development. B cell development initiates in the bone marrow where the B cell receptor (BCR,) is rearranged and expressed on the surface of immature B cells (Imm. = Immature). The developing BCR pairs with signaling molecules at this early stage (). Cells with appropriate BCR affinity (neither too high nor too low) exit the bone marrow and traffic to the secondary lymphoid organs (2° = Secondary). Here, the transitional B cell completes the maturation process to become a naïve B cell, expressing both IgM () and IgD (). Upon activation by antigen, and with Follicular T cell (TFH) help, the naïve B cell forms a germinal center. The BCR is rearranged further and plasmablasts and memory B cells (Mem. = Memory) are formed, expressing IgG, IgA or IgE (). Plasma cells are the final stage of differentiation, secreting soluble Ig () and homing to the bone marrow. Exceptions to this paradigm are noted in the text

If an optimal survival niche is not found, plasma cells are short lived. The plasma cell is optimally designed to produce large amounts of antibody molecules - somewhat analogous to the manufacturing capabilities of a biotechnology company. It should be noted that, in some cases where multivalent antigens can cross-link the BCR efficiently, T cell help is not required for antibody production, although germinal centers are not typically formed. Throughout this dynamic differentiation process, autoreactive B cells are kept in check by 1) direct deletion through apoptosis, 2) receptor editing of the BCR, and 3) through anergic BCR-driven signals, rendering the B cell unresponsive to stimulation. It is the dysregulation of these tolerance mechanisms that is thought to contribute to the survival of pathogenic autoreactive B cells and possibly result in autoimmunity.

3. B cell classification by flow cytometry

The flow cytometer is a useful instrument for the study of B cell differentiation, maturation and development. At any moment in time, the cellular composition of our bodies reflects a balance between the input of new cells versus the expansion and death of existing cells. Taken in whole, cells are transported to their tissue sites via the bloodstream and any given sample is a snapshot in time of the constituents of the biologic highway. Cells continuously enter and exit the extravascular space making blood a convenient and minimally invasive sample that captures the diversity of cells as they traverse the body to interact with other cells to mediate their effector functions. With respect to B cells, the antigens displayed on the cell surface are indicative of their developmental stage and may also reflect ongoing pathologic processes. Indeed, the paradigm of B cell classification has evolved to the extent that different B cell types have been awarded descriptive names. However, caution is advised to those that rely solely upon naming convention without functional validation of those immunophenotypic descriptions. As flow cytometers continue to advance in their ability to detect more antigens simultaneously, and as investigators continue to link functional readouts to phenotypic identities the exact definition of a given cell type is subject to change.

For those new to B cell investigations via flow cytometry, it is advisable to start with "anchor" markers and to devise a strategy to establish a B cell gate. For example, CD45 identifies all leukocytes in peripheral blood and can clearly separate this population from debris or dying cells and erythrocytes (Figure 2). The B lineage markers most commonly used to identify B cells in the blood are CD19 and CD20 and additional markers can characterize a variety of distinct subsets. Using this approach at least seven circulating B cell sub-populations can be identified: 1) immature, 2) transitional, 3) mature naïve, 4) non class-switched memory, 5) class-switched memory, 6) CD27- memory, 7) plasmablasts/cells. These B cell populations are identified by markers that are now well established; we can describe them as "pillars" of B cell biology and are expanded in more detail below.

Antigenic pillars of B cell biology – classification and caveats

Two classification systems originated in the early 1990's (Maurer et al., 1990; Maurer et al., 1992; Pascual et al., 1994), both demonstrating discrete populations that could be reliably measured over time. In the classification scheme described by Maurer et al., a combination of CD19, IgD and CD27 provide a means for describing three circulating mature B cell populations where "cB" refers to "circulating B cell": "cB1 naïve" (IgD+CD27-), "cB2 non-class switched memory" (IgD+CD27+) and "cB3 class-switched memory" (IgD-CD27+) (Figure 3A). The characterization of a "double negative (DN)" (IgD-CD27-) memory B cell population was introduced later (Wei et al., 2007; Jacobi et al., 2008). This population has been shown to be elevated in some patients with lupus and has become commonplace in the classification system using IgD and CD27. Therefore, DN memory B cells are also included in Figure 3A. This system is still routinely used to monitor changes in peripheral B cell composition in patients with SLE treated with investigational agents (Belouski et al., 2010).

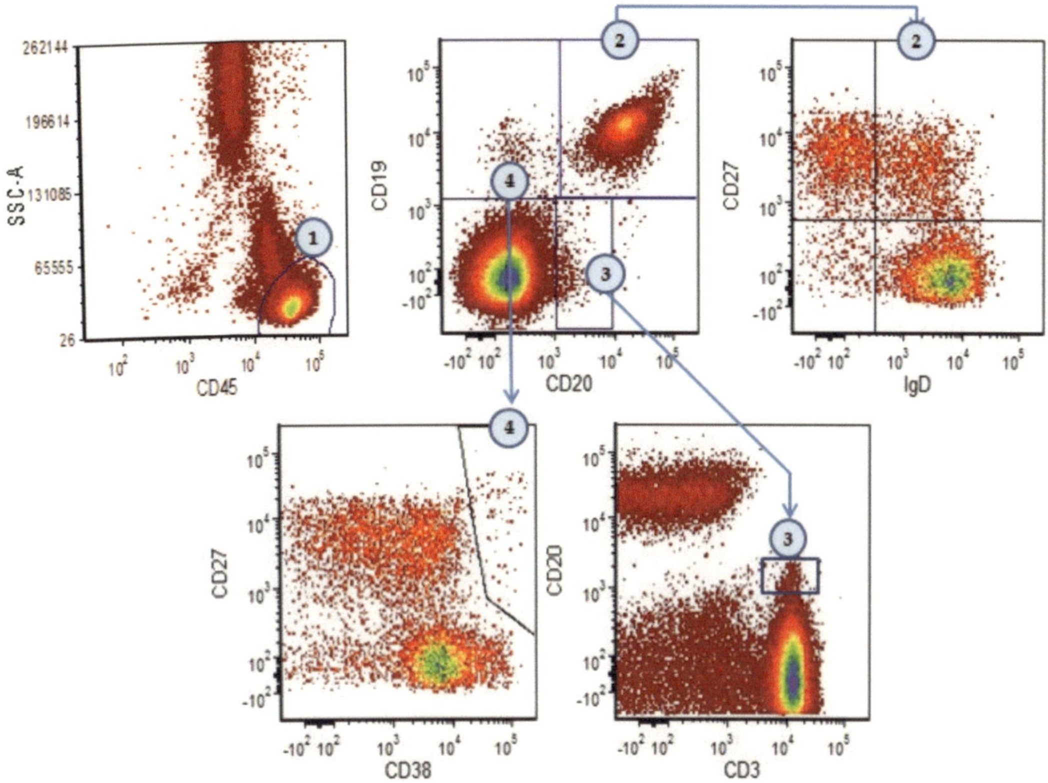

Fig. 2. Establishing the B cell gate. Blood from one healthy donor with recent influenza vaccination is shown to demonstrate B cell lineage gate. CD45 is used to discriminate leukocytes (1) from red blood cells and debris. Co-staining with CD19 and CD20 separates B cells (2) from dim CD20 expressing T cells (3) and CD20 negative plasmablasts/cells (4)

In 1994, Pascual et al. introduced additional markers to further study mature B cells. In the tonsil, B cells were characterized by activation states using CD38, CD23, and CD77 expression in addition to IgD. This resulted in a classification scheme whereby "mature B cells" were binned into categories Bm1 through Bm5 (Figure 3B) (Pascual et al., 1994). However, the focus of this classification system was on B cells involved in germinal centers formed in lymphoid tissue and was not correlated with peripheral blood populations. Mature naïve B cells were classified by surface IgD and CD38 expression (Bm1 naïve: IgD+CD38-, Bm2 naïve/activated: IgD+CD38+intermediate) and somatic mutation status in V_H region genes of the BCR. These populations were shown to have virtually no mutations.

However, it is relevant to note that IgG+ cells were depleted prior to gene rearrangement studies. Germinal center founder B cells were identified as Bm3: IgD-CD38++CD77+ (dark zone centroblasts) and Bm4: IgD-CD38++CD77- (light zone centrocytes) and showed elevated proliferation by ki-67 and increased mutational status and class switching to IgG+. Memory B cells were identified as Bm5 (IgD-CD38+/-) and demonstrated somatic hypermutation and class switching to IgG+. Bohnhorst et al. showed a correlation between tonsil and blood in healthy and primary Sjögren's syndrome donors for most of the Bm subpopulations; Bm1-2 (naïve/activated) and Bm5 (memory: early CD38+ and late CD38-). Germinal center founder cells identified as Bm3 and Bm4 (IgD-/CD38++) were not present in Bohnhorst's dataset (Bohnhorst et al., 2001). CD27 was also added to further discriminate memory B cell status. Once again, cells were sorted using cell surface markers (IgD, CD38,CD27) to study the somatic mutation status in V_H region genes of the BCR. These studies demonstrated that the "Bm1" population included both un-mutated BCR (CD27-) and mutated BCR (CD27+) populations; whereas "Bm2" showed no gene rearrangement, thus bolstering the paradigm that IgD+CD38+CD27- cells are antigen inexperienced B cells.

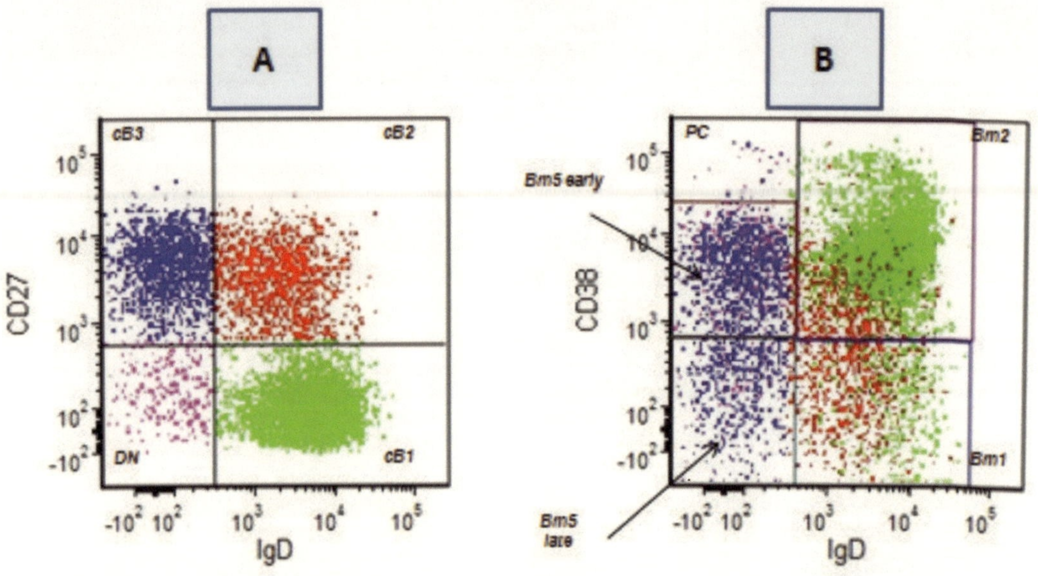

Fig. 3. B cell subset classification. Blood from one healthy donor is shown to demonstrate classification using IgD, CD27, and CD38. B cells are initially gated using CD45+ and co-expression of CD19+ and CD20+. A) cB1-cB3 and DN are defined using IgD and CD27. Mature Naïve B cells (IgD+CD27-) are designated cB1 (green), non-class switched memory B cells (IgD+CD27+) are designated cB2 (red), class-switched memory B cells (IgD-CD27+) are designated cB3 (blue), and CD27- memory B cells (IgD-CD27-) are designated DN (purple). B) Bm1-Bm5 are defined using IgD and CD38. Naïve B cells (IgD+CD38-) are designated Bm1, naïve/activated B cells (IgD+CD38+intermediate) are designated Bm2. Germinal center founder B cells (IgD-CD38++) in tonsil are defined as Bm3 (CD77+) and Bm4 (CD77-) (data not shown). In blood, this population (IgD-CD38++) is comprised of plasma blast/cells and designated PC. Memory B cells are classified as Bm5early (IgD-CD38+intermediate) and Bm5late (IgD-CD38-). The color schemes listed in A) are maintained in B) to demonstrate the location of each cB/DN population in the Bm scheme

The cB and Bm classification systems have limitations if used in isolation. For example, naïve B cells have been defined as cB1 or Bm1/2, depending on the investigator. However, with a more comprehensive arsenal of surface markers (Table 1), the heterogeneity of each B cell population becomes evident. As an example of this heterogeneity, Figure 4 demonstrates that the cB1 population also includes transitional CD10+ cells and the Bm1/2 population is muddled by CD10+ transitional cells and IgD+ non-class switched CD27+ memory cells. Indeed, more discrete populations have been described (Wei et al., 2007; Sanz et al., 2008).

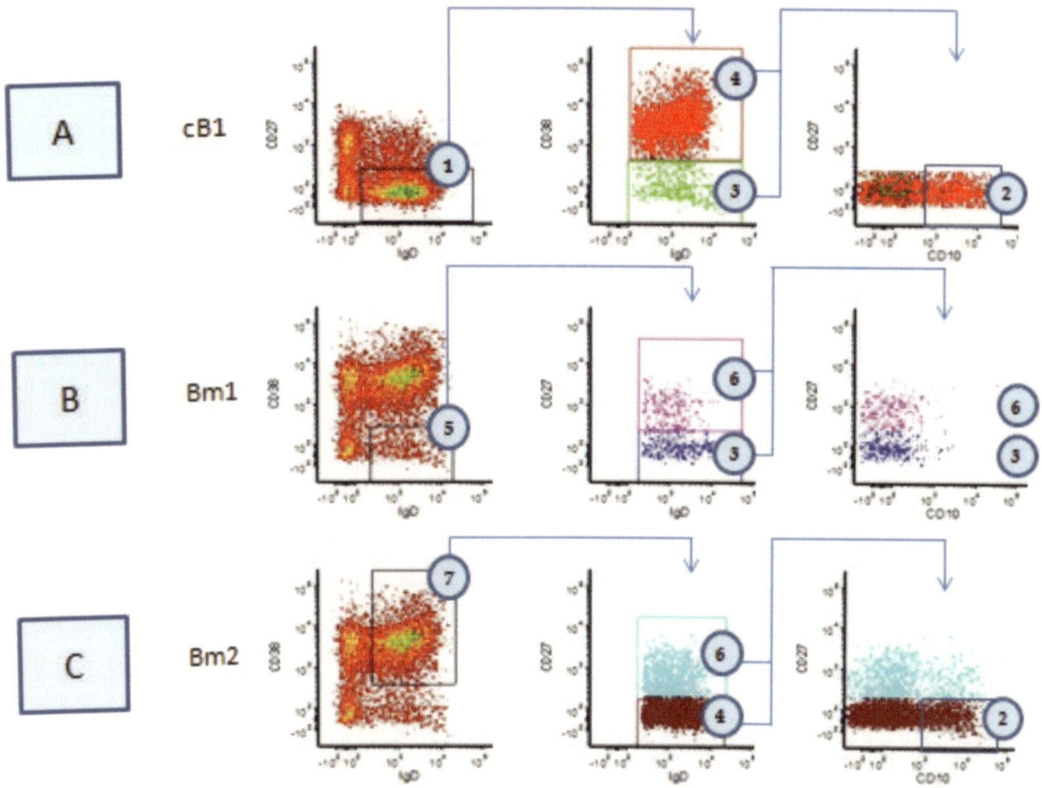

Fig. 4. Limitations of using cB1 and Bm1/2 in isolation to define the naïve B cell population. Blood from one healthy subject with recent influenza vaccination is shown. B cells are initially gated using CD45+ and co-expression of CD19+ and CD20+. IgD, CD27, CD38 are used to capture naïve B cells using both classification systems. Subpopulations are backgated to visualize heterogeneity in reciprocal classification schemes. Additionally, each classification scheme (cB1, Bm1, Bm2) is shown using CD10 and CD27 to identify CD10+CD27- transitional B cells. A) cB1 ① (IgD+CD27-) consists of transitional cells (CD10+CD27-) ② as well as mature naïve (IgD+CD27-CD38-CD10-) B cells ③ and activated naïve (IgD+CD27-CD38+CD10-) B cells ④. B) Bm1 ⑤ (IgD+CD38-) consists of mature naïve (IgD+CD27-CD38-CD10-) B cells ③ and non-class switched memory (IgD+CD27+CD10-) B cells ⑥. C) Bm2 ⑦ (IgD+CD38+) consists of transitional cells (CD10+CD27-) ② as well as activated naïve (IgD+CD27-CD38+CD10-) B cells ④ and non-class switched memory (IgD+CD27+CD10-) B cells ⑥

Marker	Antigen Specificity on B cells*	Function
IgM	First heavy chain immunoglobulin isotype expressed by B cells	Eliminates pathogens in the early stages of B cell mediated immunity, often referred to as the "natural antibody"
IgD	Second heavy chain immunoglobulin isotype expressed by B cells	Acts as receptor for antigen inexperienced B cells, stimulates basophils to release anti-microbial help
IgG	Immunoglobulin isotype expressed B cells after differentiation in the germinal center, secreted by plasma cells	Provides the majority of antibody-based immunity against invading pathogens, provides passive immunity to fetus
HLA-DR	Major histocompatibility complex class II, expressed on all mature B cells except non-proliferating plasma cells	Plays key role in antigen presentation
CD10	Expressed on immature and transitional B cells and possibly post germinal center B cells	Important in B cell development
CD19	One of the core components of the BCR expressed early in development, retained throughout maturation process, down-modulated in bone marrow resident plasma cells	Acts as signaling complex throughout life of B cell
CD20	Expressed on B cells from late pro-B cell phase to mature memory cell, down-modulated in plasma blast/cells	Acts as calcium channel in cell membrane and important in B cell activation and proliferation
CD22	Expressed cytoplasmically early in B cell development (late pro-B), surface expression coordinated with IgD, down-modulated in plasma cells	Regulates B cell adhesion and signaling functions
CD27	Expressed on memory B cells and plasma blasts/cells	Involved with memory differentiation, upregulated on plasma blasts
CD38	Expressed on various activated B cell developmental stages	Thought to indicate activation status of cell
CD45	Expressed on all nucleated hematopoietic cells	Essential for antigen receptor signal transduction and lymphocyte development
CD138	Expressed on plasma cells	Important for plasma cell adhesion to bone marrow stromal matrix

*Please refer to (Neil Barclay et al., 1997) for additional details

Table 1. Description of B cell related markers. Description of the marker's specificity on B cells only. The marker may be expressed on other cell populations with other functions

The markers most commonly used in our laboratory to analyze peripheral blood B cells are CD45, CD19, CD20, IgD, CD10, CD38, CD27 and CD138. With this strategy, using CD19 and CD20 as our anchor gate, we define the following populations within the IgD positive B cell population: transitional (IgD+CD27-CD38+CD10+), quiescent and activated naïve (IgD+CD27-CD38-/+CD10-), and non class-switched memory (IgD+CD27+CD38-/+CD10-).

The IgD negative B cells are comprised of immature (IgD-CD27-CD38+CD10+), class-switched memory (IgD-CD27+CD38-/+ and IgD-CD27-CD38-/+) and plasma blast/cell (CD20-IgD-CD27++CD38++ CD138-/+). These markers may not be appropriate in all situations and a number of caveats should be noted: [1] In clinical situations where a B-cell monoclonal therapy is used, an alternate B lineage marker may be required. For example, CD19 is used in most Rituximab trials since CD20 is the therapeutic target, [2] If CD20 is used in isolation to identify B lineage cells, a T cell marker is recommended as some T cells express low levels of CD20 (Figure 2) (Hultin et al., 1993), [3] Caution should be exercised when using CD20 to establish the initial B cell gate, as plasma cells lose expression of this marker upon terminal differentiation (Figure 2), [4] With regard to naïve B cell populations, while most IgD+ cells in the periphery co-express IgM, and IgD negative populations are assumed to express class-switched immunoglobulins (Klein et al., 1998), rare populations that are exclusively IgM+ or IgD+ have been described (Belouski et al., 2010; Weller et al., 2004), [5] CD38 is continuously expressed on B cells with frequent modulation of fluorescence intensity throughout development and therefore defining CD38$^{+bright}$ and CD38^{+dim} can be subjective without proper controls and finally, [6] CD19 expression on B cells can be quite dim in patients with SLE, so selecting a bright fluorochrome is important.

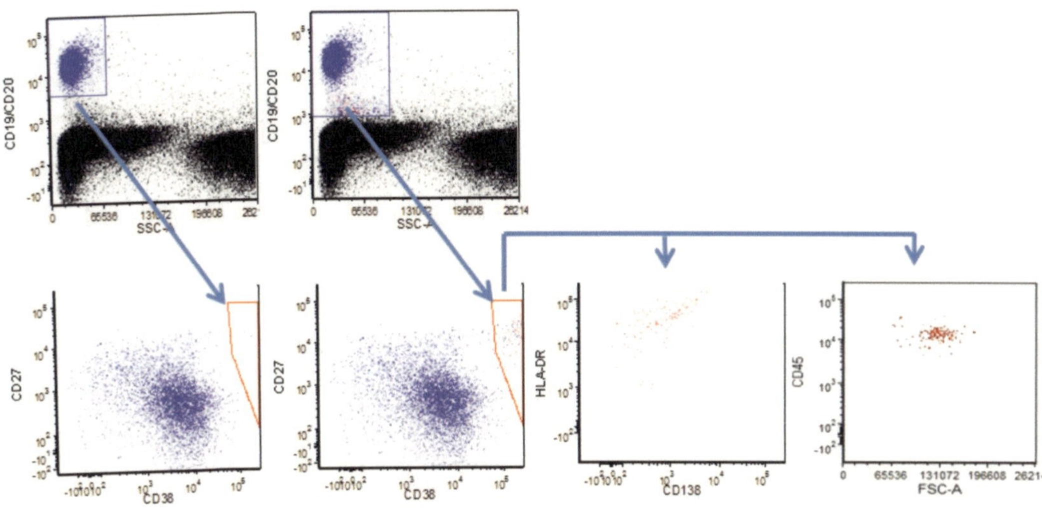

Fig. 5. Impact of gating strategy of B cells. Restricting the B cell lineage anchor gate can result in exclusion of plasma cells. Blood from one healthy subject with recent influenza vaccination is shown. B cells are initially gated using CD45+

There is still considerable debate on the phenotypic classification and nomenclature of antibody secreting cells. Uncertainties in classification most likely reflect the variety of surface antigens that can be modulated on the basis of their maturation and activation state, residence in bone marrow, blood or tissue compartments as well as the relative age of the individual (Caraux et al., 2010). A particular challenge is the differentiation of plasma cell precursors, aka plasmablasts, from the terminally differentiated, non-proliferating plasma cells. Growing evidence suggests that plasmablasts can be distinguished from plasma cells by their expression of MHC class II, elevated chemokine receptor expression (CXCR4,

CXCR3; suggestive of homing to inflamed tissues or bone marrow), and proliferative capacity (as measured by ki-67) (Odendahl et al., 2005; Jacobi et al., 2010b). In healthy subjects plasmablasts appear in the blood as a transient population that arises in response to antigen challenge (Chaussabel et al., 2008) and can be studied in this setting. Although tissue resident plasma cells downmodulate CD45, we are comfortable using CD45 to gate on plasma cells in peripheral blood (Figure 5) (Pellat-Deceunynck and Bataille, 2004; Schneider et al., 1997). Overall, we recommend that each lab carefully evaluate their schema for phenotyping plasmablast and plasma cells and generate data to support their decisions prior to embarking on tests with clinical specimens.

To further understand B cell heterogeneity and for better comparison of data across laboratories, it will be important for investigators to work toward more comparable data sets, and bring together data from many individuals for comparisons. An array of antigens could be summarized into a proteomic array of surface phenotypes and be analyzed in a comparable manner to transcription analysis by microarray. Some investigators are using complex multi-color panels (e.g. 20+ colors) to address these challenges (Lugli et al., 2010b; Lugli et al., 2010a; Gattinoni et al., 2011; Qian et al., 2010), but the impact of fluorescent overlap on the quality of these measurements is still a concern for everyday use, and may be limited to specialized laboratories. One new instrument that holds promise in approaching this kind of global standard is the elemental cytometer (Bendall et al., 2011), capable of analyzing a large array of data (e.g. 50+ parameters) and is not limited by overlapping fluorescence like more traditional flow cytometric platforms.

Dysregulated B cell Phenotypes in SLE

Methods to detect deviation from healthy development patterns have provided information for the diagnosis and monitoring of B cell aberrancies, especially in the field of oncology (Craig and Foon, 2008). Likewise, in autoimmune diseases such as SLE, the cellular composition of the B cell compartment is notably skewed. This dysregulation may provide insight into the steps that contribute to a break in tolerance observed in autoimmune diseases. Some SLE patients have a higher proportion of circulating T follicular helper (TFH) cells (CD4+CXCR5+ ICOS+) and plasmablast/cells (CD19dimCD27+CD38++) compared with healthy individuals (Hutloff et al., 2004; Illei et al., 2010). Increased frequency of TFH cells correlate with anti-dsDNA titer (Simpson et al., 2010) and increased plasma cell numbers correlate with disease activity (Dorner and Lipsky, 2004). The high number of TFH cells could reflect aberrantly high number of germinal centers; this could trigger the development of more plasma cells, and, later-on, pathogenic auto-antibodies. Likewise, on peripheral B cells, CD38 expression can be increased and conversely, CD19 expression decreased. Unusually high numbers of transitional cells have also been reported. Elevation of specific memory cell subsets (CD27-IgD-CD95+) have also been reported by many investigators as well as our own experience (Wei et al., 2007; Jacobi et al., 2008b). Finally, it is worth noting that dysregulation of B cells could potentially lead to high affinity auto-antibodies. For example, SLE patients exhibit an increase in antibody and complement deposition on circulating reticulocytes and platelets, correlating with disease activity (Navratil et al., 2006; Batal et al., 2011). Study of these deviations may provide clues to disease status and the potential efficacy of established or experimental therapeutics.

4. Technical considerations

Flow Cytometry is a powerful analytical tool yet insufficient care in technical considerations can lead to data that is difficult to interpret or worse, data that is misleading or incorrect. When establishing an immunophenotyping assay, all analytical aspects that might contribute to variability must be considered.

Specimen stability

Biological material, regardless of origin, begins to change and degrade once removed from the body. This presents a unique challenge in flow cytometric assays where accurately enumerating and measuring cellular components is dependent on maintaining the integrity of the specimen. Choice of specimen (i.e. whole peripheral blood, isolated and cryopreserved peripheral blood mononuclear cells (PBMCs)), blood collection tube, anti-coagulant, and shipping/storage conditions all play a critical role and should all be considered. Various whole blood stabilization products, such as Cyto-Chex® BCT, TransFix®, and CellSave have become available in the last few years, purporting to provide improved stability of surface marker expression and light scatter properties of lymphocytes and circulating tumor cells in whole blood. These products can be divided into two categories: 1) cell preservative solutions that are added to blood after collection into standard anticoagulant blood collection tubes or 2) direct-draw blood collection tubes that include both anticoagulant and a cell preservative solution. Although these products were initially approved by the FDA for use in extending the stability of blood for CD4 counts in remote laboratory HIV testing and maintaining integrity of fragile circulating tumor cells, there is promise that other surface markers may be stabilized as well. There is growing evidence that the use of blood collection tubes with cell preservative formulation may preserve some surface antigen expression superior to that of blood collected with anticoagulant alone (Plate et al., 2009; Warrino et al., 2005; Davis et al., 2011). However, a cell stabilization formula that truly extends the stability of blood without impacting resolution of dim markers has yet to be brought forward. Peripheral (whole) blood is the specimen of choice in our laboratory because the composition of cells in the unseparated and unfrozen state is most likely to resemble the *in vivo* state of the blood donor (Belouski et al., 2010). Peripheral blood analysis also has the advantage that the cells are exposed to the biologic matrix throughout the assay. This is particularly important in clinical trials because the therapeutic compound is retained in the specimen.

Establishing the antibody panel

The expansion of commercially available monoclonal antibodies conjugated to an ever-increasing list of fluorescent dyes has provided the opportunity for higher complexity multiplexed assays. However, to establish the optimal panel, one must consider: [1] expected antigen density and frequency of the cell population of interest, [2] interaction of reagents within the panel (spectral overlap between fluorochromes), [3] stability and sensitivity to assay conditions (temperature, pH, cell concentration), and [4] the sensitivity limitations of the flow cytometer.

Once the theoretical panel has been constructed, it is good practice to test the features of the cocktail of fluorochrome-conjugated antibodies under the conditions that you will use in your study. Questions worth answering include: [1] determination of antibody clone(s) and conjugate(s) that correctly identify the population of interest (different clones can generate markedly different staining patterns), [2] The optimal titration of each antibody for its intended purpose (the density of antigen in the target population may exceed that of the healthy range and require a higher antibody concentration to saturate the target), [3] whether compensation controls accurately address spectral overlap for each antibody-fluorochrome, based on expected dynamic range of the data (a fluorescence-minus-one (FMO) matrix experiment (example in Table 2) can provide valuable insight during the development phase and may identify potentially troublesome compensation issues and/or markers with dim or heterogeneous expression), [4] How stable are the fluorochromes in the matrix (some fluorescent dyes are sensitive to pH, fixation and photobleaching (e.g. tandem dyes))?, [5] Whether antibody cocktails with demonstrated stability and extended shelf life (>1 month) can be produced and used. With information about these biochemical components, it is now appropriate to develop the assay.

	FITC	PE	PerCP	APC	Pacific Blue
Panel	**IgD**	**CD38**	**CD45**	**CD27**	**CD19**
FMO FITC	--	CD38	CD45	CD27	CD19
FMO PE	IgD	--	CD45	CD27	CD19
FMO PerCP	IgD	CD38	--	CD27	CD19
FMO APC	IgD	CD38	CD45	--	CD19
FMO Pacific Blue	IgD	CD38	CD45	CD27	--

Table 2. Example of Fluorescence Minus One (FMO) Matrix Experiment. In this 5-color panel, each antibody-fluorochrome is removed from the matrix, one by one to determine spectral overlap issues and establish negative thresholds

Assay development

Numerous assay parameters should be tested. These include the evaluation of: [1]the impact of sample type (e.g. peripheral blood, PBMC), [2] red blood cell lysis (recipe, temperature and timing of lysis), [3] antibody-cell incubation time and temperature, [4] washing and acquisition buffers, and [5] the number of cells needed to acquire meaningful data. This is particularly true when targeting rare cell populations. Many of the cell populations that have been suggested as contributing to chronic inflammation in autoimmune diseases, such as TFH and plasmablast/cells, are quite rare in circulation. Advances in the technology of rare event detection are warranted and enrichment technologies, such as magnetic bead sorting prior to flow cytometry, may provide an improvement. The impact of enrichment on phenotype and function will need to be characterized for each population of interest.

Setting up and maintaining instrument

A key aspect to generating reliable and accurate data is ensuring that the instrument is properly set up and maintained. There is a wealth of information on how to optimize, validate, and maintain flow cytometers so the scope of this chapter will not include instrumentation specifics (Green et al., 2011). In brief, the instrument must be first properly aligned and characterized. Next, a good routine quality control system must be implemented and adhered to. Some clinical trials persist for years, making it even more important to maintain data integrity and reduce longitudinal variability. Beads with known fluorescent quantities (e.g., MESF, QuantiBRITE) can be used to establish a standard curve by which fluorescent intensity can be converted into semi-quantitative measurements, thus reducing the impact of longitudinal variability (Schwartz et al., 2004; Wang et al., 2008). Ensuring that the flow cytometer has optimal sensitivity for the panel is critical. This is especially true if the expected density of the marker is very dim. Figure 6 is an example of using standardized beads with known fluorescent properties to test these parameters, where Instrument C is inferior in the APC channel, compared with Instruments A and B.

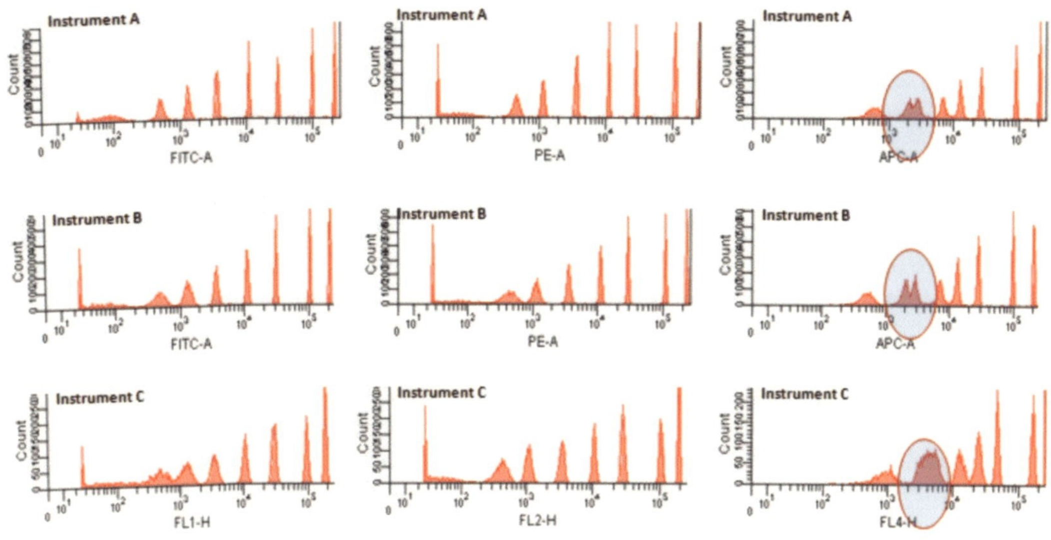

Fig. 6. Sensitivity varies between instruments. SPHERO™ Ultra Rainbow beads were acquired using optimal instrument settings on 3 different flow cytometers. Resolution of the dim peaks in the APC channel on Instrument C is inferior to Instrument A and B

Data analysis and Interpretation

Many software programs are available for post-acquisition analysis of flow cytometry data files, including instrument associated acquisition software and stand alone third party analysis software. While this flexibility provides the researcher with many tools to customize analysis for a specific purpose, caution is advised when establishing the analysis template. Electronic listmode/FCS files that are imported from various instruments into third party software may display quite differently based on hardcoded meta-data in the raw data and user preferences set within each software. While the actual electronic files have not changed, variation in data display can significantly impact the final results. Likewise, the technical detail of gating strategy represents another source of variance from standardized definitions because differences in gating can easily result in different data output regarding a given cell type. For example, a stringent CD19/CD20 gate could exclude circulating plasmablast/ cells (Figure 5).

Another component of data analysis entails understanding the reliability of each measurement. Performing validation exercises to establish: [1] the stability of whole blood for intended analytes, [2] assay precision (replicates), and [3] inter- and intra-subject variability is paramount to interpretation of meaningful changes in phenotype or composition after treatment with clinical therapeutics. Although flow cytometric datasets are not inherently different than any other regarding statistical analyses, applications in the setting of early phase clinical trials incorporate cohort sizes that are not always amenable to population-based statistical approaches. We have chosen to highlight one approach to this problem that can prove useful in this setting that is referred to as the coefficient of reliability (CoR) (Taylor et al., 1989b).

The CoR tethers reliability to the consistency of repeat measurements in an individual over a window of time, calibrating a meaningful change after treatment with a therapeutic agent as one compared against each person's baseline measurement. For this analysis scheme to work and reveal a treatment effect in a clinical trial, the within-person variability must be well characterized such that one can call-out a change after treatment that exceeds the intrinsic variability of the assay.

A CoR can be determined by dividing inter-subject variability by the total variability (inter+intra), resulting in a number from 0.00 (least reliable) to 1.00 (most reliable) (Belouski et al., 2010; Taylor et al., 1989a). Using the CoR, one can determine what analytical parameter contributes most variance (Table 3). For example, an analyte that shows very little intra-subject variability but exhibits high variability between subjects can still be considered "reliable". If more variability is seen within repeat measures from the same subject than is observed between subjects on a single draw, the analyte could be considered "unreliable". The reliability of a given measurement can reflect variability that is introduced as a function of specimen stability or specimen processing/analysis or can reflect bona-fide biologic variability. If one takes care to minimize laboratory variability, datasets with high CoR can be attained (Table 3, with discussion below).

We typically begin our investigations by estimating inter-subject variability (donor-to-donor) and intra-subject variability across three repeat blood draws in a group of healthy and/or diseased donors, and use a threshold of 0.64 as a guide to differentiate between a reliable (≥0.64) and unreliable (<0.64) measure; this reflects the original publication from Taylor et al (Taylor et al., 1989b)that examined the CoR for CD4 counts in HIV-infected persons. As an example using data generated in our laboratory (Table 3), we show the CoR of common B cell subsets for nine healthy donors (HD) and five SLE donors with mild disease severity. As shown in the Table, nearly all of the measures as expressed in this analysis exhibited a high CoR, with many approaching a value of 1.00. Such analyses would be promoted for application in a clinical trial, but we caution the reader in assuming that

CoR values such as these are typical (we have failed a variety of assays based on CoR measures that are not shown here).

Analyte	Parent Gate	HD (N=9)	SLE (N=5)
%CD3+	CD45+ Lymphocytes	0.87	0.97
%CD19+CD20+		0.91	0.96
%CD27+CD38++	B lineage	0.83	0.81
%CD138+ CD38++		0.76	0.79
IgD+/CD27-%		0.96	0.96
IgD+/CD27+%		0.96	0.97
IgD-/CD27+%		0.96	0.94
IgD-/CD27-%		0.66	0.94

Cell populations <200 events

$$\text{CoR:} \quad \frac{\text{inter-subject variability}}{\text{(inter- + intra-subject variability)}}$$

0.00 least reliable
1.00 most reliable

Table 3. Coefficient of Reliability of B cell subsets

Populations with an average of less than 200 events in Table 3 are highlighted in blue, as low event counts are a common laboratory source of low CoR scores. As depicted in the Table, it can be seen that not all flagged values fail CoR; only the cell types of lowest relative frequency in the blood, i.e., IgD-CD27- B cells in HD appear as (low) outliers in the Table. Interestingly, CoR increased as a function of a disease marked by increased frequencies of IgD-CD27- B cells in SLE (as much as 3X healthy range), that is, the higher CoR in SLE patients most likely reflected the expansion of this cell type in the blood. It is important to perform validation exercises in persons that exhibit a targeted pathology to fully characterize and understand each assay deployed in the clinical setting (Belouski et al., 2010).

Maximizing resources

It is becoming clear that for the medical community to truly leverage the information garnered by such flow cytometric investigations, consensus protocols and proficiency testing will be required. In lieu of that greater goal, it is important for any given investigator to bring forward all details of their immunophenotyping methodologies and to take time to understand the potential differences in reporting that exist between investigators and laboratories. In this regard, the ISAC (International Society for Analytical Cytometry) guidance document "Minimum Information about a Flow Cytometry Experiment" is of great value (Lee et al., 2008). Likewise, it would be inappropriate to discount the impact of resources to the implementation of a flow cytometric program. Instruments are highly technical and provide a service unique to the biomarker portfolio. However, instruments are priced accordingly, and the reagents to detect antigens, especially the 'cutting edge' fluorochromes, can be quite expensive. Two products would therefore help to reduce the cost of flow cytometry by allowing batch analysis: [1] lyophilized antibody panels with extended shelf-lives that could detect the "leukocyte proteomic array" of phenotypes and [2] collection tubes formulated to extend the window of time for processing whole blood.

Balancing the needs of the biologist (which is the best population to follow?), the technical considerations of the cytometrist (what is the most precise and accurate way to do the assay?) and resources (is it worth it?) are a few of the challenges encountered in flow cytometry biomarker programs. However, as evidenced in the next section, it is well worth the effort. The flow cytometer can provide essential decision-enabling data that unlocks evidence of therapeutic efficacy, mechanism-of-action and provide a fascinating snapshot into the dynamics of the immune system.

5. B cell flow cytometry in contemporary biomarker campaigns

Flow cytometry undeniably offers great insight into B cell biology in health and disease by enabling researchers with the ability to identify cells and understand their representation in the immune repertoire. The impact of flow cytometry based evaluations becomes even greater in the clinical settings because it allows one to understand the pharmacodynamic effects of a given treatment and when paired with biomarkers testing functional aspects of B cell biology (e.g. the vaccine response). We review some of the more common examples that have emerged from integrated assessment of B cells and B cell subsets during clinical intervention as examples of the value of understanding B cells in the context of therapeutic treatments in the clinic. In particular, we have reported in Table 4 on the phenotype as described by the investigator in each study, heterogeneity notwithstanding, and have summarized the key findings in Table 5. It is within the reach of these efforts to someday use these strategies to measure B cell-related biomarkers for patient selection, or to be leveraged in therapeutic co-development as companion diagnostic assays.

Pharmacodynamic activity of B cell-directed therapeutics

Strategies that deplete B cells to varying degrees are now commonly applied in the clinic. Initially tested in oncology, Rituximab is a chimeric monoclonal antibody that binds the B cell surface antigen CD20, leading to depletion of this population (reviewed in Boumans et al., 2011; Dorner et al., 2009). Rituximab was first approved in non-Hodgkin's lymphoma (NHL) and has now been approved in many other indications, including chronic lymphocytic leukemia, rheumatoid arthritis (RA), and two forms of vasculitis. The successful depletion of oncologic B cells in NHL was encouraging enough to trigger the study of Rituximab in autoimmune scenarios. Rituximab proved successful in the treatment of TNF-resistant RA (in combination with methotrexate) and firmly established the B cell as a central player in the *autoimmune* immune system. Investigators also reported success of Rituximab in numerous autoimmune diseases including SLE. Controlled trials of Rituximab in SLE (with and without nephritis), however, failed to meet the primary and secondary efficacy endpoints although a beneficial effect was observed in some ethnic groups (Merrill et al., 2010; Looney, 2010). Rituximab is still used often to treat SLE off-label, and that impact on B cells in SLE still provides interesting insights. Most recently, Rituximab was approved for two forms of vasculitis associated with anti-neutrophil cytoplasmic antibodies (ANCAs), Wegener's Granulomatosis and Microscopic Polyangiitis.

Marker System or Study	Transitional (T) / Immature (Im)	Naïve	Non class-switched Memory	Class-switched Memory	Plasmablasts (PB) Plasma cells (PC)	Reference
cB1-4	nd	CD19+ IgD+ CD27-	CD19+ IgD+ CD27+	CD19+ IgD- CD27+	nd	Maurer et al. 1990, Maurer et al. 1992
Bm1-5	nd	IgD+ CD27- CD38+/-	IgD-/+ CD27+ CD38+/-		nd	Pascual et al. 1994 Bohnhorst et al. 2001
Rituximab in SLE	nd	CD19+ CD27- CD38-	CD19+ CD27++ CD38-		CD19+ CD20+/- CD27++ CD38++(PB)	Vital et al. 2011
	CD38++IgD+ CD10+CD24+ (Im)	CD19+ IgD+CD38+	CD19+ IgD+/- CD27+		IgD-CD38++CD27+ CD20- (PC)	Roll et al. 2008
	nd	CD19+ CD24+ IgD+ CD38- CD10-	nd	CD19+ CD1c+/- IgD- CD27+ IgM +/-	nd	Pescovitz et al 2011
	CD38^{high}CD24^{high}IgD- (Im) CD38^{high}CD24^{high}IgD+ (T)*	CD38^{intermediate} CD24^{low} IgD+CD27-	IgD+CD27+	IgD-CD27+	CD19^{low} CD20- CD38^{high} IgD- CD27+ (PB)	Anolik et al. 2004 Anolik, et al. 2007
Belimumab in SLE	CD19+ IgD+ CD27- CD10+ (T)	CD19+ IgD+ CD27- CD10-	CD19+ IgD+ CD27+	CD19+ IgD- CD27-/+	CD19+ IgD- CD27++ CD38++ (PB/PC)	Jacobi et al 2010a
Atacicept in RA	nd	CD19+ IgD+ CD27-	CD19+ CD27+ CD38-		CD19^{dim} CD38^{bright}(PC)	Van Vollenhoven et al. 2011
Tocilizumab in SLE	nd	nd	nd	nd	CD19^{low} IgD- CD38+++ (PC)	Illei et al 2010
Our system	CD19+CD20+ IgD- CD27- CD38+ CD10+ (Im) CD19+CD20+ IgD+ CD27- CD38+ CD10+ (T)	CD19+ CD20+ IgD+ CD27- CD38+/- CD10-	CD19+ CD20+ IgD+CD27+ CD38+/- CD10-	CD19+ CD20+ IgD-CD27-/+ CD38+/- CD10-/+	CD19+CD20- IgD- CD27++ CD38++ CD138+/- (PB/PC)	

Table 4. Identification of B cell populations-common marker systems and examples from clinical literature. Phenotypes summarized in this table are not all inclusive. As emerging technologies are developed and implemented, it is likely that characterization schemes will change. *Subsets are further described by investigator

Mechanism	Example	Transitional	Naïve	Memory	Plasmablast / cell
Anti-CD20 (depleting)	Rituximab	nd	↓	↓	↔
Anti-BAFF	Belimumab	↓	↓	↑	↔
TACI-Ig	Atacicept	nd	↓	↑	↓
Anti-IL-6R	Tocilizumab	nd	↔	↔	↓

Table 5. Summary of changes in B cell populations in response to B cell therapeutics. Nomenclature varies for each study and this summary is based on the phenotype as described by the investigator. Please refer to the text for more details. nd = not determined

The effects of Rituximab mediated depletion and repletion of the B cell compartment have been carefully characterized using flow cytometry (Anolik et al., 2004; Anolik et al., 2007). In most subjects, Rituximab leads to the rapid depletion of CD19+ B cells in the peripheral blood (Merrill et al., 2010; Edwards et al., 2004), with fewer than 5 cells/µL by two weeks post dose. In a Phase 2 efficacy trial of general SLE, approximately 9.5% of treated subjects did not reach this level of depletion in the peripheral blood. [Removing these subjects from the efficacy analysis did not change the result in SLE.] Interestingly, approximately 26% of subjects had developed anti-therapeutic antibodies (Merrill et al., 2010) at week 52, during the early stages of B cell repletion.

The functional impact of B cell repletion was recently described in a study of neo-antigen (phiX174) and recall (tetanus toxoid) responses in Rituximab-treated patients. Peripheral B cell depletion was achieved (fewer than 5 cells/µL) in all subjects treated with Rituximab. The Rituximab-treated group had significantly lower anti-phiX174 responses compared to placebo during the window of B cell depletion (weeks 6-8) (Pescovitz et al., 2011). However, when re-immunized at weeks 52 and 56, after naïve (CD19+ CD24+ IgD+ CD38-CD10-) but not memory (CD19+ CD1c+/- IgD- CD27+ IgM-/+) B cell repletion had begun, the anti-phiX174 response returned to nearly normal levels. The vaccine memory response was tested at 52 weeks and although the memory B cell compartment had not returned to normal levels, all subjects mounted a response, albeit weaker in the Rituximab group. The impact of this study is important to note. The kinetics of Rituximab depletion and repletion of B cells, the half-life of the tetanus titer in healthy individuals (~11 years (Amanna et al., 2007)) and the new knowledge that Rituximab-treated individuals can rebuild their serologic titers once naïve B cell repletion begins will help physicians estimate when to begin re-vaccination on a patient-specific basis.

Resistance to depletion and repletion of B cells may also help identify those patients most likely to benefit from Rituximab or when to re-treat therapeutic responders. In SLE, Rituximab depletes peripheral naive and memory B cells (CD19+CD27-CD38- and CD19+CD27++CD38-, respectively) and circulating plasmablasts (CD19+ CD20+/- CD27++ CD38++) (Vital et al., 2011). However, the plasmablast level at 26 weeks may predict relapse of the clinical response, as subjects with more than 0.8 plasmablast cells/µL were more likely to relapse then subjects with fewer than 0.8 plasmablast cells/µL. In RA, subjects had a more favorable outcome with delayed B cell repletion (both naïve (CD19+IgD+) and memory (CD19+ CD27+) cells) (Teng et al., 2009; Roll et al., 2008) and reduced plasma cells (CD79a+ CD20-) in the synovium (Teng et al., 2009). A second study of RA demonstrated early relapse was characterized by higher non-class switched memory B cells (CD19+ IgD+ CD27+) before therapy (Roll et al., 2008). These studies suggest that the efficacy of Rituximab could be related to pre-treatment levels of unusual memory B cells, plasmablasts or plasma cells. Leveraging these studies, but using transcript analysis, a recent report suggests that plasmablast levels can identify those patients most likely to respond to anti-CD20 depletion therapies (Owczarczyk et al., 2011).

The effects of Belimumab (anti-BAFF) can be differentiated from those of Rituximab, where Belimumab selectively leads to the reduction in naïve (CD19+ IgD+ CD27- CD10-) and transitional (CD19+ IgD+ CD27- CD10+) B cells but leaves the memory (CD19+ CD27+ IgD-) B cell compartment intact (Jacobi et al., 2010a; Jacobi et al., 2010b). Non-class switched memory B cells (CD19+ CD27+ IgD+) cells and the compartment containing plasmablasts and plasma cells (CD19+ IgD- CD27++ CD38++) decreased after much longer exposure to therapy (~1.5 years). The phase III studies of Belimumab used a novel SLE Responder Index (SRI) (Furie et al., 2009) based on Belimumab's clinical phase II experience. With this strategy, Belimumab demonstrated efficacy in SLE and was approved by the FDA in 2011. Further studies of agents targeting BAFF have been initiated. Two phase III studies of Lilly's LY2127399 in patients with SLE are currently recruiting (Clinical Trials identifiers: NCT01196091, NCT01205438) and a phase III study of Anthera's Blisibimod (A-623) is scheduled to study safety and efficacy in SLE (NCT01395745).

The effects of Atacicept treatment (TACI-Ig) are distinct from Rituximab and Belimumab as well. Atacicept is a fusion protein of the extracellular portion of the TACI receptor and the Fc portion of human IgG. The TACI receptor binds BAFF and APRIL, two proteins with numerous functions (Davidson, 2010), including providing homeostatic survival signals to naïve B cells (BAFF) and plasma cells (APRIL) (Mackay and Schneider, 2008). Atacicept reduces the level of circulating naive B cells (CD19+ IgD+ CD27-) and plasma cells ($CD19^{dim}$ $CD38^{bright}$). Memory B cells (CD19+CD27+CD38-) exhibit a transient increase in the peripheral blood (van Vollenhoven et al., 2011). Atacicept additionally reduces total immunoglobulin levels (IgM, IgG and IgA) (Dall'Era et al., 2007; van Vollenhoven et al., 2011). In RA, Atacicept did not meet the primary endpoint in two studies - in subjects with inadequate responses to methotrexate (van Vollenhoven et al., 2011) and subjects with inadequate response to TNF antagonist therapy (Genovese et al., 2011). By impacting a broad spectrum of B cell subsets, BAFF/APRIL blockade may deplete long lived tissue resident plasma cells that produce pathogenic autoantibodies; however, BAFF/APRIL blockade may carry a greater infectious risk due to the depletion of protective antibody titers as well.

Finally, we discuss a molecule that significantly decreases the frequency of circulating plasma cells, Tocilizumab (anti-IL-6R). IL-6 has numerous roles in immune regulation, hematopoiesis, inflammation and oncogenesis (reviewed in (Kishimoto, 2010)) as well as providing survival signals to plasmablasts and plasma cells. Tocilizumab was efficacious in RA patients in several Phase 3 trials and has been approved in the US for patients who have failed TNF-blockers (Yazici et al., 2011) and in small studies of other autoimmune disorders (Kishimoto, 2010). In an open-label study of SLE subjects, Tocilizumab led to a significant decrease in circulating plasma cells ($CD19^{low}$ IgD- CD38+++), a decrease in serum IgG levels and a promising clinical response (Illei et al., 2010). There were no other changes in peripheral T or B cells.

More traditional therapies like cyclophosphamide may result in B cell depletion to a degree not as fully appreciated in the past. For example, cyclophosphamide induced significant B cell depletion in a trial compared with Rituximab in ANCA-associated vasculitis (Stone et al., 2010).

Modulation of B cell function

CD22 is an important signaling molecule for the homeostasis of early B lineage cells (Tedder et al., 2005). CD22 is expressed on developing pro- and pre- B cells as well as naïve B cells and is lost after activation; i.e. memory B cells, plasmablasts and plasma cells do not express CD22 (Dorken et al., 1986; Tedder et al., 2005). Epratuzumab is an anti-CD22 monoclonal antibody that modulates B cell function although the mechanism of action *in vivo* is unclear. *In vitro*, Epratuzumab leads to the rapid internalization of the CD22/antibody complex, resulting in significant CD22 phosphorylation (Carnahan et al., 2003) as well as a change in adhesion molecule cell surface expression and migration (Daridon et al., 2010). Epratuzumab is not thought to mediate ADCC or complement-dependent cytotoxicity (CDC) *in vivo*. In SLE, however, Epratuzumab leads to a significant reduction in CD27-negative B cells (primarily naïve and transitional populations) (Dorner et al., 2006; Jacobi et al., 2008a). The recent hypothesis that Epratuzumab alters B cell migration is compelling (Daridon et al., 2010) and may shed light on the mechanism of action, but has yet to be tested in the clinic. Epratuzumab has shown promising results in combination with Rituximab in oncology (Grant, 2010); SLE trials were terminated early due to insufficient drug supply. An interim report of the data suggested that Epratuzumab was effective (Wallace, 2010), however this study was not powered to detect statistical differences between treatment groups. A new set of phase III studies in severe general SLE (NCT01262365 and NCT01261793) will provided a clearer picture soon.

Additional molecules such as those targeting JAK3 kinase, mTOR and Syk (Changelian et al., 2008; Fernandez and Perl, 2010; Weinblatt et al., 2008) have been shown preliminarily to modulate B cell function in autoimmune subjects. Ongoing trials continue to evaluate the effectiveness and safety of these agents in various autoimmune disorders.

Pharmacodynamic activity of indirect B cell therapeutics

Therapeutic blockade of T cell help also removes essential B cell survival signals. In such circumstances a "T cell therapeutic" may also be considered a "B cell therapeutic"; or an *indirect* B cell target. A number of molecular interactions are required to form the germinal center reaction and to produce high affinity antibodies. Costimulation through CD28:CD80, CD28:CD86 or ICOS:ICOSL is required for naive T cell activation. T cell help to B cells requires CD40:CD40L interactions as well as ICOS:ICOSL and IL-21 signaling. Therapeutic blockade of each of these signaling nodes could reduce the generation of high affinity autoreactive antibodies.

Abatacept is a fusion protein of the extracellular domain of CTLA4 and the Fc portion of human IgG. CTLA4 binds CD80 and CD86 with higher affinity than CD28, thus making a fusion protein a good therapeutic candidate for blocking early steps in T cell activation.

A controlled trial of Abatacept in SLE (in patients with arthritis, serositis, or discoid lupus) did not reach the primary endpoints, however a post-hoc analysis demonstrated a significant benefit in certain SLE subgroups and issues with the study design, including the relatively high dose of glucocorticoids mandated during the trial, may have obscured the trial results (Lateef and Petri, 2010). Abatacept increases the proportion of monocytes in RA subjects (Bonelli, 2010) and baseline numbers of CD28+ T cells may predict remission (Scarsi et al., 2011).

Another approach is to block signaling in established, autoreactive germinal centers. BG9588, a monoclonal anti-CD40L antibody, showed initial clinical success in renal SLE (Boumpas et al., 2003). Safety concerns led to the discontinuation of this program due to thrombotic events due to platelet CD40L expression (Buchner et al., 2003; Henn et al., 2001). A second generation anti-CD40L antibody (IDEC-131) showed initial benefit in SLE subjects, however in a large phase II IDEC-131 study failed to show efficacy over the placebo group. Additional clinical study of IDEC-131 was initiated in other autoimmune settings but halted after a thromboembolic event in a Crohn's trial (Sidiropoulos and Boumpas, 2004). Of interest to the flow cytometry expert, in a study of four renal SLE patients, BG9588 in combination with prednisone was capable of modulating effector B cell populations and return components of the dysregulated phenotype to normal. Highly activated naïve and memory B cells (expressing CD38++) and intracellular Ig+ plasma cells (CD19+ CD38++) were reduced following two treatments of BG9588 (Grammer et al., 2003), although they returned to high baseline levels after treatment. This in combination with a reduction in proteinuria and anti-dsDNA antibodies (Grammer et al., 2003; Sidiropoulos and Boumpas, 2004) suggested that CD40:CD40L interactions contribute to the generation of autoreactive plasmablast and plasma cell populations and that perhaps other, safer, therapeutics that target the GC reaction could provide benefit in SLE.

Recent advances in T cell immunology have identified a specialized subset of CD4 T cells that provide help to B cells attempting to form a germinal center. This population has been called T follicular helper cells (TFH) (Crotty, 2011). Naïve CD4 T cells become activated in the T cell zone of the secondary lymphoid organ. The inducible costimulator, ICOS, is expressed, and ICOS engagement drives the upregulation of CXCR5 and BcL6, migration toward the B cell zone and differentiation into a TFH (Choi et al., 2011). Phenotypically, TFH are characterized by their high expression of CXCR5, ICOS and PD-1, and location (if possible). Patients with an ICOS-null mutation do not develop TFH and have significantly reduced serum IgG concentrations (Bossaller et al., 2006; Warnatz et al., 2006; Grimbacher et al., 2003).

MEDI-570 is a monoclonal antibody that depletes ICOS-bearing T cells and is currently being tested in a phase I study of SLE (NCT01127321). AMG 557 is a monoclonal antibody that binds ICOSL and blocks the ICOS:ICOSL interaction; AMG 557 is currently being studied in SLE (NCT00774943), Subacute Cutaneous Lupus Erythematosus (NCT01389895), Psoriasis (NCT01493518), and SLE with Lupus Arthritis. NN8828 is a monoclonal antibody that binds the cytokine IL-21, which has many effects including the prolongation of the germinal center reaction; NN8828 is being studied in RA (NCT01208506). It will be intriguing to see these data come forth over the next few years – does safe blockade of the GC reaction with anti-ICOS, anti-ICOSL or anti-IL-21 lead to similar effects on the immunophenotype as anti-CD40L?

Patient selection

One of the goals of personalized medicine is to identify biomarkers for patient selection. An elegant example of this is the recent description of a peripheral blood plasmablast biomarker to identify non-response to anti-CD20 depleting therapy in RA (Owczarczyk et al., 2011). Many studies had shown that the level of plasmablasts (or pre-plasma cells) were high in non-responders (Boumans et al., 2011). Behrens et al. demonstrated that two mRNA biomarkers of plasmablast levels in peripheral blood ($IgJ^{hi}FCRL5^{lo}$) identify a group of one in five RA subjects who are not likely to respond to anti-CD20 depletion therapy. Peripheral blood B cells were identified flow cytometrically (CD19+) and whole blood RNA samples were assayed for CD20 mRNA expression by RT-qPCR. Levels of the FCRL5 transcript in whole blood correlated with the proportion of naïve B cells while the IgJ transcript was anti-correlated with the levels of naïve and memory B cells. Therefore, the $IgJ^{hi}FCRL5^{lo}$ whole blood transcript could identify subjects with high levels of plasmablasts and plasma cells and low levels of naïve cells.

For other therapeutic programs, data is more preliminary. For example, baseline numbers of CD28+ T cells have been shown, in a small study, to predict remission of RA treated with Abatacept (Scarsi et al., 2011). One thing that is clear is that flow cytometry has utility in patient selection in its own right but can also enable utilization of other platforms towards this goal.

6. Conclusion

In summary, the clinical flow cytometer has provided decision-enabling data in the monitoring of therapeutic impact (e.g., B cell depletion and repletion, normalization to the healthy phenotype), and is beginning to be used to identify biomarkers for patient selection. We hope to help clarify the context of flow cytometry in clinical development and provide some of our insight into successful implementation of immunophenotyping biomarker programs. However, to those new to B cell investigations via flow cytometry, caution should be utilized - it should be acknowledged that "*anyone can get dots*" on the flow cytometer but that it is up to the investigators to truly understand their assay. With this rigor, it will be possible to generate meaningful biomarker data and help guide decision-making on the next generation of B cell therapeutics.

7. Acknowledgements

We gratefully thank our executive management, David Reese and Steven J. Swanson (Amgen Medical Sciences), for support of this work. We also thank James Chung (Amgen Early Development), Ajay Nirula (Amgen Global Development) and Stephen Zoog (Amgen Clinical Immunology) for critical comments and technical discussions. We gratefully thank the healthy and SLE donors that provided whole blood samples with informed consent for these studies.

8. References

[1] Amanna, I.J., Carlson, N.E. and Slifka, M.K., 2007. Duration of humoral immunity to common viral and vaccine antigens. N. Engl. J. Med. 357, 1903.

[2] Anolik, J.H., Barnard, J., Cappione, A., Pugh-Bernard, A.E., Felgar, R.E., Looney, R.J. and Sanz, I., 2004. Rituximab improves peripheral B cell abnormalities in human systemic lupus erythematosus. Arthritis Rheum. 50, 3580.

[3] Anolik, J.H., Barnard, J., Owen, T., Zheng, B., Kemshetti, S., Looney, R.J. and Sanz, I., 2007. Delayed memory B cell recovery in peripheral blood and lymphoid tissue in systemic lupus erythematosus after B cell depletion therapy. Arthritis Rheum. 56, 3044.

[4] Batal, I., Liang, K., Bastacky, S., Kiss, L.P., McHale, T., Wilson, N.L., Paul, B., Lertratanakul, A., Ahearn, J.M., Manzi, S.M. and Kao, A.H., 2011. Prospective assessment of C4d deposits on circulating cells and renal tissues in lupus nephritis: a pilot study. Lupus.

[5] Belouski, S.S., Wallace, D., Weisman, M., Ishimori, M., Hendricks, L., Zack, D., Vincent, M., Rasmussen, E., Ferbas, J. and Chung, J., 2010. Sample stability and variability of B-cell subsets in blood from healthy subjects and patients with systemic lupus erythematosus. Cytometry B Clin. Cytom. 78, 49.

[6] Bendall, S.C., Simonds, E.F., Qiu, P., Amir, e., Krutzik, P.O., Finck, R., Bruggner, R.V., Melamed, R., Trejo, A., Ornatsky, O.I., Balderas, R.S., Plevritis, S.K., Sachs, K., Pe'er, D., Tanner, S.D. and Nolan, G.P., 2011. Single-cell mass cytometry of differential immune and drug responses across a human hematopoietic continuum. Science 332, 687.

[7] Bohnhorst, J.O., Bjorgan, M.B., Thoen, J.E., Natvig, J.B. and Thompson, K.M., 2001. Bm1-Bm5 classification of peripheral blood B cells reveals circulating germinal center founder cells in healthy individuals and disturbance in the B cell subpopulations in patients with primary Sjogren's syndrome. J. Immunol. 167, 3610.

[8] Bonelli, E.F.A.S.S.B.C.-W.S.E.R.J.S.S.C.S. Effects of abatacept on monocytes in patients with rheumatoid arthritis . Ann Rheum Dis 69(A67). 2010. Ref Type: Abstract

[9] Bossaller, L., Burger, J., Draeger, R., Grimbacher, B., Knoth, R., Plebani, A., Durandy, A., Baumann, U., Schlesier, M., Welcher, A.A., Peter, H.H. and Warnatz, K., 2006. ICOS deficiency is associated with a severe reduction of CXCR5+CD4 germinal center Th cells. J. Immunol. 177, 4927.

[10] Boumans, M.J., Thurlings, R.M., Gerlag, D.M., Vos, K. and Tak, P.P., 2011. Response to rituximab in patients with rheumatoid arthritis in different compartments of the immune system. Arthritis Rheum.

[11] Boumpas, D.T., Furie, R., Manzi, S., Illei, G.G., Wallace, D.J., Balow, J.E. and Vaishnaw, A., 2003. A short course of BG9588 (anti-CD40 ligand antibody) improves serologic activity and decreases hematuria in patients with proliferative lupus glomerulonephritis. Arthritis Rheum. 48, 719.

[12] Buchner, K., Henn, V., Grafe, M., de Boer, O.J., Becker, A.E. and Kroczek, R.A., 2003. CD40 ligand is selectively expressed on CD4+ T cells and platelets: implications for CD40-CD40L signalling in atherosclerosis. J. Pathol. 201, 288.

[13] Caraux, A., Klein, B., Paiva, B., Bret, C., Schmitz, A., Fuhler, G.M., Bos, N.A., Johnsen, H.E., Orfao, A. and Perez-Andres, M., 2010. Circulating human B and plasma cells. Age-associated changes in counts and detailed characterization of circulating normal C. Haematologica 95, 1016.

[14] Carnahan, J., Wang, P., Kendall, R., Chen, C., Hu, S., Boone, T., Juan, T., Talvenheimo, J., Montestruque, S., Sun, J., Elliott, G., Thomas, J., Ferbas, J., Kern, B., Briddell, R.,

Leonard, J.P. and Cesano, A., 2003. Epratuzumab, a humanized monoclonal antibody targeting CD22: characterization of in vitro properties. Clin. Cancer Res. 9, 3982S.

[15] Carsetti, R., Kohler, G. and Lamers, M.C., 1995. Transitional B cells are the target of negative selection in the B cell compartment. J. Exp. Med. 181, 2129.

[16] Changelian, P.S., Moshinsky, D., Kuhn, C.F., Flanagan, M.E., Munchhof, M.J., Harris, T.M., Whipple, D.A., Doty, J.L., Sun, J., Kent, C.R., Magnuson, K.S., Perregaux, D.G., Sawyer, P.S. and Kudlacz, E.M., 2008. The specificity of JAK3 kinase inhibitors. Blood 111, 2155.

[17] Chaussabel, D., Quinn, C., Shen, J., Patel, P., Glaser, C., Baldwin, N., Stichweh, D., Blankenship, D., Li, L., Munagala, I., Bennett, L., Allantaz, F., Mejias, A., Ardura, M., Kaizer, E., Monnet, L., Allman, W., Randall, H., Johnson, D., Lanier, A., Punaro, M., Wittkowski, K.M., White, P., Fay, J., Klintmalm, G., Ramilo, O., Palucka, A.K., Banchereau, J. and Pascual, V., 2008. A modular analysis framework for blood genomics studies: application to systemic lupus erythematosus. Immunity. 29, 150.

[18] Choi, Y.S., Kageyama, R., Eto, D., Escobar, T.C., Johnston, R.J., Monticelli, L., Lao, C. and Crotty, S., 2011. ICOS receptor instructs T follicular helper cell versus effector cell differentiation via induction of the transcriptional repressor Bcl6. Immunity. 34, 932.

[19] Craig, F.E. and Foon, K.A., 2008. Flow cytometric immunophenotyping for hematologic neoplasms. Blood 111, 3941.

[20] Crotty, S., 2011. Follicular helper CD4 T cells (TFH). Annu. Rev. Immunol. 29, 621.

[21] Crotty, S., Felgner, P., Davies, H., Glidewell, J., Villarreal, L. and Ahmed, R., 2003. Cutting edge: long-term B cell memory in humans after smallpox vaccination. J. Immunol. 171, 4969.

[22] Dall'Era, M., Chakravarty, E., Wallace, D., Genovese, M., Weisman, M., Kavanaugh, A., Kalunian, K., Dhar, P., Vincent, E., Pena-Rossi, C. and Wofsy, D., 2007. Reduced B lymphocyte and immunoglobulin levels after atacicept treatment in patients with systemic lupus erythematosus: results of a multicenter, phase Ib, double-blind, placebo-controlled, dose-escalating trial. Arthritis Rheum. 56, 4142.

[23] Daridon, C., Blassfeld, D., Reiter, K., Mei, H.E., Giesecke, C., Goldenberg, D.M., Hansen, A., Hostmann, A., Frolich, D. and Dorner, T., 2010. Epratuzumab targeting of CD22 affects adhesion molecule expression and migration of B-cells in systemic lupus erythematosus. Arthritis Res. Ther. 12, R204.

[24] Davidson, A., 2010. Targeting BAFF in autoimmunity. Curr. Opin. Immunol. 22, 732.

[25] Davis, C., Wu, X., Li, W., Fan, H. and Reddy, M., 2011. Stability of immunophenotypic markers in fixed peripheral blood for extended analysis using flow cytometry. J. Immunol. Methods 363, 158.

[26] Dorken, B., Moldenhauer, G., Pezzutto, A., Schwartz, R., Feller, A., Kiesel, S. and Nadler, L.M., 1986. HD39 (B3), a B lineage-restricted antigen whose cell surface expression is limited to resting and activated human B lymphocytes. J. Immunol. 136, 4470.

[27] Dorner, T., Kaufmann, J., Wegener, W.A., Teoh, N., Goldenberg, D.M. and Burmester, G.R., 2006. Initial clinical trial of epratuzumab (humanized anti-CD22 antibody) for immunotherapy of systemic lupus erythematosus. Arthritis Res. Ther. 8, R74.

[28] Dorner, T. and Lipsky, P.E., 2004. Correlation of circulating CD27high plasma cells and disease activity in systemic lupus erythematosus. Lupus 13, 283.

[29] Dorner, T., Radbruch, A. and Burmester, G.R., 2009. B-cell-directed therapies for autoimmune disease. Nat. Rev. Rheumatol. 5, 433.

[30] Edwards, J.C., Szczepanski, L., Szechinski, J., Filipowicz-Sosnowska, A., Emery, P., Close, D.R., Stevens, R.M. and Shaw, T., 2004. Efficacy of B-cell-targeted therapy with rituximab in patients with rheumatoid arthritis. N. Engl. J. Med. 350, 2572.

[31] Fernandez, D. and Perl, A., 2010. mTOR signaling: a central pathway to pathogenesis in systemic lupus erythematosus? Discov. Med. 9, 173.

[32] Furie, R.A., Petri, M.A., Wallace, D.J., Ginzler, E.M., Merrill, J.T., Stohl, W., Chatham, W.W., Strand, V., Weinstein, A., Chevrier, M.R., Zhong, Z.J. and Freimuth, W.W., 2009. Novel evidence-based systemic lupus erythematosus responder index. Arthritis Rheum. 61, 1143.

[33] Gattinoni, L., Lugli, E., Ji, Y., Pos, Z., Paulos, C.M., Quigley, M.F., Almeida, J.R., Gostick, E., Yu, Z., Carpenito, C., Wang, E., Douek, D.C., Price, D.A., June, C.H., Marincola, F.M., Roederer, M. and Restifo, N.P., 2011. A human memory T cell subset with stem cell-like properties. Nat. Med. 17, 1290.

[34] Genovese, M.C., Kinnman, N., de La, B.G., Pena, R.C. and Tak, P.P., 2011. Atacicept in patients with rheumatoid arthritis and an inadequate response to tumor necrosis factor antagonist therapy: results of a phase II, randomized, placebo-controlled, dose-finding trial. Arthritis Rheum. 63, 1793.

[35] Grammer, A.C., Slota, R., Fischer, R., Gur, H., Girschick, H., Yarboro, C., Illei, G.G. and Lipsky, P.E., 2003. Abnormal germinal center reactions in systemic lupus erythematosus demonstrated by blockade of CD154-CD40 interactions. J. Clin. Invest 112, 1506.

[36] Grant, L.J.K.H.B.J.J.a.C. Combination biologic therapy as initial treatment for follicular lymphoma: Initial results from CALGB 50701 - a Phase II trial of extended induction Epratuzumab (anti-CD22) and Rituximab (anti-CD20). Blood (ASH Annual Meeting Abstracts) 116(Abstract 427). 2010.

[37] Green, C.L., Brown, L., Stewart, J.J., Xu, Y., Litwin, V. and Mc Closkey, T.W., 2011. Recommendations for the validation of flow cytometric testing during drug development: I instrumentation. J. Immunol. Methods 363, 104.

[38] Grimbacher, B., Hutloff, A., Schlesier, M., Glocker, E., Warnatz, K., Drager, R., Eibel, H., Fischer, B., Schaffer, A.A., Mages, H.W., Kroczek, R.A. and Peter, H.H., 2003. Homozygous loss of ICOS is associated with adult-onset common variable immunodeficiency. Nat. Immunol. 4, 261.

[39] Henn, V., Steinbach, S., Buchner, K., Presek, P. and Kroczek, R.A., 2001. The inflammatory action of CD40 ligand (CD154) expressed on activated human platelets is temporally limited by coexpressed CD40. Blood 98, 1047.

[40] Hultin, L.E., Hausner, M.A., Hultin, P.M. and Giorgi, J.V., 1993. CD20 (pan-B cell) antigen is expressed at a low level on a subpopulation of human T lymphocytes. Cytometry 14, 196.

[41] Hutloff, A., Buchner, K., Reiter, K., Baelde, H.J., Odendahl, M., Jacobi, A., Dorner, T. and Kroczek, R.A., 2004. Involvement of inducible costimulator in the exaggerated memory B cell and plasma cell generation in systemic lupus erythematosus. Arthritis Rheum. 50, 3211.

[42] Illei, G.G., Shirota, Y., Yarboro, C.H., Daruwalla, J., Tackey, E., Takada, K., Fleisher, T., Balow, J.E. and Lipsky, P.E., 2010. Tocilizumab in systemic lupus erythematosus: data on safety, preliminary efficacy, and impact on circulating plasma cells from an open-label phase I dosage-escalation study. Arthritis Rheum. 62, 542.

[43] Jacobi, A.M., Goldenberg, D.M., Hiepe, F., Radbruch, A., Burmester, G.R. and Dorner, T., 2008a. Differential effects of epratuzumab on peripheral blood B cells of patients with systemic lupus erythematosus versus normal controls. Ann. Rheum. Dis. 67, 450.

[44] Jacobi, A.M., Huang, W., Wang, T., Freimuth, W., Sanz, I., Furie, R., Mackay, M., Aranow, C., Diamond, B. and Davidson, A., 2010a. Effect of long-term belimumab treatment on B cells in systemic lupus erythematosus: extension of a phase II, double-blind, placebo-controlled, dose-ranging study. Arthritis Rheum. 62, 201.

[45] Jacobi, A.M., Mei, H., Hoyer, B.F., Mumtaz, I.M., Thiele, K., Radbruch, A., Burmester, G.R., Hiepe, F. and Dorner, T., 2010b. HLA-DRhigh/CD27high plasmablasts indicate active disease in patients with systemic lupus erythematosus. Ann. Rheum. Dis. 69, 305.

[46] Jacobi, A.M., Reiter, K., Mackay, M., Aranow, C., Hiepe, F., Radbruch, A., Hansen, A., Burmester, G.R., Diamond, B., Lipsky, P.E. and Dorner, T., 2008b. Activated memory B cell subsets correlate with disease activity in systemic lupus erythematosus: delineation by expression of CD27, IgD, and CD95. Arthritis Rheum. 58, 1762.

[47] Kishimoto, T., 2010. IL-6: from its discovery to clinical applications. Int. Immunol. 22, 347.

[48] Klein, U., Rajewsky, K. and Kuppers, R., 1998. Human immunoglobulin (Ig)M+IgD+ peripheral blood B cells expressing the CD27 cell surface antigen carry somatically mutated variable region genes: CD27 as a general marker for somatically mutated (memory) B cells. J. Exp. Med. 188, 1679.

[49] Krutzik, P.O. and Nolan, G.P., 2006. Fluorescent cell barcoding in flow cytometry allows high-throughput drug screening and signaling profiling. Nat. Methods 3, 361.

[50] Lateef, A. and Petri, M., 2010. Biologics in the treatment of systemic lupus erythematosus. [Review]. Current Opinion in Rheumatology 22, 504.

[51] Lee, J.A., Spidlen, J., Boyce, K., Cai, J., Crosbie, N., Dalphin, M., Furlong, J., Gasparetto, M., Goldberg, M., Goralczyk, E.M., Hyun, B., Jansen, K., Kollmann, T., Kong, M., Leif, R., McWeeney, S., Moloshok, T.D., Moore, W., Nolan, G., Nolan, J., Nikolich-Zugich, J., Parrish, D., Purcell, B., Qian, Y., Selvaraj, B., Smith, C., Tchuvatkina, O., Wertheimer, A., Wilkinson, P., Wilson, C., Wood, J., Zigon, R., Scheuermann, R.H. and Brinkman, R.R., 2008. MIFlowCyt: the minimum information about a Flow Cytometry Experiment. Cytometry A 73, 926.

[52] Looney, R.J., 2010. B cell-targeted therapies for systemic lupus erythematosus: an update on clinical trial data. Drugs 70, 529.

[53] Lugli, E., Goldman, C.K., Perera, L.P., Smedley, J., Pung, R., Yovandich, J.L., Creekmore, S.P., Waldmann, T.A. and Roederer, M., 2010a. Transient and persistent effects of IL-15 on lymphocyte homeostasis in nonhuman primates. Blood 116, 3238.

[54] Lugli, E., Roederer, M. and Cossarizza, A., 2010b. Data analysis in flow cytometry: the future just started. Cytometry A 77, 705.

[55] Mackay, F. and Schneider, P., 2008. TACI, an enigmatic BAFF/APRIL receptor, with new unappreciated biochemical and biological properties. Cytokine Growth Factor Rev. 19, 263.

[56] Maurer, D., Fischer, G.F., Fae, I., Majdic, O., Stuhlmeier, K., Von, J.N., Holter, W. and Knapp, W., 1992. IgM and IgG but not cytokine secretion is restricted to the CD27+ B lymphocyte subset. J. Immunol. 148, 3700.

[57] Maurer, D., Holter, W., Majdic, O., Fischer, G.F. and Knapp, W., 1990. CD27 expression by a distinct subpopulation of human B lymphocytes. Eur. J. Immunol. 20, 2679.

[58] Maxwell, D., Chang, Q., Zhang, X., Barnett, E.M. and Piwnica-Worms, D., 2009. An improved cell-penetrating, caspase-activatable, near-infrared fluorescent peptide for apoptosis imaging. Bioconjug. Chem. 20, 702.

[59] Merrill, J.T., Neuwelt, C.M., Wallace, D.J., Shanahan, J.C., Latinis, K.M., Oates, J.C., Utset, T.O., Gordon, C., Isenberg, D.A., Hsieh, H.J., Zhang, D. and Brunetta, P.G., 2010. Efficacy and safety of rituximab in moderately-to-severely active systemic lupus erythematosus: the randomized, double-blind, phase II/III systemic lupus erythematosus evaluation of rituximab trial. Arthritis Rheum. 62, 222.

[60] Michael R.Betts, R.A.K. Detection of T-Cell Degranulation: CD107a and b. 75. 2004. Methods in Cell Biology.

[61] Monroe, J.G., Bannish, G., Fuentes-Panana, E.M., King, L.B., Sandel, P.C., Chung, J. and Sater, R., 2003. Positive and negative selection during B lymphocyte development. Immunol. Res. 27, 427.

[62] Navratil, J.S., Manzi, S., Kao, A.H., Krishnaswami, S., Liu, C.C., Ruffing, M.J., Shaw, P.S., Nilson, A.C., Dryden, E.R., Johnson, J.J. and Ahearn, J.M., 2006. Platelet C4d is highly specific for systemic lupus erythematosus. Arthritis Rheum. 54, 670.

[63] Neil Barclay, Marion Brown, S.K.Alex Law, Andrew J.McKnight, Michael G.Tomlinson and P.Anton van der Merwe, 1997. The Leucocyte Antigen Facts Book. Elsevier Inc.

[64] Nemazee, D., 2006. Receptor editing in lymphocyte development and central tolerance. Nat. Rev. Immunol. 6, 728.

[65] Odendahl, M., Mei, H., Hoyer, B.F., Jacobi, A.M., Hansen, A., Muehlinghaus, G., Berek, C., Hiepe, F., Manz, R., Radbruch, A. and Dorner, T., 2005. Generation of migratory antigen-specific plasma blasts and mobilization of resident plasma cells in a secondary immune response. Blood 105, 1614.

[66] Owczarczyk, K., Lal, P., Abbas, A.R., Wolslegel, K., Holweg, C.T., Dummer, W., Kelman, A., Brunetta, P., Lewin-Koh, N., Sorani, M., Leong, D., Fielder, P., Yocum, D., Ho, C., Ortmann, W., Townsend, M.J. and Behrens, T.W., 2011. A Plasmablast Biomarker for Nonresponse to Antibody Therapy to CD20 in Rheumatoid Arthritis. Sci. Transl. Med. 3, 101ra92.

[67] Pascual, V., Liu, Y.J., Magalski, A., de, B.O., Banchereau, J. and Capra, J.D., 1994. Analysis of somatic mutation in five B cell subsets of human tonsil. J. Exp. Med. 180, 329.

[68] Pellat-Deceunynck, C. and Bataille, R., 2004. Normal and malignant human plasma cells: proliferation, differentiation, and expansions in relation to CD45 expression. Blood Cells Mol. Dis. 32, 293.

[69] Pescovitz, M.D., Torgerson, T.R., Ochs, H.D., Ocheltree, E., McGee, P., Krause-Steinrauf, H., Lachin, J.M., Canniff, J., Greenbaum, C., Herold, K.C., Skyler, J.S. and Weinberg,

A., 2011. Effect of rituximab on human in vivo antibody immune responses. J. Allergy Clin. Immunol.

[70] Plate, M.M., Louzao, R., Steele, P.M., Greengrass, V., Morris, L.M., Lewis, J., Barnett, D., Warrino, D., Hearps, A.C., Denny, T. and Crowe, S.M., 2009. Evaluation of the blood stabilizers TransFix and Cyto-Chex BCT for low-cost CD4 T-cell methodologies. Viral Immunol. 22, 329.

[71] Qian, Y., Wei, C., Eun-Hyung, L.F., Campbell, J., Halliley, J., Lee, J.A., Cai, J., Kong, Y.M., Sadat, E., Thomson, E., Dunn, P., Seegmiller, A.C., Karandikar, N.J., Tipton, C.M., Mosmann, T., Sanz, I. and Scheuermann, R.H., 2010. Elucidation of seventeen human peripheral blood B-cell subsets and quantification of the tetanus response using a density-based method for the automated identification of cell populations in multidimensional flow cytometry data. Cytometry B Clin. Cytom. 78 Suppl 1, S69-S82.

[72] Roll, P., Dorner, T. and Tony, H.P., 2008. Anti-CD20 therapy in patients with rheumatoid arthritis: predictors of response and B cell subset regeneration after repeated treatment. Arthritis Rheum. 58, 1566.

[73] Sanz, I., Wei, C., Lee, F.E. and Anolik, J., 2008. Phenotypic and functional heterogeneity of human memory B cells. Semin. Immunol. 20, 67.

[74] Scarsi, M., Ziglioli, T. and Airo', P., 2011. Baseline Numbers of Circulating CD28-negative T Cells May Predict Clinical Response to Abatacept in Patients with Rheumatoid Arthritis. J. Rheumatol. 38, 2105.

[75] Schneider, U., van, L.A., Huhn, D. and Serke, S., 1997. Two subsets of peripheral blood plasma cells defined by differential expression of CD45 antigen. Br. J. Haematol. 97, 56.

[76] Schwartz, A., Gaigalas, A.K., Wang, L., Marti, G.E., Vogt, R.F. and Fernandez-Repollet, E., 2004. Formalization of the MESF unit of fluorescence intensity. Cytometry B Clin. Cytom. 57, 1.

[77] Sidiropoulos, P.I. and Boumpas, D.T., 2004. Lessons learned from anti-CD40L treatment in systemic lupus erythematosus patients. Lupus 13, 391.

[78] Simpson, T.R., Quezada, S.A. and Allison, J.P., 2010. Regulation of CD4 T cell activation and effector function by inducible costimulator (ICOS). Curr. Opin. Immunol. 22, 326.

[79] Stone, J.H., Merkel, P.A., Spiera, R., Seo, P., Langford, C.A., Hoffman, G.S., Kallenberg, C.G., St Clair, E.W., Turkiewicz, A., Tchao, N.K., Webber, L., Ding, L., Sejismundo, L.P., Mieras, K., Weitzenkamp, D., Ikle, D., Seyfert-Margolis, V., Mueller, M., Brunetta, P., Allen, N.B., Fervenza, F.C., Geetha, D., Keogh, K.A., Kissin, E.Y., Monach, P.A., Peikert, T., Stegeman, C., Ytterberg, S.R. and Specks, U., 2010. Rituximab versus cyclophosphamide for ANCA-associated vasculitis. N. Engl. J. Med. 363, 221.

[80] Taylor, J.M., Fahey, J.L., Detels, R. and Giorgi, J.V., 1989a. CD4 percentage, CD4 number, and CD4:CD8 ratio in HIV infection: which to choose and how to use. J. Acquir. Immune. Defic. Syndr. 2, 114.

[81] Taylor, J.M., Fahey, J.L., Detels, R. and Giorgi, J.V., 1989b. CD4 percentage, CD4 number, and CD4:CD8 ratio in HIV infection: which to choose and how to use. J. Acquir. Immune. Defic. Syndr. 2, 114.

[82] Tedder, T.F., Poe, J.C. and Haas, K.M., 2005. CD22: a multifunctional receptor that regulates B lymphocyte survival and signal transduction. Adv. Immunol. 88, 1.

[83] Teng, Y.K., Levarht, E.W., Toes, R.E., Huizinga, T.W. and van Laar, J.M., 2009. Residual inflammation after rituximab treatment is associated with sustained synovial plasma cell infiltration and enhanced B cell repopulation. Ann. Rheum. Dis. 68, 1011.

[84] Toda, T., Kitabatake, M., Igarashi, H. and Sakaguchi, N., 2009. The immature B-cell subpopulation with low RAG1 expression is increased in the autoimmune New Zealand Black mouse. Eur. J. Immunol. 39, 600.

[85] van Vollenhoven, R.F., Kinnman, N., Vincent, E., Wax, S. and Bathon, J., 2011. Atacicept in patients with rheumatoid arthritis and an inadequate response to methotrexate: results of a phase II, randomized, placebo-controlled trial. Arthritis Rheum. 63, 1782.

[86] Vital, E.M., Dass, S., Buch, M.H., Henshaw, K., Pease, C.T., Martin, M.F., Ponchel, F., Rawstron, A.C. and Emery, P., 2011. B cell biomarkers of rituximab responses in systemic lupus erythematosus. Arthritis Rheum. 63, 3038.

[87] Wallace, K.P.S.K.K.a.G. Epratuzumab demonstrates clinically meaningful improvements in patients with moderate to severe systemic lupus erythematosus (SLE): Results from EMBLEMTM, a phase IIb study. Ann Rheum Dis. 69 (Suppl3)(558). 2010.

[88] Wang, L., Gaigalas, A.K., Marti, G., Abbasi, F. and Hoffman, R.A., 2008. Toward quantitative fluorescence measurements with multicolor flow cytometry. Cytometry A 73, 279.

[89] Warnatz, K., Bossaller, L., Salzer, U., Skrabl-Baumgartner, A., Schwinger, W., van der Burg, M., van Dongen, J.J., Orlowska-Volk, M., Knoth, R., Durandy, A., Draeger, R., Schlesier, M., Peter, H.H. and Grimbacher, B., 2006. Human ICOS deficiency abrogates the germinal center reaction and provides a monogenic model for common variable immunodeficiency. Blood 107, 3045.

[90] Warrino, D.E., DeGennaro, L.J., Hanson, M., Swindells, S., Pirruccello, S.J. and Ryan, W.L., 2005. Stabilization of white blood cells and immunologic markers for extended analysis using flow cytometry. J. Immunol. Methods 305, 107.

[91] Wei, C., Anolik, J., Cappione, A., Zheng, B., Pugh-Bernard, A., Brooks, J., Lee, E.H., Milner, E.C. and Sanz, I., 2007. A new population of cells lacking expression of CD27 represents a notable component of the B cell memory compartment in systemic lupus erythematosus. J. Immunol. 178, 6624.

[92] Weinblatt, M.E., Kavanaugh, A., Burgos-Vargas, R., Dikranian, A.H., Medrano-Ramirez, G., Morales-Torres, J.L., Murphy, F.T., Musser, T.K., Straniero, N., Vicente-Gonzales, A.V. and Grossbard, E., 2008. Treatment of rheumatoid arthritis with a Syk kinase inhibitor: a twelve-week, randomized, placebo-controlled trial. Arthritis Rheum. 58, 3309.

[93] Weller, S., Braun, M.C., Tan, B.K., Rosenwald, A., Cordier, C., Conley, M.E., Plebani, A., Kumararatne, D.S., Bonnet, D., Tournilhac, O., Tchernia, G., Steiniger, B., Staudt, L.M., Casanova, J.L., Reynaud, C.A. and Weill, J.C., 2004. Human blood IgM "memory" B cells are circulating splenic marginal zone B cells harboring a prediversified immunoglobulin repertoire. Blood 104, 3647.

[94] Wrammert, J., Miller, J., Akondy, R. and Ahmed, R., 2009. Human immune memory to yellow fever and smallpox vaccination. J. Clin. Immunol. 29, 151.

[95] Wu, S., Jin, L., Vence, L. and Radvanyi, L.G., 2010. Development and application of 'phosphoflow' as a tool for immunomonitoring. Expert. Rev. Vaccines. 9, 631.

[96] Yazici, Y., Curtis, J.R., Ince, A., Baraf, H., Malamet, R.L., Teng, L.L. and Kavanaugh, A., 2011. Efficacy of tocilizumab in patients with moderate to severe active rheumatoid arthritis and a previous inadequate response to disease-modifying antirheumatic drugs: the ROSE study. Ann. Rheum. Dis.

5

Evaluation of the Anti-Tumoural and Immune Modulatory Activity of Natural Products by Flow Cytometry

Susana Fiorentino, Claudia Urueña, Sandra Quijano,
Sandra Paola Santander, John Fredy Hernandez and Claudia Cifuentes
Immunobiology and Cell Biology Group, Microbiology Department,
Pontificia Universidad Javeriana,
Bogotá,
Colombia

1. Introduction

Flow cytometry has shown to be a very useful tool in the assessment of plant-derived compounds, having potential anti-tumour activity. Our group has focused in the study of fractions and isolated compounds with biological activity over tumour cells and regulatory immune cells, such as dendritic cells. Also we have implemented a flow cytometry screening tests for estimating the biological activity of plant-derived fractions.

The present chapter will discuss important and useful facts to be taken into account for effectively carrying out biological assays in this area. We will start with recommendations about the production of plant fractions and continue with the biological assessment of cell lines or monocyte-derived dendritic cells. Since these protocols are constantly evolving, herein we describe our current experience.

2. Natural product specifications

Natural product specifications will differ depending upon the type of plant material in which the study is to be undertaken: complex fractions or isolated compounds. Similarly, settings will differ depending upon the biological target assigned for the assay e.g. primary tumour cells, tumour cell lines, dendritic cells or antigen presenting cells. Our group has developed plant complex fractions enriched in secondary metabolites, using conventional organic solvent fractionation methods, and primary metabolites-enriched fractions using fractionation of aqueous solutions. Both types of fractions contain a vast variety of compounds, as well as structure diversity.

Our group has been working with fractions enriched in secondary metabolites from *Petiveria alliacea* and *Caesalpinia spinosa* plants. The chemical complexity of the fractions is analysed by dereplication, by comparing the molecular weights of the compounds within the fraction with the molecular weights of compounds known to be present in the plant under study. Among the difficulties we have run into is the autofluorescence display by compounds present in our fractions, as well as in many other natural products, a condition that interferes with flow cytometry lectures. The autofluorescence displayed by many secondary metabolites, such as flavonoids, covers most of the visible spectrum overlapping the emission range of many flow cytometry fluorochromes. We have overcome such interference by making fraction dilutions and estimating fluorescence values at the overlapping wavelengths. Those values are used as background in the flow cytometry estimations.

Another critical condition to be aware of is the fraction sterility condition with regard to cell culture contamination hazards. The presence of microorganisms in the plant material, such as viruses, bacteria or fungi, must be controlled. Chemical agents such as benzyl chloride, lauryl dimethyl ammonium (benzalkonium chloride) in concentrations between 50 and 100 ppm could be used to prevent the microorganisms' occurrence. Similarly, treatment with short wave ultraviolet radiation (UVC) within the range of 200-280 nm can reduce microbial load. In the case of stock solutions, membrane filtration (0.22 microns) is suggested, taking the precaution to previously check membrane solvent compatibility. The use of high-pressure pasteurisation (600mPa, 20°C) has also been proposed to attain microorganism safe plant material. Chen et al, established that high-pressure pasteurisation for 2 to 5 minutes in *Echinacea purpurea* plant reduced microbial load without affecting biological activity. In addition, the presence of lipopolysaccharide (LPS) in plant-derived fractions must be avoided, since LPS is a major membrane component of gram-negative bacteria. LPS is recognised by macrophages and endothelial cells through CD14-TLR4 (toll like receptor) - MD2 complex, triggering cytokine secretion and expression of co-stimulatory molecules. LPS may appear in the plant material from pathogenic bacteria (*Pseudomonas, Xanthomonas,* Burkholderia and Agrobacterium), or beneficial symbiotic Rhizobiaceae (*Pseudomonas fluorescens*).

To estimate LPS presence in the fractions, a limulus amebocyte lysate (LAL) test is commonly used, although detection of 3β-hydroximiristate (a LPS component) can also be used. For LPS removal, an anti-endotoxin synthetic peptide -SAEP- cross-linked with polymyxin B (POLB), can be used to neutralise it. In relation to the fractions eluents, especially in non-polar fractions, it is advisable to use as first choice ethanol then secondly dimethyl sulfoxide (DMSO) for the stock solution preparation. Then proceed to dilute the fraction or isolated compound until the ethanol concentration in the cell culture does not exceed 0,02%.

3. Instrument setup and colour compensation

To ensure data analysis quality in multicolour flow cytometry, daily adjustments are necessary to acquire standard intensity peaks and build up adequate follow-up curves. Currently, there are several quality controls commercially available that can be used to monitor reagents' performance, reproducibility, cell preparation and cell staining. Among the most commonly used are the beads of known concentration and a stable number of fluorochromes per bead (> 6-colour). Also they control parameters such as laser alignment, optics, fluidics, mean fluorescence intensity (MFI) (each bead in solution produces equal amounts of fluorescence), fluorescence signal coefficient variation, autofluorescence threshold and colour compensation. Standardisation of cytometer measurements is essential to accurately make comparisons between experiments.

On the other hand, biological samples (including normal peripheral blood) should be stained with the fluorochrome of interest to compensate the cytometer. The positive cell population must be set as the brightest signal for each fluorochrome. As a negative control, cells without antibody and marked with an irrelevant antibody or isotype control can be used. For tandem fluorochromes, it is important to compensate separately each reagent containing a tandem fluorochrome, because spectral emission properties can vary from lot to lot, between manufacturers and over time. Once the flow cytometer is adjusted and the immunophenotypic panels have been selected, it is essential to optimise and evaluate each reagent in terms of fluorescence intensity to exclude unwanted interactions between them. It is highly recommended to use normal peripheral blood as a sample control since positive and negative cell populations are needed to test the antibody under study.

Using different fluorochromes at the same phenotypic panel can produce fluorescence spectral overlapping. In consequence the emitted light of one fluorochrome may appear in the other detector. To correct overlapping, a compensation protocol could be used. Herein, is the basic protocol that can be used for compensation adjustment using BD™ CompBeads set anti-mouse Igκ (binds mouse Kappa light chain-bearing immunoglobulin) and the BD™ CompBeads negative control (no binding capacity). Before starting the experiment it is necessary to prepare tubes with each conjugate antibody to compensate fluorescence. Briefly, pretitrated monoclonal antibody (MAb) amounts are added to stain buffer aliquots (e.g. phosphate-buffered saline, pH 7.6), the CompBeads anti-mouse Igκ and the CompBeads negative control. In this example: fluorocrome conjugated-fluorescein isothiocyanate (FITC)/phycoerythrin (PE)/peridinin chlorophyll protein-cyanin 5.5 (PerCPCy5.5)/allophycocyanin (APC)/APCCy7- combinations of MAb are used. In addition, a tube containing the CompBeads negative control is used to adjust the photomultipliers voltage settings. After gentle mixing, the different bead aliquots are incubated for 30 min at room temperature (RT) under dark conditions. Then, the beads are washed with 2 mL of staining buffer/aliquot (10 min at 200 g). Immediately after the sample preparation is complete, data acquisition is performed on a FACS Canto II flow cytometer using the FACS DIVA software programme (BD Biosciences). For each MAbs combination with CompBeads, $5x10^3$ events are acquired and stored. The flow cytometer compensation strategy employed is shown in Figures 1, 2 and 3.

4. Cell lines selection

Biological activity of plant complex fractions or isolated compounds is selective; their effect depends upon the nature of the cell line used at the assay. Our research interest has mostly been on compounds with activity on breast cancer cells, e.g. human breast adenocarcinoma (MCF7) from the American Type Culture Collection (ATCC, Rockville, MD) and mammary murine adenoma carcinoma (4T1), kindly donated by Dr. Alexander Asea, Texas A & M University. Similarly, we have used human melanoma cells (A375) kindly donated by La Universidad del Rosario (Bogotá, Colombia) and murine melanoma (Mel-Rel) donated by Armelle Prevost (Institute Curie, France). We have also used chronic myeloid leukaemia (HL60), human promyelocytic K562 cell lines from the ATCC and finally pancreatic cancer cells (Panc28 and L.3.6PL) donated by Dr. Steven Safe from Texas A & M University as biological agents. In addition we have some others cell lines, obtained from ATCC.

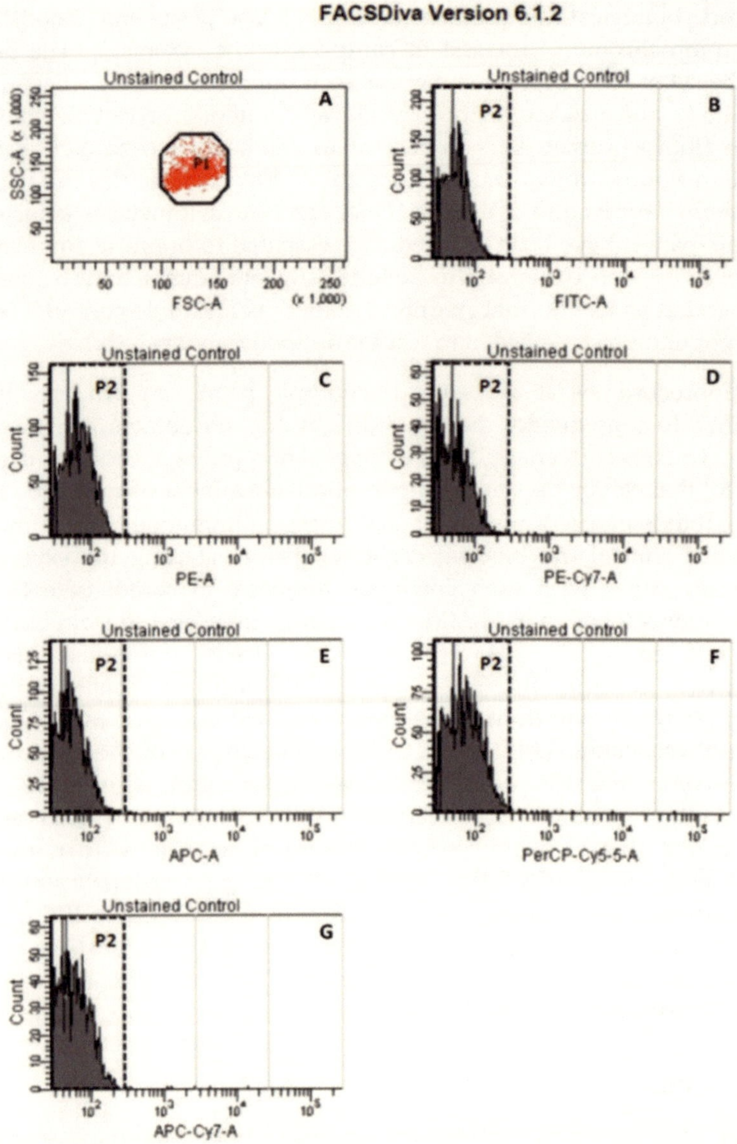

Fig. 1. Dot plot histograms for FACS Canto II cytometer compensation using the commercial BD™ CompBeads negative control (uncoupled with anti-mouse IgG) for voltage adjustment (parameters: Forward Scatter –FSC- and Side-Scatter-SSC- (panel A) and fluorescence detectors (FITC, PE, PERCPCY5.5, APC, APCCy7 and PECY7) (panels B-G). Histogram represents the negative value area for each parameter. The beads are gated on FSC and SSC (red dots in P1 region). Acquisition is done only in the P1 region verifying histograms for each fluorochrome and simultaneously adjusting the voltages for each fluorescent channel, so that the peak areas are located in the negative area (region P2 in each histogram). The adjusted minimum voltages in the photomultipliers are used for the BD™ CompBeads set anti-mouse Igκ and the BD™ CompBeads negative control acquisition mixture. *Y* axes units correspond to relative fluorescence intensity

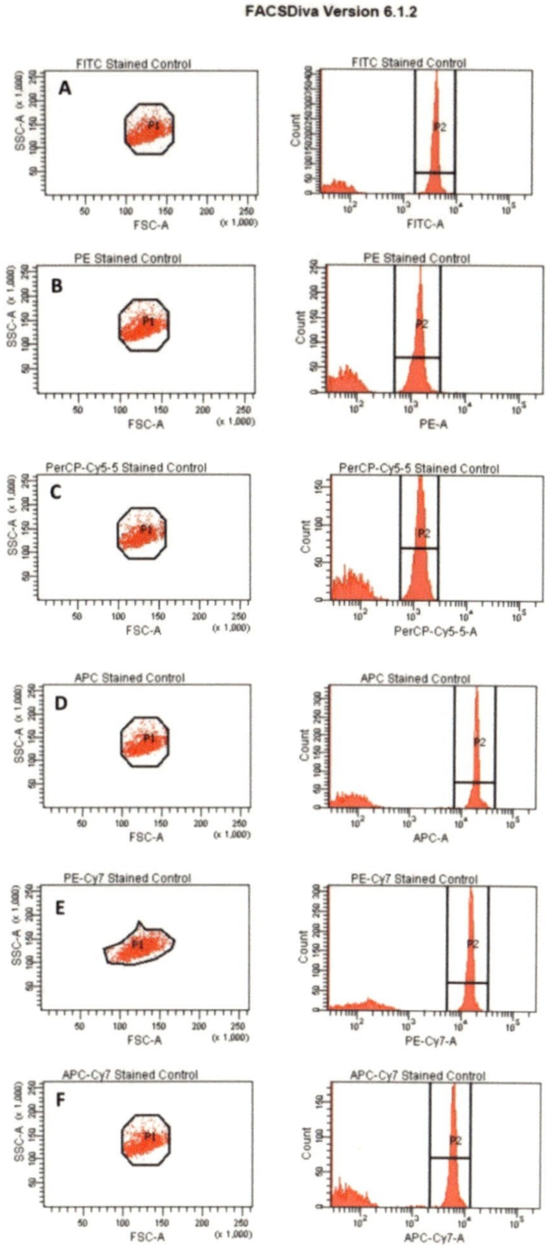

Fig. 2. Dot plot histograms for FACS Canto II cytometer compensation using BD™ CompBeads set anti-mouse Igκ and the BD™ CompBeads negative control commercial mixture. After P1 region acquisition (containing the spheres mixture), histograms have two fluorescence emission peaks, a negative (no fluorescence emission) and a positive (fluorescence emission; P2 region) (panels A –F). The cytometer automatically discriminates positive and negative peaks and calculates the compensation for each and between fluorochromes. The compensation values are stored in the software for future experiments containing the same fluorochrome

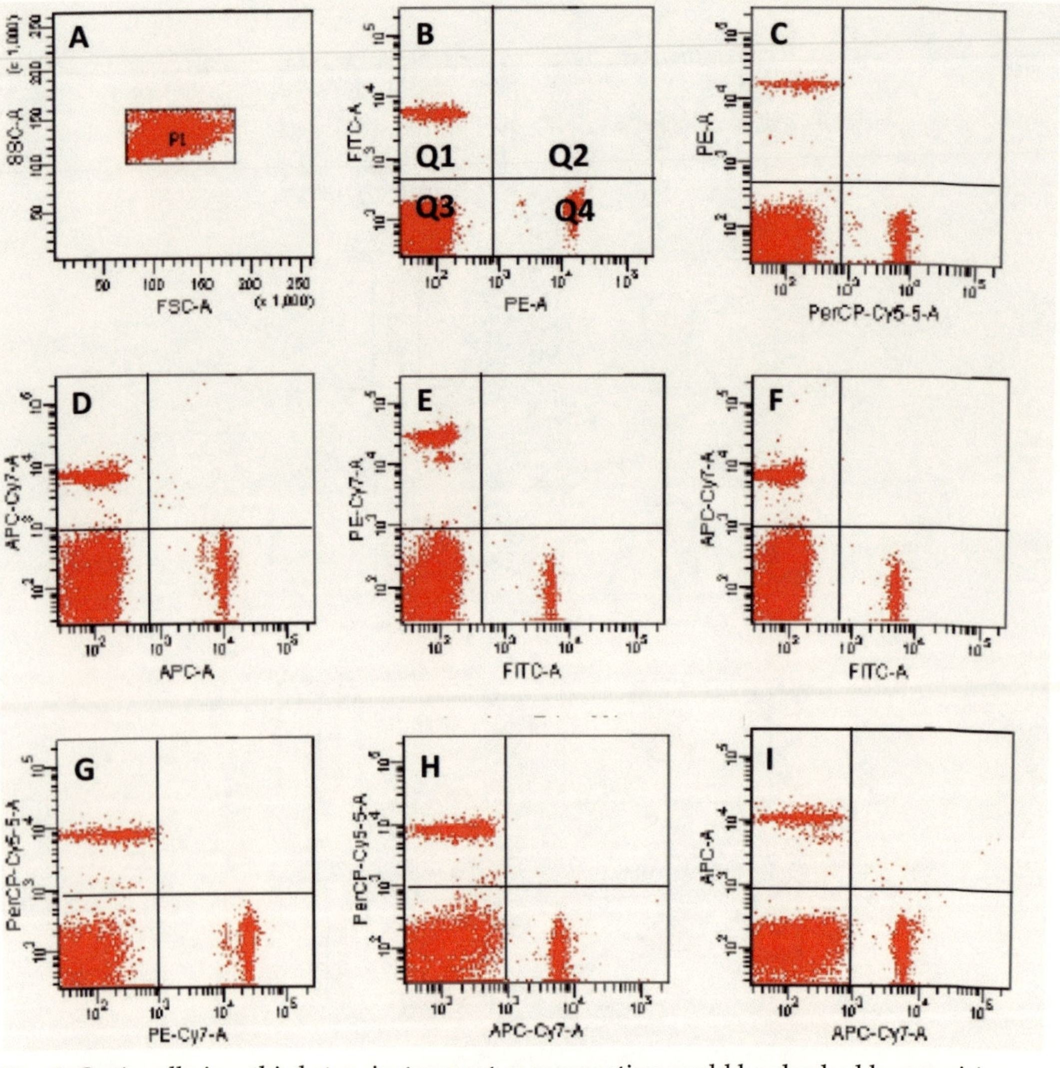

Fig. 3. Optionally in a third step, instrument compensation could be checked by acquiring the bead mixture attached to each antibody conjugate and using the same compensation values calculated by the software as described in figure 2. Creating different two-dimensional dot plots with each fluorochrome on the x-axis and y-axis respectively and verifying that there is no fluorescence overlapping (panels B-I) (e. g. FITC vs PE, PE vs PercPC y 5.5, etc). If the fluorochrome signal is uncompensated, voltage manual adjustment is required

Cells are cultured under humidified conditions with 5% CO_2 in RPMI 1640 media, supplemented with 10% foetal bovine serum (FBS), 0.01 M Hepes, 100 µg/ml penicillin, 100 U/ml streptomycin, 2 mM glutamine and 0.01 M of sodium pyruvate (Eurobio, France). It is important to determine if the fraction activity displays selectivity on highly proliferating cells, or to the contrary, if its activity can also affect normal cells. Lymphocytes derived from human peripheral blood, separated with Ficoll-Hypaque, or human gingival mucosa fibroblasts can be used as normal cell samples.

4.1 Mononuclear cell isolation by Ficoll-Hypaque gradient

Mononuclear cells can be separated from heparin, EDTA, sodium citrate or defibrinated anti-coagulated blood. Equal parts of phosphate buffered saline (PBS) are used to dilute the blood sample at RT. In a 15 ml conical tube, 3 ml of ficoll are carefully placed and 4 ml of diluted blood are placed on top, avoiding damage to the gradient (the sample must be poured slowly along the tube walls). The tube is centrifuged (300 × g) for 30-40 minutes at RT. After centrifugation, four layers should appear in the tube. Granulocytes and erythrocytes are the cells found at the bottom of the tube, next is the ficoll hypaque layer, monocytes, lymphocytes and platelets are at the upper intermediate phase, and finally, at the top layer is the plasma. The layer containing the lymphocytes has to be carefully removed, transferred into a new tube, diluted with three parts of PBS (6 ml) and centrifuged (100 × g) for 10 min at RT. The latter washing procedure should be done twice and at the end cells must be suspended in supplemented culture medium.

4.2 Gingival fibroblast generation

Gingival fibroblasts are obtained from the gingival tissue of healthy volunteers. Briefly, a gingival sample is cut into small pieces and cultured in RPMI 1640 supplemented media with 10% FBS, 0.01 M Hepes, 100 µg/ml penicillin, 100 U/ml streptomycin, 2 mM glutamine and 0.01 M sodium pyruvate (Eurobio, France) under humidified conditions and 5% CO_2. The culture medium is replaced every three days until the fibroblasts are derived from the tissue. After two weeks of culture, a confluent fibroblast culture is obtained.

5. Determination of fraction concentration and anti-tumour bioassays

5.1 Fraction's cytotoxic activity on tumour cells

The fraction's cytotoxic effect is evaluated by trypan blue and MTT assays (Sigma, St. Louis MO, USA) using tumour and normal cell cultures. Suspension or adherent tumour cells ($5x10^3$ cells/well or 3 x 10^3 cells/well, respectively) and fibroblasts (3 x 10^3 cells/well) are cultured in 96-well plates at different plant fraction concentrations (from 125 to 0.975 µg /ml) in ethanol (0.02% final concentration). Aqueous ethanol solution is used as a negative control and doxorubicin, etoposide, vincristine, taxol and camptothecin (10 µM) as positive controls, during 48 h at 37°C. Peripheral blood mononuclear cells (2 x 10^5 cells/well) are incubated for 12 h with phytohemagglutinin (Invitrogen Corp, Grand Island, NY, USA) before treatment. At the end of the incubation time, the culture media of the tumour and normal cells is removed and replaced with new RPMI 1640 media lacking phenol red dye (Eurobio, Toulouse, FR). 50 µl of MTT (1 mg/ml) [3-(4,5-dimethylthiazol-2-yl)-2,5-diphenyl tetrazolium bromide] (Sigma, St. Louis MO, USA), is placed in each well and incubated for 4 h at 37°C. The formazan crystals are dissolved with DMSO and their optical density at 540 nm is measured in a MultiskanMCC/340 (Labsystems, Thermo Fisher Scientific, Waltham, USA). Probit analysis is used to calculate the inhibitory concentration 50 (IC50) (MINITAB ® Release14.1 Statistical Software Minitab Inc. 2003). In addition, cell viability is determined using Newbauer haemocytometer and trypan blue dye.

For these types of procedures the preparation of negative controls is extremely important. Since some plant fractions can reduce MTT reagent, a negative control containing plant fraction, culture media and MTT without cells, should be prepared.

5.2 Tumour cells' mitochondrial membrane potential assessment

For many years mitochondria was considered only as the cell energy source, generating ATP through oxidative phosphorylation and lipid oxidation. Now, is clear that this organelle has a pivotal role in apoptosis, a form of cell death characterised by morphological and biochemical specific changes. The mitochondrial membrane potential ($\Delta\Psi$), addresses the oxidative phosphorylation process and mitochondrial calcium uptake. If the electron transport ceases, as happens in ischemia, the inner mitochondrial membrane potential is developed at the expense of ATP hydrolysis. A decrease in $\Delta\Psi$ is often considered as an early apoptotic signal, an event that can be detected by flow cytometry. Nonetheless, the relationship between the mitochondrial membrane depolarisation and apoptosis is still controversial Some researchers even consider a decrease in $\Delta\Psi$ an irreversible sign of apoptosis, while others say it is an apoptotic late event.

Changes in mitochondrial membrane potential can be assessed using a lipophilic cationic probe JC-1 (5,5',6,6'-tetrachloro-1,1',3,3'-tetraethylbenzimidazolylcarbocyanine iodide). The probe potential depends on its mitochondrial accumulation, which is indicated by a change in green fluorescence (525nm) to red (590 nm) emission. The mitochondrial membrane depolarisation is indicated by a decrease in fluorescence intensity through the red/green ratio. The change in colour is due to the "red fluorescent J aggregates" accumulation which in turn depends on the concentration. One advantage of JC-1 dye is the possibility to be used in a wide variety of cell types, including myocytes, neurons and tumour cells, among others.

For optimal results tumour cell concentration in the culture should be one in which confluence is reached only after incubation for 48 hours. Usually, 2.5 x 10^5 cells/well are placed in 12-well plates. Adherent cells should be allowed to adhere before the treatment begins. Cells are tested with different plant fraction concentrations, using ethanol aqueous solution as a negative control and valinomycin as a positive inductor of membrane

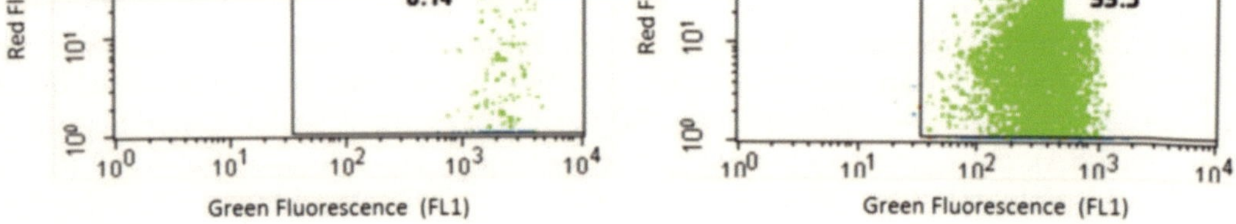

Fig. 4. *C. spinosa*-derived fraction induces mitochondrial membrane depolarisation. K562 cells treated with the fraction or the negative control. The left panel shows the eluent effect (ethanol), the right panel shows the fraction effect on the cell mitochondrial membrane depolarisation

depolarisation. The assay is carried out in kinetics of 4, 8, 12, 24 and/or 48 h. At the end of the treatment, cells are collected in cytometry tubes and JC-1 dye (2.5 mg/ml in PBS) is added for 10 minutes at 37°C. JC-1 fluorescence intensity is quantified in a flow cytometer FACSDiVa (Becton Dickinson, New Jersey, USA) and data analysis is performed using FlowJo software (Tree Star Inc., Ashland, USA). All treatments are done in triplicate and results are expressed as mean +/- SEM. Figure 4.

5.3 Analysis of apoptosis vs necrosis - annexin V/PI staining

There are two main cell death mechanisms: apoptosis or programmed cell death and necrosis or trauma cell death. Both types of cell death have different morphological and biochemical characteristics. Changes as phosphatidylserine (PS) externalisation, chromatin and nuclear condensation, appearance of apoptotic bodies, among others, can be seen in apoptotic cells. Necrotic cells show nuclear swelling, chromatin flocculation, loss of nuclear basophilia, breakdown of the cytoplasmic structure, organelle function and swelling cytolysis.

Plasma membrane phospholipids display asymmetrical distribution. Most of the phosphatidylcholine and sphingomyelin are mainly located at the outer side, while PS is mostly located at the inner side of the plasma membrane. During apoptotic cell death, phospholipid asymmetry is disturbed and PS begins to expose at the membrane outer side. Annexin V is an anticoagulant protein with the property of binding PS with high affinity; in conjugation with fluorochromes it is used to detect apoptotic cells by flow cytometry. Since apoptotic cells begin to react with annexin V before the plasma membrane loses the ability to exclude cationic dyes as propidium iodide (PI), marking the cells with a combination of annexin V-FITC/PI, allows us to distinguish four populations: non-apoptotic cells (annexin V-FITC negative/PI negative), early apoptotic cells (annexin V-FITC positive/PI negative), late apoptotic cells (annexin V-FITC positive/PI positive) and necrotic cells (annexin V-FITC negative/PI positive).

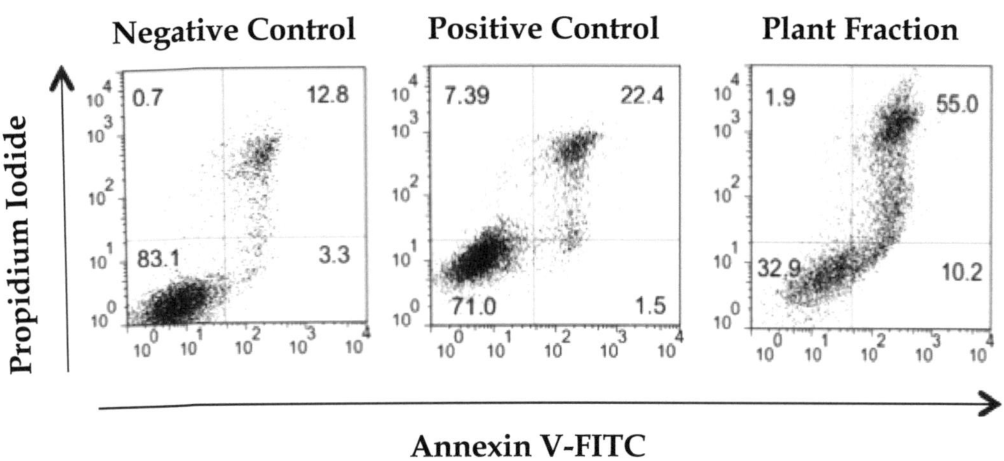

Fig. 5. 4T1 cells marked with annexin V and PI after treatment with *C. spinosa* fraction. Ethanol solution is used as a negative control and doxorubicin as a positive control

Tumour cells (3×10^5) are treated with plant fractions at different concentrations, or doxorubicin (positive control) or ethanol solutions (negative control), for 24 or 48 h. After the treatment, cells are suspended in an annexin V buffer (Hepes 100 mM, NaCl 140 mM, $CaCl_2$ 2.5mM), incubated with annexin V-Alexa fluor 488 for 8 min at 37°C and then incubated with IP for 2 min at 37°C. Assays are made in triplicate. Cells are acquired in a FACSAria I (Becton Dickinson, New Jersey, USA) and FlowJo (Tree Star Inc, Ashland, USA) software for analysis (Figure 5).

5.4 Cell cycle analysis

Cell division is an evolutionarily conserved process involving series of molecular events. The mammalian cell cycle has five phases: three gaps, a G0 phase where the quiescent or resting cells are; G1 and G2 phases were RNA and protein synthesis takes place, the S phase is where DNA replicates and the M phase is where mitosis and cytokinesis happens. G0, G1, S and G2 are collectively known as interphase. Cell cycle control is a fundamental cell process. The progression from G1 to S to G2 and mitosis is coordinated at checkpoints. Before mitosis begins, the cell must check if the DNA is fully replicated and free of damage. The spindle mitotic control stops the cell cycle if the spindle is not properly formed or if the chromosomes are not properly attached. DNA aneuploidy or mutations are the result if the cell avoids these controls. A gap in any of the control sites allows the cell to repair DNA and enter mitosis, otherwise it goes into apoptosis. In cancer, the control repair of the cell cycle is damaged and this is precisely where new drugs based on natural products or their derivatives can achieve a stop in tumour cell division and perhaps induced apoptosis.

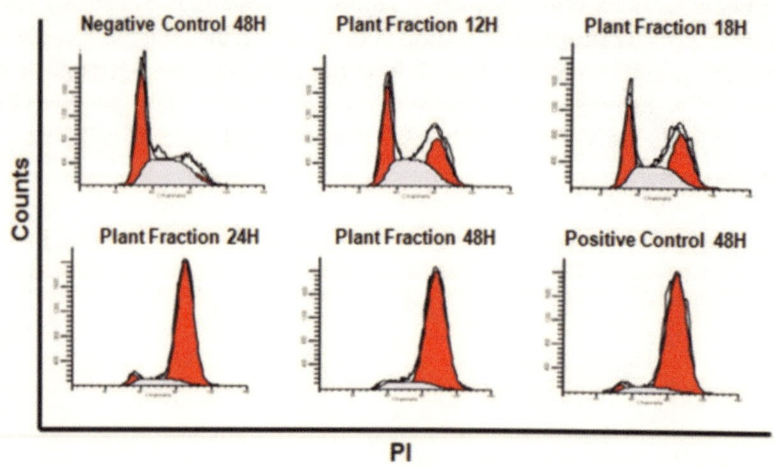

Fig. 6. Effect of a *P alliacea*-derived fraction on cell cycle distribution. A375 cells treated with plant fractions during 12, 18, 24 and 48 h. Ethanol is used as a negative control and vincristine as a positive control

A common and simple way to evaluate cell cycle phases is to measure the DNA cell content. DNA cell content allows the discrimination between cell populations in G0/G1, S and G2/M cell cycle phases. The DNA can be labelled with fluorescent dyes and cell fluorescence can be measured by flow cytometry. Dyes such as PI, Hoechst, 7-AAD and DAPI can be used for this purpose. To start, cells must be synchronised in the G1 phase, a process that can be done by depriving the cells of serum. Mel Rel, A375 and K562 cells are deprived of FBS for 72 h are seeded in 12-well plate (4x10^5 cells/well) and treated with different plant fraction concentrations or vincristine (positive control) or ethanol (negative control) for 12, 18, 24 and 48 h under humidified conditions 37°C and 5% CO_2. Next cells are washed and fixed with ethanol (70% ice-cold) for 18 h, then suspended in PBS 1X with 100 U/ml RNAse A, 50 µg/ml PI (Sigma, St Louise, MO, USA) at RT for 30 min. DNA cell content is measured by flow cytometry using a FACSAria I (Becton Dickinson, New Jersey, USA). The cell cycle distribution percentages are calculated by FlowJo (Tree Star Inc., Ashland, USA) and ModFit LT software. Treatments are done in triplicate (Figure 6).

6. Immunomodulatory evaluation on human-derived dendritic cells

Natural products are good immunostimulating agents and can be evaluated using human monocyte-derived dendritic cells. Although the model cannot be used as a screening test, once standardised, it allows a large number of compounds to be tested in a more physiological way. The test measures the plant fractions real activity on normal human cells. Following we will describe the procedures carried out in our laboratory which includes dendritic cell separation and flow cytometry measurements of the biological activity of plant-derived fractions.

6.1 Monocyte-derived dendritic cell differentiation

Peripheral blood monocytes are attained from concentrated packs (15 ml) of leukocytes from healthy volunteers attending the blood bank and who previously gave informed consent. The mononuclear cells are separated from the peripheral blood using the Ficoll Hypaque density gradient (Amercham, GE Healthcare Europe GmbH). $CD14^+$ population cells are separated with a MiniMACS positive selection kit, using the protocol suggested by the manufacturer, without any modifications (Miltenyi Biotech GmbH, Bergisch, Gladbach, United Kingdom). Cell purity is determined by flow cytometry. Eluted cells (10 µl) are labelled with anti-CD14-APC (Pharmingen, San Diego, CA, USA). Monocytes with purity over 98% are grown for five days in 24-well plates in RPMI 1640 (1 ml) supplemented with 5% FBS, 2 mM glutamine and 100 IU/ml penicillin/streptomycin (Eurobio, Paris, France). The differentiation stimulus used is 800 UI/ml of Granulocyte-Macrophage colony-stimulating factor and 1000 IU/ml of interleukin 4 (R & D Systems, Minneapolis, MN, USA). After three days of differentiation, one half of the media culture is replaced with fresh medium and supplemented with half of the stated cytokines concentration.

At day five, monocyte-derived dendritic cells (MDDC) are stimulated with different concentrations of the plant fractions dissolved in ethanol, DMSO or culture medium, depending upon the fraction solubility, for 48 h. Control DCs (immature) are incubated without stimulus or with the plant fractions eluents. As maturation control, DCs are stimulated with LPS 1µg/ml in PBS (Sigma, St Louis, MO, USA). Additionally, plant fractions are pre-treated with agarose beads coated with POLB (Sigma, St Louis, MO, USA) to eliminate possible LPS contamination. To discard LPS presence in the plant fractions, all reagents are tested with LAL (Bio Whittaker Inc., Walkersville, MD, USA) and used according to manufacturer's instructions. Cell viability is estimated to monitor the fractions' or compounds' potential toxicity using the trypan blue exclusion test.

6.2 Dendritic cell phenotype analysis

Expression of membrane surface markers in immature DCs or those treated with LPS, or with compounds or fractions, are assessed after seven days. Phenotypic analysis is performed using anti-CD1a Pacific Blue, anti-CD86 PE, anti-CD83 FITC, anti-HLA-DR APC-H7, anti-CD209 PerCP-Cy5 and anti-CD206 APC (BD Biosciences). The cells are suspended in a PBS buffer (0.1% sodium azide and 2% FBS) at 4°C. To discriminate living from dead, cells are marked with LIVE/DEAD®Fixable Aqua Dead Cell Stain (Invitrogen. Carlsbad, CA. USA). Also 5 to 20 µl of each antibody is added according to the manufacturer's instructions and incubated for 30 min at RT. After incubation, cells are washed twice with buffer and suspended in 400 µl, to be read on the FACSAria. The analysis is carried out with FACSDiva ™ 6.1(BD Immunocytometry Systems, BD Biosciences, Franklin Lakes, NJ, USA) and FlowJo 8.7 (Tree Star Inc., Ashland, USA). As an example, Figure 7 shows how a galactomannan derived from the *C.spinosa* plant, induces maturation of human dendritic cells shown by the increase in expression of surface membrane markers such as CD86 and HLA-DR.

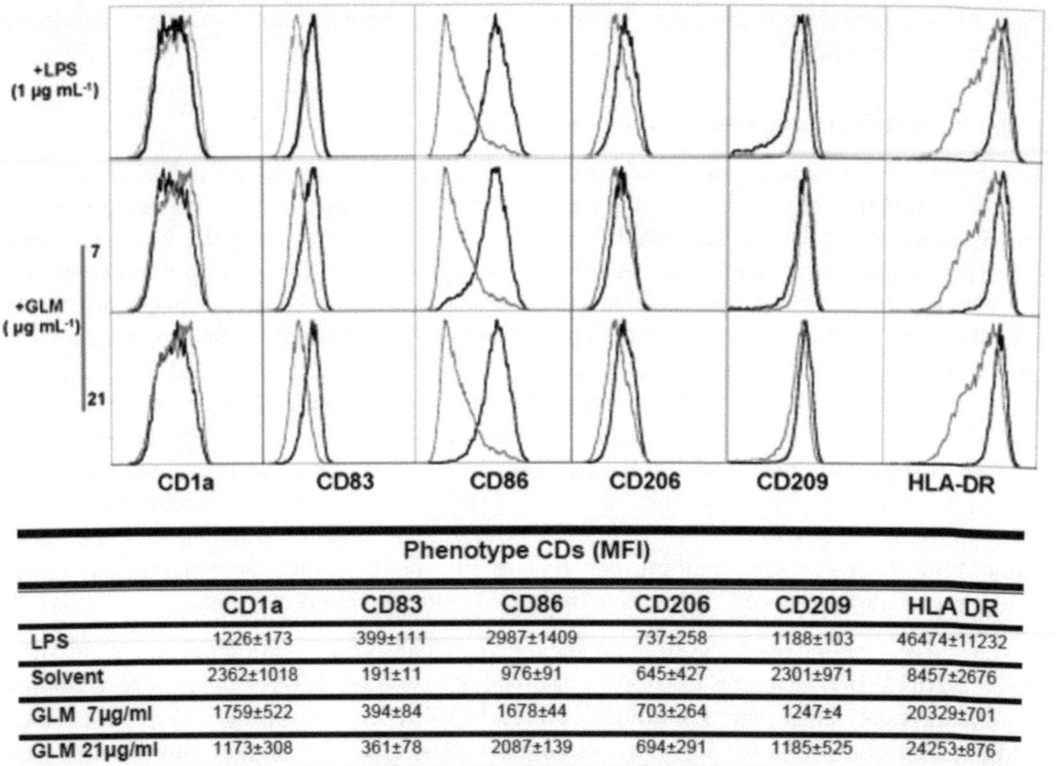

Phenotype CDs (MFI)

	CD1a	CD83	CD86	CD206	CD209	HLA DR
LPS	1226±173	399±111	2987±1409	737±258	1188±103	46474±11232
Solvent	2362±1018	191±11	976±91	645±427	2301±971	8457±2676
GLM 7µg/ml	1759±522	394±84	1678±44	703±264	1247±4	20329±701
GLM 21µg/ml	1173±308	361±78	2087±139	694±291	1185±525	24253±876

Fig. 7. Galactomannan induces phenotypic and functional maturation of DCs. DC cultured for 48 h with LPS (1 µg/mL) and galactomannan (7 and 21 µg/mL). An increase in expression of membrane surface molecules such as HLA-DR, CD86 and CD83 is shown after treatment with galactomannan (black) as compared to the controls (grey). Histograms represent one of four independent experiments. Differences on the mean fluorescence are shown on the table

6.3 Phagocytosis assays

To examine DC's phagocytic capacity, 100,000 DCs/well are grown in RPMI medium supplemented with 5% FBS and stimulated for 48 h with the different treatments. Immature and stimulated DCs are washed with Hanks buffer and suspended in 100 µl (0.5 µg/ml) of E. coli pHrodo™ (Invitrogen) bioparticles, for 3 h at 37°C. Bio-particles fluorescence is read in a fluorometer using an excitation filter of 535 nm and an emission filter of 595 nm (Dynex Technologies, Chantilly, VA, USA). The phagocytic cell percentage is estimated by flow cytometry. DCs are labelled with anti-CD11c-APC and the double labelled cell population is analysed. Assays are performed in triplicate and the analysed as previously described. Figure 8 illustrates the phagocytic activity induced by a galactomannan derived from *C. spinosa*.

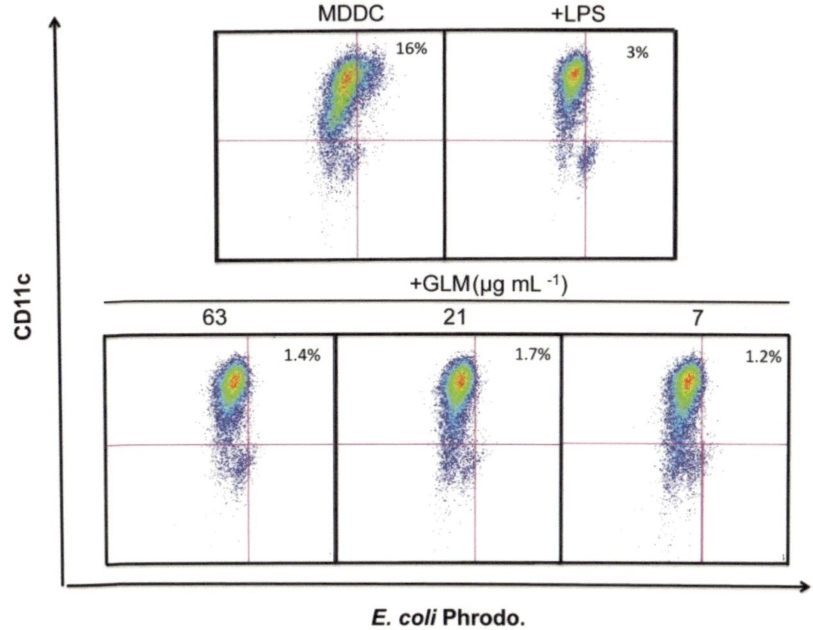

Fig. 8. Phagocytosis is evaluated by staining DCs (MDDC) with CD11c-APC antibody. The scatter plots show the cells after the treatments. DCs (MDDC), DCs (MDDC) plus LPS, DCs with galactomanan (GLM) 63, 21 and 7 ($\mu g\ mL^{-1}$). Dot plots are representing one of four independent experiments

6.4 Mixed leukocyte reaction

Immunostimulatory activity of natural products can be evaluated by measuring the DCs' ability to induce allogeneic response in an assay named mixed leukocyte reaction. Human monocyte-derived DCs are stimulated for 48 h with LPS (1µg/ml) or plant-derived fractions at different concentrations in RPMI supplemented medium. The stimulated DCs are recovered, washed and cultured in fresh RPMI medium supplemented with 5% of human AB serum GemCell™ (Gemini Bio-Products, West Sacramento, CA). 500,000 CDs/well are cultured at different ratios of allogeneic peripheral blood mononuclear cells (PBMC) (1:2, 1:5 and 1:10) previously obtained through Ficoll Hypaque gradient and labelled with

2.5 μM of carboxyfluorescein succinimidylester (CFSE) according to the manufacturer's recommendations (Invitrogen). Cells are collected after five days of co-culture; the first cells are marked with fluorescent viability marker aqua reactive dye (Invitrogen) and the second with anti-CD3 PerCP, anti-CD4 APC-H7 and anti-CD8 Pacific Blue (BD Biosciences). Samples are acquired on a FACSAria (BD Biosciences) and analysed as described above. As an example, Figure 9 shows T cell proliferation after treating DCs with a galactomannan derived from *C. spinosa*.

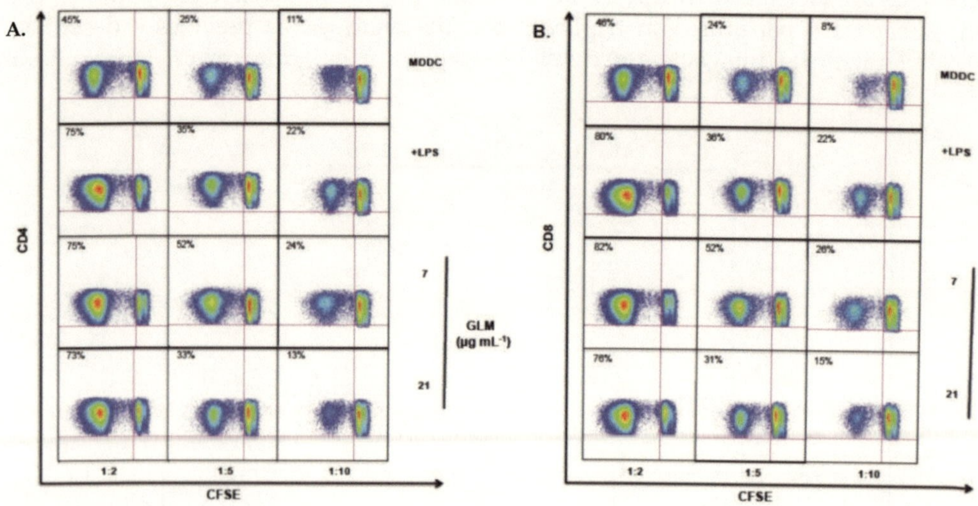

Fig. 9. (A) Dendritic cells (MDDCs) induce allogenic CD4 and CD8 T cell proliferation after treatment with a galactomannan derived from *C. spinosa*. Antigen presenting DCs (MDDC) after stimulation with LPS (1μg mL $^{-1}$) or GLM (7 or 21 μg mL $^{-1}$) determined by T cell proliferation assays. PBMCs stained with CFSE (2,5 μM) and co-cultured with DCs (MDDC) in ratios 1:2, 1:5 and 1:10 (DCs: PBMC) over five days. CD4+ and CD8+ (B) cell proliferation is determined by specific antibodies and analysed through flow cytometry. Dot plots are representing one of four independent experiments

6.5 Cytokine secretion measurement

Cytokine secretion can be assessed by flow cytometry after stimulating with sterile and LPS-free plant fractions or compounds for 48 h as indicated above. The CBA kit (human inflammation cytometric bead array kit) (BD Biosciences) is used to evaluate levels of proinflammatory cytokines such as IL-1, IL-6, IL-8, IL-10, IL-12p70, and TNF-α, in the culture supernatant according to the manufacturer's instructions (CBA, BD Biosciences). The CBA application allows flow cytometry users to quantify simultaneously multiple proteins based on the cytometer capability to detect fine levels of fluorescence. The beads are coupled to antibodies that can capture different substances. Each bead has a unique fluorescence intensity allowing them to mix and record all bead signals at the same time and in a single tube. The analysed supernatants are obtained from $1x10^6$ cells/per well and can be stored at -80°C until analysis. Marking is done according to the supplier instructions and the tubes are analysed as described above.

7. Conclusion

In general terms, flow cytometry constitutes a powerful tool to evaluate the anti-tumour and immunomodulatory activities of natural products, always keeping in mind the correct use of the controls and the instrument settings.

8. Acknowledgment

This work had been supported by grants of The Instituto Colombiano para el Desarrollo de la Ciencia y la Tecnología, Francisco Jose de Caldas (COLCIENCIAS), Pontificia Universidad Javeriana Bogotá, Colombia and the ECOS NORD programme (France-Colombia). We thank Tito Sandoval for his valuable help in the editing, to the sample donors and all of the group students for their help in the development of the techniques. We also thank Carolina Avila for her help in the laboratory logistics.

9. References

Bossy-Wetzel, E., D. D. Newmeyer & D. R. Green (1998). "Mitochondrial cytochrome c release in apoptosis occurs upstream of DEVD-specific caspase activation and independently of mitochondrial transmembrane depolarization." The EMBO Journal 17(1): 37-49.

Chen, X. M., C. Hu, E. Raghubeer & D. D. Kitts (2010). "Effect of High Pressure Pasteurization on Bacterial Load and Bioactivity of Echinacea Purpurea." Journal of Food Science 75(7): C613-C618.

Fadok, V. A., D. R. Voelker, P. A. Campbell, J. J. Cohen, D. L. Bratton & P. M. Henson (1992). "Exposure of phosphatidylserine on the surface of apoptotic lymphocytes triggers specific recognition and removal by macrophages." The Journal of Immunology 148(7): 2207.

Greig, B., T. Oldaker, M. Warzynski & B. Wood (2007). "2006 Bethesda International Consensus recommendations on the immunophenotypic analysis of hematolymphoid neoplasia by flow cytometry: Recommendations for training and education to perform clinical flow cytometry." Cytometry Part B: Clinical Cytometry 72(S1): S23-S33.

Guerrero-Beltran, J. & G. Barbosa-C (2004). "Advantages and limitations on processing foods by UV light." Food science and technology international 10(3): 137.

Humphrey, T. C. & G. Brooks (2005). The Mammalian Cell Cycle: An Overview. Cell cycle control: mechanisms and protocols. T. C. Humphrey & G. Brooks, Humana Pr Inc. 296.

Koopman, G., C. Reutelingsperger, G. Kuijten, R. Keehnen, S. Pals & M. Van Oers (1994). "Annexin V for flow cytometric detection of phosphatidylserine expression on B cells undergoing apoptosis." Blood 84(5): 1415.

Kraan, J., J. W. Gratama, C. Haioun, A. Orfao, A. Plonquet, A. Porwit, S. Quijano, M. Stetler-Stevenson, D. Subira & W. Wilson (2008); Chapter 6: Unit 6.25. Flow Cytometric Immunophenotyping of Cerebrospinal Fluid. Current Protocols in Cytometry, John Wiley & Sons, Inc.

López, L., J. Romero & F. Duarte (2003). "Calidad microbiológica y efecto del lavado y desinfección en vegetales pretrozados expendidos en chile." Arch Latinoam Nutr 53(4): 383-388.

Maecker, H. T. & J. Trotter (2006). "Flow cytometry controls, instrument setup, and the determination of positivity." Cytometry Part A 69(9): 1037-1042.

Mitchell, P. & J. Moyle (1967). "Chemiosmotic hypothesis of oxidative phosphorylation." Nature 213: 137-139.

Nigg, E. A. (2001). "Mitotic kinases as regulators of cell division and its checkpoints." Nature Reviews Molecular Cell Biology 2(1): 21-32.

Paulovich, A. G., D. P. Toczyski & L. H. Hartwell (1997). "When checkpoints fail." Cell 88(3): 315-321.

Raetz, C. R. H. & C. Whitfield (2002). "Lipopolysaccharide endotoxins." Annual Review of Biochemistry 71: 635.

Roa-Higuera, D. C., S. Fiorentino, V. M. Rodríguez-Pardo, A. M. Campos-Arenas, E. A. Infante-Acosta, C. C. Cardozo-Romero & S. M. Quijano-Gómez (2010). "Immunophenotypic analysis of normal cell samples from bone marrow: applications in quality control of cytometry laboratories." Universitas Scientiarum 15(3): 206-223.

Santander, S., M. Aoki, J. Hernandez, M. Pombo, H. Moins-Teisserenc, N. Mooney & S. Fiorentino (2011). "Galactomannan from Caesalpinia spinosa induces phenotypic and functional maturation of human dendritic cells." International Immunopharmacology 11(6): 652-660.

Schepetkin, I. A. & M. T. Quinn (2006). "Botanical polysaccharides: macrophage immunomodulation and therapeutic potential." International Immunopharmacology 6(3): 317-333.

Sugár, I. P., J. González-Lergier & S. C. Sealfon (2011). "Improved compensation in flow cytometry by multivariable optimization." Cytometry Part A.

Urueña, C., C. Cifuentes, D. Castañeda, A. Arango, P. Kaur, A. Asea & S. Fiorentino (2008). "Petiveria alliacea extracts uses multiple mechanisms to inhibit growth of human and mouse tumoral cells." BMC Complementary and Alternative Medicine 8(1): 60.

Van Engeland, M., L. J. W. Nieland, F. C. S. Ramaekers, B. Schutte & C. P. M. Reutelingsperger (1998). "Annexin V-affinity assay: a review on an apoptosis detection system based on phosphatidylserine exposure." Cytometry 31(1): 1-9.

Zamzami, N., S. A. Susin, P. Marchetti, T. Hirsch, I. Gómez-Monterrey, M. Castedo & G. Kroemer (1996). "Mitochondrial control of nuclear apoptosis." The Journal of Experimental Medicine 183(4): 1533.

Zhivotosky, B. & S. Orrenius (2001). Chapter 18: Unit 8.3. "Assessment of apoptosis and necrosis by DNA fragmentation and morphological criteria." Current Protocols in Cell Biology, John Wiley & Sons, Inc.

6

Identification and Characterization of Cancer Stem Cells Using Flow Cytometry

Yasunari Kanda
Division of Pharmacology, National Institute of Health Sciences
Japan

1. Introduction

Tumors are heterogeneous in their cellular morphology, proliferation rate, differentiation grade, genetic lesions, and therapeutic response. The cellular and molecular mechanisms that cause tumor heterogeneity are largely unknown. Growing evidence suggests that tumors are organized in a hierarchy of heterogeneous cell populations and are made and maintained from a small population of stem/stem-like cells called cancer stem cells (CSCs). CSCs are defined on the basis of characteristics such as high tumorigenicity, self-renewal, and differentiation that contribute to heterogeneity. Cancer recurrence is thought to be due to CSCs that are resistant to chemotherapy and radiation.

Dick and his coworkers first reported that all cancer phenotypes present in acute myeloid leukemia (AML) were derived from a few rare populations (0.1–1% of total cells) (Bonnet & Dick, 1997). These leukemic stem cells were isolated from the peripheral blood of AML patients by the surface markers $CD34^{+}/CD38^{-}$, which are similar to those in normal hematopoietic stem cells. These CSCs had a much higher rate of self-renewal than normal stem cells and recapitulated the morphological features of the original malignancy when engrafted in immunodeficient mice. CSCs are thought to have the ability to self-renew and to produce heterogeneous tumors.

This discovery paved the way for the study of CSCs in solid tumors. Based on a similar approach of combined flow cytometry and xenotransplantation, many researchers attempted to isolate CSCs from other tumors. Since the isolation of rare CSCs is a crucial step, the method of CSC isolation using flow cytometry has been improved by using surface markers, side populations, and the ALDEFLUOR assay, as described below. Thus far, CSCs have been found in various solid tumors, including breast, brain, colon, pancreas, prostate, and ovarian tumors (Collins et al., 2005; Curley et al., 2009; Dalerba et al., 2007; Ponti et al., 2005; Singh et al., 2004).

It is still unclear how CSCs are generated. It has been speculated that normal stem cells in various tissues are malignantly transformed by multiple steps such as genetic and epigenetic mutations (Visvader & Lindeman, 2008). A recent study suggests that the dedifferentiation of transformed malignant cells results in the production of CSCs (Gupta et al., 2011). Although there is still a lot of controversy regarding CSCs, a CSC model might provide a potential screening strategy for drug discovery (Gupta et al., 2009). Given the variation of CSCs both in primary specimens and established cancer cell lines, it is essential to characterize CSCs and to optimize the isolation protocol.

This review focuses on the current protocols to identify and characterize CSCs by flow cytometry. In particular, the isolation of CSCs from established breast cancer cell lines is used as a simple model. These protocols would provide new insights into the targeting of CSCs and the implications for cancer therapy.

2. Sphere formation

Normal stem cells have the ability to proliferate in suspension as non-adherent spheres. Neural stem cells and their derived progenitor cells can be enriched and expanded in vitro by their ability to form floating aggregates called neurospheres (Reynolds & Weiss, 1992). These non-adherent spheres were enriched in stem/progenitor cells and were able to differentiate into neurons and glia. In these spheres, between 4% and 20% of the cells were stem cells whereas the other cells represented progenitor cells in different phases of differentiation (Weiss et al., 1996), suggesting that stem cells had been successfully enriched. The markers and receptors that regulate neural stem cell growth have been identified using this cell culture system (Hiramoto et al., 2007; Holmberg et al., 2005; Nagato et al., 2005).These non-adherent culture conditions were also adapted to other normal stem cells. Mammary stem cells that are grown in suspension form mammospheres, which are the equivalent of neurospheres (Dontu et al., 2003).

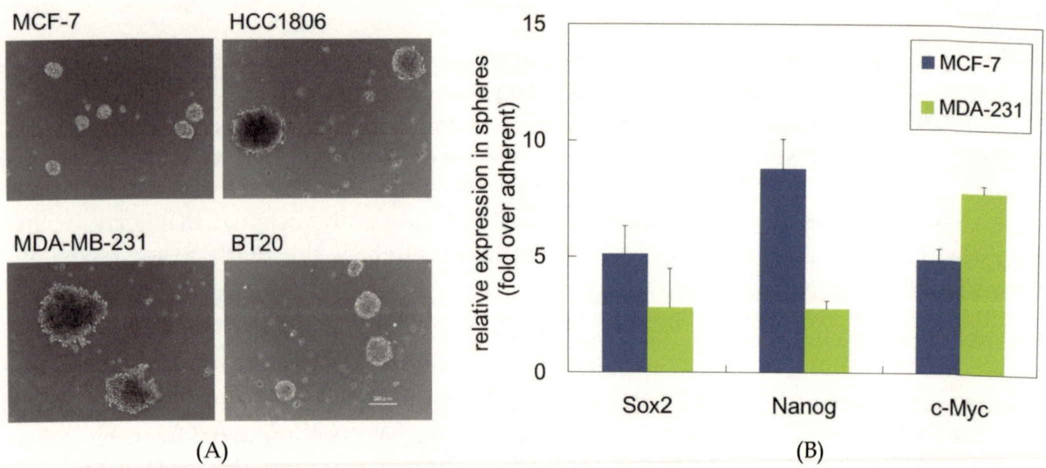

Fig. 1. Mammosphere culture in established breast cancer cell lines (A) ER-positive (MCF-7, HCC1806) and ER-negative (MDA-MB-231, BT20) breast cancer cell lines were seeded in stem cell medium in ultra-low attachment dishes (Corning). After 7 days, mammospheres were observed in MCF-7, HCC1806, and BT20 cells. MDA-MB-231 cells produced loosely adherent cell clumps. (B) Expression of stemness markers in sphere culture from MCF-7 and MDA-MB-231 cells

Subsequently, the sphere culture technique was applied to grow stem cell populations from a variety of clinical cancer samples or cancer cell lines, such as brain cancers (Galli et al., 2004; Singh et al., 2003, 2004). We also applied this approach to form non-adherent mammospheres using established human cancer cell lines, such as MCF-7 (Hirata et al., 2010). As shown in Fig. 1A, both estrogen receptor (ER)-positive and ER-negative breast cancer cell lines can grow as mammospheres in stem cell medium without serum that is supplemented with growth factors such as basic FGF and N_2.Compared with adherent cells, sphere cells from MCF-7 and MDA-MB-231 cells exhibited higher expression of stemness markers such as Nanog, Sox2, and c-Myc, suggesting that they have self-renewal properties (Fig. 1B). In addition, sphere cells have shown high tumorigenicity when injected in immunodeficient mice (Fillmore & Kuperwasser, 2008).

Thus, the sphere assay might represent a potentially valid and useful technique for enrichment of CSCs from clinical specimens or cell lines. However, the stem cell population cannot be purified completely by the sphere technique because CSCs from primary tumors are highly variable (Visvader & Lindeman, 2008) and it is possible that the stem cell population is contaminated with more differentiated cells. Therefore, further purification of CSCs by flow cytometry would be required for CSC characterization.

3. Surface markers

Expression of cell surface markers has been widely used to isolate normal stem cells and the choice of markers varies among tissues and species. As shown in Table 1, CSCs have been isolated by various markers from many types of cancers and these cell surface markers are similar to their normal counterparts.

Tumor type	Surface markers	References	Year
Acute myeloid leukemia	$CD34^+/CD38^-$	Bonnet & Dick	1997
Breast	$CD44^+/CD24^-$	Al-Hajj et al.	2003
Brain	$CD133^+$	Singh et al.	2003
Prostate	$CD133^+$	Miki et al.	2004
Colon	$CD133^+$	O'Brien et al.	2005
Melanoma	$CD20^+$	Fang et al.	2005
Head and neck	$CD44^+$	Prince et al.	2007
Pancreas	$CD133^+/CXCR4^+$	Hermann et al.	2007
Ovary	$CD44^+/CD24^+/ESA^+$	Zhang et al.	2008
Glioblastoma	$CD49f^+$	Lathia et al.	2010

Table 1. Distinct surface markers for isolation of CSCs from different cancer types

3.1 $CD34^+/CD38^-$

As described in the Introduction, $CD34^+/CD38^-$ cell population has been identified as a cell surface marker on leukemic CSCs. This $CD34^+/CD38^-$ cell population had the capacity to initiate leukemia in NOD-SCID mice when compared with $CD34^-$ and $CD34^+/CD38^+$ cell population (Bonnet & Dick, 1997). Although the identification of leukemic CSCs was a major advancement in stem cell field, this subpopulation is still considered heterogeneous (Sarry et al., 2011). A strict definition of leukemic CSCs is necessary to further target these cells.

3.2 CD44$^+$/CD24$^-$

Al-Hajj et al. found CSCs in human solid tumors by using CD44$^+$CD24$^{-/low}$ in breast cancer cells (Al-Hajj et al., 2003). As few as 200 cells from this subpopulation were able to form tumors when injected into NOD/SCID mice, whereas tens of thousands of other cells did not form tumors (Al- Hajj et al., 2003). The tumors from this subpopulation recapitulated the phenotypic heterogeneity of the initial tumor, containing a minority of CD44$^+$CD24$^{-/low}$ cells. The CD44$^+$CD24$^{-/low}$ phenotype has been used to identify and isolate CSCs from breast cancer specimens after in vitro expansion (Ponti et al., 2005) and from breast cancer cell lines (Fillmore & Kuperwasser, 2008). In addition to breast cancer, CSCs in ovarian cancer cells have been isolated by using CD44$^+$/CD24$^-$ (Zhang et al., 2008).

Cancer cell lines that are enriched in CD44$^+$CD24$^{-/low}$ cells are not more tumorigenic than cell lines that contain only 5% of cells with the same phenotype (Fillmore & Kuperwasser, 2008), suggesting that CD44$^+$/CD24$^{-/low}$ cells are heterogeneous and only a subgroup within the CD44$^+$CD24$^{-/low}$ cells is self-renewing.

3.3 CD133

CD133, also known as PROML1 or prominin, is a transmembrane glycoprotein that was identified in mouse neuroepithelial stem cells (Weigmann et al., 1997) and human hematopoietic stem cells (Miraglia et al., 1997). CD133 was also found on progenitor cells in endothelial cells (Peichev et al., 2000), lymphangiogenic cells (Salven et al., 2003) and myoangiogenic cells (Shmelkov et al., 2005). Although its biological function is still unclear, CD133 has been recognized as a putative CSC marker for brain, colon, and prostate cancers (Miki et al., 2007; O'Brien et al., 2007; Ricci-Vitiani et al., 2007; Richardson et al., 2004; Singh et al., 2004). In addition, CD133$^+$CXCR4$^+$ CSCs were found at the invasive front of pancreatic tumors and possibly determine the metastatic phenotype of individual tumors (Hermann et al., 2007).

However, several reports have shown that CD133$^-$ cells have properties of self-renewal. For example, the CD133$^-$ population in colon cancer cells was capable of self-renewal and tumorigenicity (Shmelkov et al., 2008). CD133$^-$ cells derived from several glioma patients were tumorigenic in nude rats and several of the resulting tumors contained CD133$^+$ cells (Wang et al., 2008). Taken together, these data suggest that CD133 is not an appropriate marker for isolation of CSCs in some solid tumors.

3.4 ATP-binding cassette sub-family B member 5 (ABCB5)

Schatton et al. identified an ABCB5$^+$ subpopulation of melanoma cells that showed a high capacity for re-establishing malignancy after xenotransplantation into mice (Schatton et al., 2008). In addition, this group reported that systemic administration of monoclonal antibodies against ABCB5 induces antibody-dependent cell-mediated cytotoxicity in ABCB5$^+$ malignant melanoma initiating cells and exerts tumor-inhibitory effects in a xenograft model. Quintana et al. showed that the frequency of CSCs in human melanoma might depend on the conditions of the xenotransplantation assay using NOD/SCID/IL2Rγc^{null} mice (Quintana et al., 2008). Further investigation is required to elucidate the phenotypic differences between tumorigenic and non-tumorigenic cell populations.

3.5 Integrin α6/CD49f

Integrin α6 (CD49f) is expressed in the stem cells of several tissues including epidermal, keratinocyte, and mammary stem cells (Fortunel et al., 2003; Jones & Watt 1993; Li et al., 1998). A small subpopulation of mouse mammary stem cells, sorted as CD45-/Ter119-/CD31-/Sca-1^{low}/CD24^{med}/CD49f^{high}, was used to purify a rare subset of adult mouse mammary stem cells that were able to individually regenerate an entire mammary gland in vivo (Stingl et al., 2006).

Lathia et al. reported that CSCs in glioblastomas express high levels of integrin α6. In addition, targeting integrin α6 inhibits self-renewal, proliferation, and tumor formation, suggesting that it is a possible therapeutic target (Lathia et al., 2010). Another study showed that knockdown of α6-integrin causes mammosphere-derived cells to lose their ability to grow as mammospheres and abrogates their tumorigenicity in mice, suggesting that integrin α6 is a potential therapeutic target for breast cancer stem cells (Cariati et al., 2008).

As described above, surface markers are very useful tools to isolate and enrich CSCs from a variety of cancer cells. However, expression of these markers is not adequate for the complete purification of CSCs. Moreover, there are currently no universal surface markers for a pure population of CSCs. Since surface markers are also expressed on normal stem cells and these normal stem cells may contaminate the CSC population, more specific markers need to be determined.

4. Side population

In contrast to cell-type specific surface markers, the use of Hoechst 33342 dye to identify and isolate CSCs as a side population (SP) overcomes the barrier of diverse phenotype markers and replaces it with more direct functional markers (Hadnagy et al., 2006).

SP cells were identified in normal murine hematopoietic stem cells. The method is based on the efficient and specific efflux of the fluorescent DNA-binding dye Hoechst 33342 by an ATP-binding cassette (ABC) transporter. By monitoring the blue and red fluorescence emission of Hoechst 33342 following UV excitation, a very small subpopulation of cells was observed that displayed low blue and red fluorescence (Goodell et al, 1996).

Kondo et al. were the first to report SP cells in rat C6 glioma cell line (Kondo et al., 2004). Because SP cells show resistance to anti-cancer drugs due to rapid efflux of those compounds and exhibit higher tumorigenicity than non-SP cells, the SP phenotype defines a type of CSC. Following this finding, SP cells have been identified in various established cell lines (Nakanishi et al., 2010) and tumor specimens (Hirschmann-Jax et al., 2004).

Consistent with these data, we also detected SP cells in human MCF-7 breast cancer cells (Fig. 2). To determine the gate of the SP, it is important to use an ABC transporter-blocking agent such as verapamil or reserpine as a control. In the case of MCF-7 cells, reserpine was more effective than verapamil in inhibiting efflux of Hoechst 33342 by SP cells. In contrast to MCF-7 cells, SP cells have not been observed in human MDA-MB-231 breast cancer cells (data not shown). Therefore, SP cells might not be universal among cell lines. The SP technique could help to identify more specific CSC markers by comparing the expression profiles of SP and non-SP cells.

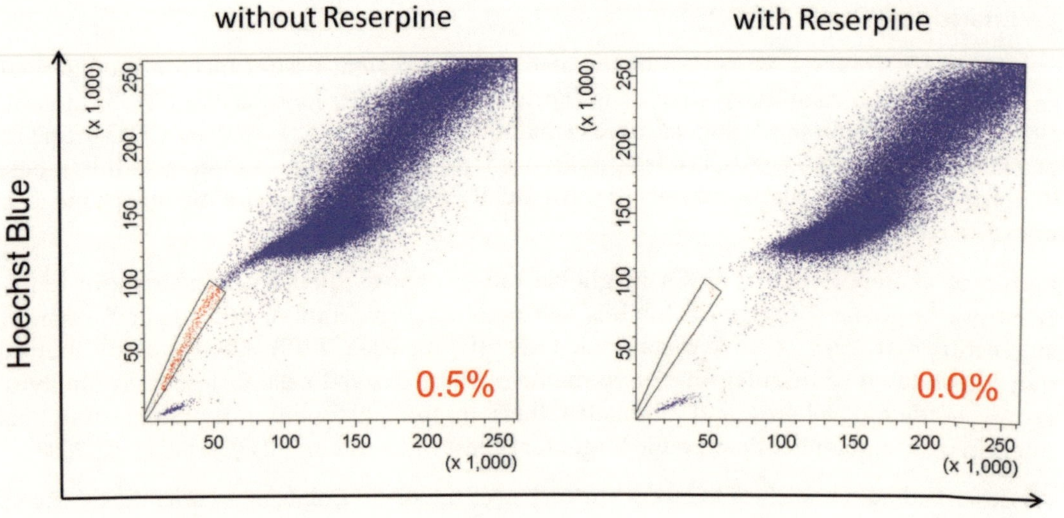

Fig. 2. Side population assay in human MCF-7 breast cancer cells MCF-7 cells were stained with Hoechst 33342 in the absence or presence of reserpine, an inhibitor of ABC transporter, and analyzed by flow cytometry

SP cells are heterogeneous and vary according to tissue type, stage of development, and method of preparation (Uchida et al., 2004). Although SP cells are usually enriched in primitive stem cells, some reports suggest that SP cells do not distinguish stem cells (Triel et al., 2004).

5. ALDEFLUOR assay

Similar to the SP assay, the ALDEFLUOR dye has been developed as a direct functional marker of CSCs. The aldehyde dehydrogenase (ALDH) family of cytosolic isoenzymes is responsible for oxidizing intracellular aldehydes, leading to the oxidation of retinol to retinoic acid. Increased ALDH activity has been described in human hematopoietic stem cells (Hess et al., 2004). As few as 10 ALDEFLUOR-positive cells isolated from the rat hematopoietic system were capable of long-term repopulation of bone marrow upon transplantation in sub-lethally irradiated animals.

ALDEFLUOR staining uses an ALDH substrate, BODIPY-aminoacetaldehyde (BAAA). BAAA is transported into living cells through passive diffusion and is converted into the reaction product BODIPY-aminoacetate (BAA^-) by intracellular ALDH. BAA^- is retained inside cells and becomes brightly fluorescent (Christ et al., 2007). A specific ALDH inhibitor, diethylaminobenzaldehyde (DEAB), is used to determine background fluorescence. Thus, the cells that have high ALDH activity can be detected in the green fluorescence channel by standard flow cytometry. As shown in Fig. 3, we have shown that both MCF-7 and MDA-MB-231 cells contain ALDEFLUOR-positive cells. The proportion of ALDEFLUOR-positive cell was varied by fetal bovine serum (FBS) concentration (unpublished data).

This method has been used to isolate CSCs from breast cancer cells as well as multiple myeloma and leukemia cells (Matsui et al., 2004; Pearce et al., 2005). CSCs with high ALDH activity have been shown to generate tumors in NOD/SCID mice with phenotypic characteristics resembling the parental tumor (Ginestier et al., 2007). In addition, ALDH expression is associated with poor prognosis in breast cancer (Ginestier et al., 2007; Marcato et al., 2011).

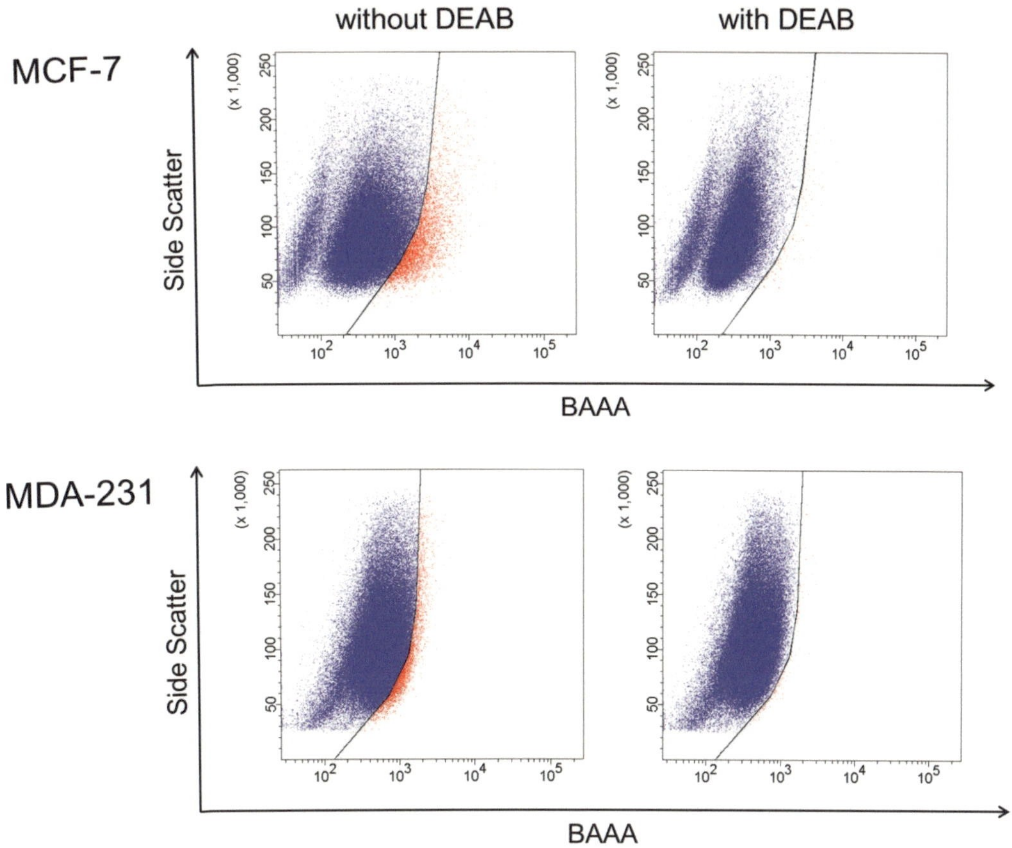

Fig. 3. ALDEFLUOR assay in human breast cancer cell lines MCF-7 and MDA-MB-231 cells were incubated with ALDEFLUOR substrate BAAA alone (left) or in the presence of the ALDH inhibitor DEAB (right), and then analyzed by flow cytometry. DEAB was used to establish the baseline fluorescence of these cells (shown in blue) and to define the ALDEFLUOR-positive region (shown in red)

Although the ALDEFLUOR assay is a potential protocol for CSC isolation, there are several limitations of this technique in certain tumors. For example, both $ALDEFLUOR^{br}$ and $ALDEFLUOR^{low}$ cells from the H522 lung carcinoma cell line were able to initiate tumors after transplantation into NOD/SCID mice. Moreover, tumors generated from $ALDEFLUOR^{low}$ cells grew faster and were larger than the tumors from $ALDEFLUOR^{br}$ cells (Ucar et al., 2009). These results suggest that the ALDEFLUOR assay is not suitable for lung CSCs.

Another problem is that the stem cell population identified using the ALDEFLUOR assay is presumably heterogeneous and must be dissected using additional surface markers. In breast cancer cell lines, cell selection using the $CD44^+/CD24^-/ALDH^+$ phenotype increases the tumorigenicity of breast cancer cells in comparison with $CD44^{+}/CD24^{-}$ or $ALDH^{+}$ cells (Ginestier et al., 2007). This suggests that CSCs obtained with a given marker can be further divided into distinct metastatic or non-metastatic subpopulations using additional markers. These data open new possibilities for cancer stem cell biology with therapeutic applications using marker combinations.

6. CSCs in human cancer cell lines

According to the CSC model, new cancer therapies should focus on targeting and eliminating CSCs, which requires the ability to characterize CSCs.

Clinical CSC samples are difficult to obtain and expand in vitro. A large number of cells should be required for high-throughput screening of lead compounds or drug development. Our experience with breast cancer cells obtained from clinical tumors indicates that a common, distinctive feature of breast CSCs is currently not available.

As described in the section 2, the capability to form non-adherent spheres has been recognized in cancer cell lines that have been established from different solid tumor types. In addition, CSCs isolated by several approaches from established cancer cell lines can be considered models of direct xenografts in immunodeficient mice. Compared with clinical CSCs, the CSCs in human cancer cell lines are easily accessible and provide a simple model for obtaining reproducible results.

For example, we have found that a concentration of nicotine closely related to the blood concentration in cigarette smokers (10 nM–10 μM) increases a proportion of $ALDH^{+}$ population in MCF-7 cells (Hirata et al, 2010). This population, which formed mammospheres, was characterized with respect to Notch signaling. Fillmore et al. reported that the estrogen/FGF/Tbx3 signaling axis has been shown to regulate CSC numbers both in vitro and in vivo by using a proportion of the $CD44^{+}/CD24^{-}/ESA^{+}$ population in MCF-7 cells (Fillmore et al., 2010). Curcumin, a phytochemical compound from the Indian spice turmeric, decreased the SP population in rat C6 glioma cells (Fong et al., 2010). Given that many human cancer cell lines have been used to test the functions of oncogenes and for anti-cancer drug screening, CSCs in human cancer cell lines can serve as a good model for both drug discovery and elucidating the mechanism of disease.

Various drug-screening platforms that were specifically designed to target CSCs have begun to identify novel anti-cancer drugs (Pollard et al., 2009; Gupta et al., 2009). RNA interference libraries also can be screened to identify factors that control CSC tumorigenicity (Wurdak et al., 2010). However, considerable effort should be made to assess the validity, optimal experimental conditions, and the genetic stability of the screening system (van Staveren et al., 2009).

7. Self-renewal pathways of CSCs

The CSC model provides therapeutic strategies beyond traditional anti-proliferative agents (Zhou et al., 2009). A potential approach to eliminating CSCs is blocking the essential self-renewal signaling pathway for CSC survival. Since self-renewal is critical for both normal stem cells and CSCs, common self-renewal pathways presumably exist among them. In addition, these self-renewal pathways might be more conserved than surface markers among CSCs. Taken together, these observations suggest that the search for drugs that target this common mechanism would be a powerful strategy for drug discovery.

It has been suggested that specific signaling pathways such as Notch, Wnt/β-catenin, and Hedgehog play a role in the self-renewal and differentiation of normal stem cells. Alterations in genes that encode signaling molecules belonging to these pathways have been found in human tumor samples (Lobo et al, 2007; Sánchez-García et al., 2007), suggesting that they are likely involved in CSC regulation (Fig. 4).

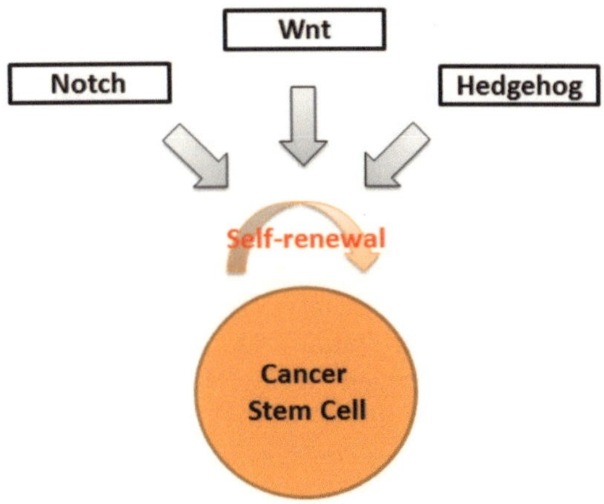

Fig. 4. Self-renewal signaling pathways in CSCs. CSCs are thought to share many molecular similarities with normal stem cells

7.1 Notch

The Notch signaling pathway plays an important role in the maintenance of a variety of adult stem cells, including breast (Dontu et al., 2004), neural (Hitoshi et al., 2002) and intestinal (Fre et al., 2005) stem cells, by promoting self-renewal.

Components of the Notch pathway reportedly act as oncogenes in a wide range of human tumors including breast cancers and gliomas (Kanamori et al., 2007; Reedijk et al., 2005; Stylianou et al., 2006). In addition, breast CSCs have been shown to exist within breast cell lines and primary samples and to self-renew via the Notch pathway (Harrison et al., 2010). Neurospheres derived from human glioblastoma specimens have been shown to grow via the Notch-dependent pathway (Fan et al., 2010).

γ-Secretase inhibitors, which inhibit cleavage of activated Notch receptors and thereby prevent Notch signaling, may be a promising approach for clinical trial. MK-0752 , one of γ-Secretase inhibitors, is currently undergoing clinical trials as a target for breast cancer stem cells after chemotherapy (ClinicalTrials.gov, number NCT00645333) and recurrent CNS malignancies (Fouladi et al., 2011).

7.2 Wnt/β-catenin

The Wnt/β-catenin signaling pathway plays an important role in embryonic development (Clevers, 2006). This pathway is considered a master switch that controls proliferation versus differentiation in both stem cell and cancer cell maintenance and growth in intestinal, epidermal, and hematopoietic tissues (Van der Wetering et al., 2002; Reya & Clevers, 2005). Wnt pathways are commonly hyperactivated in tumors and are required for sustained tumor growth (Reya & Clevers, 2005).

Several small molecule inhibitors of Wnt/β-catenin signaling have been developed. ICG-001 selectively antagonizes interactions between β-catenin and the cyclic AMP response element-binding protein (CBP), which is a transcriptional co-activator essential for β-catenin-mediated transcription (Emami et al., 2004). NSC668036 binds to the PDZ domain of the Wnt-pathway signaling molecule Disheveled and mimics the endogenous Wnt inhibitor Dapper1 (Zhang et al., 2006). XAV939 selectively inhibits β-catenin-mediated transcription. This inhibitor stimulates β-catenin degradation by stabilizing axin, which is a member of the destruction complex that induces ubiquitin-mediated degradation of β-catenin (Huang et al., 2009). Among these Wnt inhibitors, an ICG-001 analog (known as PRI-721) is currently being tested in a clinical trial in patients with gastrointestinal cancers.

7.3 Hedgehog

The Hedgehog signaling pathway was initially identified in Drosophila as a mediator of segmental patterning during development (Nusslein-Volhard & Wieschaus, 1980). This pathway is also essential for maintaining the normal adult stem cell population (Ingham & McMahon, 2001).

Xu et al. identified a Hedgehog-dependent subset of brain tumor stem cells (Xu et al., 2008). Inhibition of Hedgehog signaling has been shown to be effective in a pancreatic cancer xenograft model (Jimeno et al., 2009). Moreover, the Hedgehog pathway has also been implicated in maintaining human leukemic CSCs (Dierks et al., 2008; Zhao et al., 2009). Loss of smoothened, which is a Hedgehog pathway component, resulted in depletion of chronic myeloid CSCs.

Based on these data, many inhibitors of this pathway are currently under development (Mahindroo et al., 2009). For example, GDC-0449 was originally identified as a smoothened antagonist in a chemical compound screen (Robarge et al., 2009) and has been used in a clinical trial in solid tumor patients (Von Hoff et al., 2009). BMS-833923 (XL139) was also used in a clinical trial for uncontrolled basal cell nevus syndrome (Siu et al., 2010).

8. Conclusions

CSCs play a central role in the field of cancer biology and evidence is accumulating that CSCs are involved in tumorigenesis and response to therapy. Although the contribution of CSCs to cancer development is still unclear, targeting CSCs is a potential approach for discovering new drugs that eliminate all cancer cells and finding effective and clinically applicable therapies that prevent disease recurrence and metastasis.

CSC populations in established cancer cell lines are considered good in vitro models. These CSCs can be easily isolated with the protocols described herein and are useful for chemical screening. However, CSC isolation protocols and the efficiency of purification should be improved. The percentage of CSCs in cell lines, their capability to form tumors, and their self-renewal potential can widely vary. In addition, it is essential to investigate whether the

CSCs identified in cancer cell lines have the same properties as the CSCs obtained from patient specimens. Future studies are required to evaluate CSC phenotypes.

Development of new therapies for targeting CSCs must consider both the differences between CSCs and other tumor cells and the signaling pathways shared between CSCs and normal stem cells. Elucidation of the specific mechanisms by which CSCs regulate self-renewal will be useful for the design of new therapeutic alternatives. CSC-targeted therapies should avoid or minimize the potential toxic side effects to normal tissue stem cells.

9. Acknowledgments

This work was supported by a grant from Health Sciences of the National Institute of Biomedical Innovation (No. 09-02), a Grant-in-Aid for Scientific Research from the Ministry of Education, Culture, Sports, Science, and Technology, Japan (No. 23590322) and a Health and Labour Sciences Research Grant from the Ministry of Health, Labour and Welfare, Japan, and a grant from the Smoking Research Foundation.

10. References

Al-Hajj M., Wicha M.S., Benito-Hernandez A., Morrison S.J. & Clarke M.F. (2003). Prospective identification of tumorigenic breast cancer cells. *Proc Natl Acad Sci USA* 100, 3983-8.

Bonnet D. & Dick J.E. (1997). Human acute myeloid leukemia is organized as a hierarchy that originates from a primitive hematopoietic cell. *Nat Med* 3, 730-7.

Cariati M., Naderi A., Brown J.P., Smalley M.J., Pinder S.E., Caldas C. & Purushotham A.D. (2008). α-6 integrin is necessary for the tumourigenicity of a stem cell-like subpopulation within the MCF7 breast cancer cell line. *Int J Cancer* 122, 298-304.

Christ O., Lucke K., Imren S., Leung K., Hamilton M., Eaves A., Smith C. & Eaves C. (2007). Improved purification of hematopoietic stem cells based on their elevated aldehyde dehydrogenase activity, *Haematologica* 92, 1165-72.

Clevers H. (2006). Wnt/β-catenin signaling in development and disease. *Cell* 127, 469–80.

Collins A.T., Berry P.A., Hyde C., Stower M.J. & Maitland N.J. (2005). Prospective identification of tumorigenic prostate cancer stem cells. *Cancer Res* 65, 10946-51.

Curley M.D., Therrien V.A., Cummings C.L., Sergent P.A., Koulouris C.R., Friel A.M., Roberts D.J., Seiden M.V., Scadden D.T., Rueda B.R. & Foster R. (2009). Cd133 expression defines a tumor initiating cell population in primary human ovarian cancer. *Stem Cells* 27, 2875-83.

Dalerba P., Dylla S.J., Park I.K., Liu R., Wang X., Cho R.W., Hoey T., Gurney A., Huang E.H., Simeone D.M., Ricci-Vitiani L., Lombardi D.G., Pilozzi E., Biffoni M., Todaro M., Peschle C. & De Maria R. (2007). Identification and expansion of human colon-cancer-initiating cells. *Nature* 445, 111-5.

Dierks C., Beigi R., Guo G.R., Zirlik K., Stegert M.R., Manley P., Trussell C., Schmitt-Graeff A., Landwerlin K., Veelken H. & Warmuth M. (2008). Expansion of Bcr-Abl-positive leukemic stem cells is dependent on Hedgehog pathway activation. *Cancer Cell* 14, 238–49.

Dontu G., Abdallah W.M., Foley J.M., Jackson K.W., Clarke M.F., Kawamura M.J. & Wicha M.S. (2003). In vitro propagation and transcriptional profiling of human mammary stem/progenitor cells. *Genes Dev* 17, 1253-70.

Dontu G., Jackson K.W., McNicholas E., Kawamura M.J., Abdallah W.M. & Wicha MS. (2004). Role of Notch signaling in cell-fate determination of human mammary stem/progenitor cells. *Breast Cancer Res* 6, R605–15.

Emami K.H., Nguyen C., Ma H., Kim D.H., Jeong K.W., Eguchi M., Moon R.T., Teo J.L., Kim H.Y., Moon S.H., Ha J.R. & Kahn M. (2004). A small molecule inhibitor of β-catenin/CREB-binding protein transcription. *Proc Natl Aca Sci USA* 101, 12682-7.

Fan X., Khaki L., Zhu T.S., Soules M.E., Talsma C.E., Gul N., Koh C., Zhang J., Li Y.M., Maciaczyk J., Nikkhah G., Dimeco F., Piccirillo S., Vescovi A.L., Eberhart C.G. (2010). NOTCH pathway blockade depletes CD133-positive glioblastoma cells and inhibits growth of tumor neurospheres and xenografts. *Stem Cells* 28, 5-16.

Fang D, Nguyen TK, Leishear K, Finko R, Kulp AN, Hotz S, Van Belle PA, Xu X, Elder DE, Herlyn M. (2005). A tumorigenic subpopulation with stem cell properties in melanomas. *Cancer Res* 65, 9328-37.

Fillmore CM, Gupta PB, Rudnick JA, Caballero S, Keller PJ, Lander ES, and Kuperwasser C. Estrogen expands breast cancer stem-like cells through paracrine FGF/Tbx3 signaling. *Proc Natl Acad. Sci USA* 107, 21737-42.

Fillmore C.M. & Kuperwasser C. (2008). Human breast cancer cell lines contain stem-like cells that self-renew, give rise to phenotypically diverse progeny and survive chemotherapy. *Breast Cancer Res* 10(2), R25.

Fong D., Yeh A., Naftalovich .R, Choi T.H. & Chan M.M. (2010). Curcumin inhibits the side population (SP) phenotype of the rat C6 glioma cell line: towards targeting of cancer stem cells with phytochemicals. *Cancer Lett* 293, 65-72.

Fortunel N.O., Otu H.H., Ng H.H., Chen J., Mu X., Chevassut T., Li X., Joseph M., Bailey C., Hatzfeld J.A., Hatzfeld A., Usta F., Vega V.B., Long P.M., Libermann T.A., Lim B. (2003). Comment on " 'Stemness': transcriptional profiling of embryonic and adult stem cells" and "a stem cell molecular signature". *Science* 302, 393.

Fre S., Huyghe M., Mourikis P., Robine S., Louvard D & Artavanis-Tsakonas S. (2005). Notch signals control the fate of immature progenitor cells in the intestine. *Nature* 435, 964–8.

Fouladi M., Stewart C.F., Olson J., Wagner L.M., Onar-Thomas A., Kocak M., Packer R.J., Goldman S., Gururangan S., Gajjar A., Demuth T., Kun L.E., Boyett J.M. & Gilbertson RJ. (2011). Phase I trial of MK-0752 in children with refractory CNS malignancies: a pediatric brain tumor consortium study. *J Clin Oncol* 29, 3529-34.

Galli R., Binda E., Orfanelli U., Cipelletti B., Gritti A., De Vitis S., Fiocco R., Foroni C., Dimeco F. & Vescovi A. (2004). Isolation and characterization of tumorigenic, stem-like neural precursors from human glioblastoma. *Cancer Res* 64, 7011-21.

Ginestier C., Hur M.H., Charafe-Jauffret E., Monville F., Dutcher J., Brown M., Jacquemier J., Viens P., Kleer C.G., Liu S., Schott A., Hayes D., Birnbaum D., Wicha M.S. & Dontu G. (2007). ALDH1 is a marker of normal and malignant human mammary stem cells and a predictor of poor clinical outcome. *Cell Stem Cell* 1, 555-67.

Goodell M.A., Brose K., Paradis G., Conner A.S. & Mulligan R.C. (1996). Isolation and functional properties of murine hematopoietic stem cells that are replicating in vivo. *J Exp Med* 183, 1797-806

Gupta P.B., Onder T.T., Jiang G., Tao K., Kuperwasser C., Weinberg R.A., Lander E.S. (2009). Identification of selective inhibitors of cancer stem cells by high-throughput screening. *Cell* 138, 645-59.

Gupta P.B., Fillmore C.M., Jiang G., Shapira S.D., Tao K., Kuperwasser C., Lander E.S. (2011). Stochastic state transitions give rise to phenotypic equilibrium in populations of cancer cells. *Cell* 146, 633-44.

Hadnagy A., Gaboury L., Beaulieu R. & Balicki D. (2006). SP analysis may be used to identify cancer stem cell populations. *Exp Cell Res* 312, 3701-10.

Harrison H., Farnie G., Howell S.J., Rock R.E., Stylianou S., Brennan K.R., Bundred N.J. & Clarke R.B. (2010). Regulation of breast cancer stem cell activity by signaling through the Notch4 receptor. *Cancer Res* 70, 709–18.

Hermann P.C., Huber S.L., Herrler T., Aicher A., Ellwart J.W., Guba M., Bruns C.J. & Heeschen C. (2007). Distinct populations of cancer stem cells determine tumor growth and metastatic activity in human pancreatic cancer. *Cell Stem Cell* 1, 313–23.

Hess D.A., Meyerrose T.E., Wirthlin L., Craft T.P., Herrbrich P.E., Creer M.H. & Nolta J.A. (2004). Functional characterization of highly purified human hematopoietic repopulating cells isolated according to aldehyde dehydrogenase activity. *Blood* 104, 1648-55.

Hiramoto T., Kanda Y., Satoh Y., Takishima K. & Watanabe Y. (2007). Dopamine D2 receptor stimulation promotes the proliferation of neural progenitor cells in adult mouse hippocampus. *Neuroreport* 18, 659-64.

Hirata N., Sekino Y. & Kanda Y. (2010). Nicotine increases cancer stem cell population in MCF-7 cells, *Biochem Biophys Res Commun* 403, 138–43.

Hirschmann-Jax C., Foster A.E., Wulf G.G., Nuchtern J.G., Jax T.W., Gobel U., Goodell M.A. & Brenner M.K. (2004). A distinct "side population" of cells with high drug efflux capacity in human tumor cells. *Proc Natl Acad Sci USA* 101, 14228-33.

Hitoshi S., Alexson T., Tropepe V., Donoviel D., Elia A.J., Nye J.S., Conlon R.A., Mak T.W., Bernstein A. & van der Kooy D. (2002). Notch pathway molecules are essential for the maintenance, but not the generation, of mammalian neural stem cells. *Genes Dev* 16, 846–58.

Holmberg J., Armulik A., Senti K.A., Edoff K., Spalding K., Momma S., Cassidy R., Flanagan J.G.& Frisén J. (2005). Ephrin-A2 reverse signaling negatively regulates neural progenitor proliferation and neurogenesis. *Genes Dev* 19, 462-71.

Huang S.M., Mishina Y.M., Liu S., Cheung A., Stegmeier F., Michaud G.A., Charlat O., Wiellette E., Zhang Y., Wiessner S., Hild M., Shi X., Wilson C.J., Mickanin C., Myer V., Fazal A., Tomlinson R., Serluca F., Shao W., Cheng H., Shultz M., Rau C., Schirle M., Schlegl J., Ghidelli S., Fawell S., Lu C., Curtis D., Kirschner M.W., Lengauer C., Finan P.M., Tallarico .JA., Bouwmeester T., Porter J.A., Bauer A. & Cong F. (2009). Tankyrase inhibition stabilizes axin and antagonizes Wnt signalling. *Nature* 461, 614-20.

Ingham P.W. & McMahon A.P. (2001). Hedgehog signaling in animal development: paradigms and principles. *Genes Dev* 15, 3059-87.

Jimeno A., Feldmann G., Suárez-Gauthier A., Rasheed Z., Solomon A., Zou G.M. Rubio-Viqueira B., García-García E., López-Ríos F., Matsui W. Maitra A. & Hidalgo M. (2009). A direct pancreatic cancer xenograft model as a platform for cancer stem cell therapeutic development. *Mol Cancer Ther* 8, 310-4.

Jones PH & Watt FM. (1993). Separation of human epidermal stem cells from transit amplifying cells on the basis of differences in integrin function and expression. *Cell* 73, 713-24.

Kanamori M., Kawaguchi T., Nigro J.M., Feuerstein B.G., Berger M.S., Miele L. & Pieper R.O. (2007). Contribution of Notch signaling activation to human glioblastoma multiforme. *J Neurosurg* 106, 417-27.

Kondo T., Setoguchi T. & Taga T. (2004). Persistence of a small subpopulation of cancer stem-like cells in the C6 glioma cell line. *Proc Natl Acad Sci USA* 101, 781-6.

Lathia J.D., Gallagher J., Heddleston J.M., Wang J., Eyler C.E., Macswords J. Wu Q., Vasanji A., McLendon R.E., Hjelmeland A.B. & Rich J.N. (2010). Integrin α6 Regulates Glioblastoma Stem Cells. *Cell Stem Cell* 6, 421–32.

Li A., Simmons P.J. & Kaur P. (1998). Identification and isolation of candidate human keratinocyte stem cells based on cell surface phenotype. *Proc Natl Acad. Sci USA* 95, 3902–7.

Lobo N.A., Shimono Y., Qian D. & Clarke M.F. (2007). The biology of cancer stem cells. *Annu Rev Cell Dev Biol* 23, 675-99.

Mahindroo N., Punchihewa C. & Fujii N. (2009). Hedgehog-Gli signaling pathway inhibitors as anticancer agents. *J Med Chem* 52, 3829–45.

Marcato P., Dean C.A., Pan D., Araslanova R., Gillis M., Joshi M., Helyer L., Pan L., Leidal A., Gujar S., Giacomantonio C.A. & Lee P.W. (2011). Aldehyde dehydrogenase activity of breast cancer stem cells is primarily due to isoform ALDH1A3 and its expression is predictive of metastasis. *Stem Cells* 29, 32-45.

Matsui W., Huff C.A., Wang Q., Malehorn M.T., Barber J., Tanhehco Y., Smith B.D., Civin C.I. & Jones R.J. (2004). Characterization of clonogenic multiple myeloma cells. *Blood* 103, 2332-6.

Miki J., Furusato B., Li H., Gu Y., Takahashi H., Egawa S., Sesterhenn I.A., McLeod D.G., Srivastava S. & Rhim J.S. (2007). Identification of putative stem cell markers, CD133 and CXCR4, in hTERT-immortalized primary nonmalignant and malignant tumor-derived human prostate epithelial cell lines and in prostate cancer specimens. *Cancer Res* 67, 3153–61.

Miraglia S., Godfrey W., Yin A.H., Atkins K., Warnke R., Holden J.T., Bray R.A., Waller E.K. & Buck D.W. (1997). A novel five-transmembrane hematopoietic stem cell antigen: isolation, characterization, and molecular cloning. *Blood* 90, 5013–21.

Nagato M., Heike T., Kato T., Yamanaka Y., Yoshimoto M., Shimazaki T., Okano H. & Nakahata T. (2005). Prospective characterization of neural stem cells by flow cytometry analysis using a combination of surface markers. *J Neurosci Res* 80, 456-66.

Nakanishi T., Chumsri S., Khakpour N., Brodie A.H., Leyland-Jones B., Hamburger A.W., Ross D.D. & Burger A.M. (2010). Side-population cells in luminal-type breast cancer have tumour-initiating cell properties, and are regulated by HER2 expression and signalling. *Br J Cancer* 102, 815-26.

Nusslein-Volhard C. & Wieschaus E. Mutations affecting segment number and polarity in Drosophila. (1980). *Nature* 287, 795–801.

O'Brien C.A., Pollett A., Gallinger S. & Dick JE. (2007). A human colon cancer cell capable of initiating tumour growth in immunodeficient mice. *Nature* 445, 106–10.

Peukert S. & Miller-Moslin K. (2010). Small-molecule inhibitors of the hedgehog signaling pathway ascancer therapeutics. *Chem Med Chem* 5, 500-12.

Pearce D.J., Taussig D., Simpson C., Allen K., Rohatiner A.Z., Lister T.A. & Bonnet D. (2005). Characterization of cells with a high aldehyde dehydrogenase activity from cord blood and acute myeloid leukemia samples. *Stem Cells* 23, 752-60.

Peichev M., Naiyer A.J., Pereira D., Zhu Z., Lane W.J., Williams M., Oz M.C., Hicklin D.J., Witte L., Moore M.A. & Rafii S. (2000). Expression of VEGFR-2 and AC133 by circulating human CD34(+) cells identifies a population of functional endothelial precursors. *Blood* 95, 952-8.

Pollard S.M., Yoshikawa K., Clarke I.D., Danovi D., Stricker S., Russell R., Bayani J., Head R., Lee M., Bernstein M., Squire J.A., Smith A. & Dirks P.(2009). Glioma stem cell lines expanded in adherent culture have tumor-specific phenotypes and are suitable for chemical and genetic screens. *Cell Stem Cell* 4, 568–80.

Ponti D., Costa A., Zaffaroni N., Pratesi G., Petrangolini G., Coradini D., Pilotti S., Pierotti M.A. & Daidone M.G. (2005). Isolation and in vitro propagation of tumorigenic breast cancer cells with stem/progenitor cell properties. *Cancer Res* 65, 5506-11.

Prince M.E., Sivanandan R., Kaczorowski A., Wolf G.T., Kaplan M., Dalerba P., Weissman I.L., Clarke M.F. & Ailles L.E. (2007). Identification of a subpopulation of cells with cancer stem cell properties in head and neck squamous cell carcinoma. *Proc Natl Acad Sci USA* 104, 973-8.

Quintana E., Shackleton M., Sabel M.S., Fullen D.R., Johnson T.M. & Morrison S.J. (2008). Efficient tumor formation by single human melanoma cells. *Nature* 456, 593–8.

Reedijk M., Odorcic S., Chang L., Zhang H., Miller N., McCready D.R., Lockwood G. & Egan S.E. (2005). High-level coexpression of JAG1 and NOTCH1 is observed in human breast cancer and is associated with poor overall survival. *Cancer Res* 65, 8530-7.

Reya T. & Clevers H. (2005). Wnt signalling in stem cells and cancer. *Nature* 434, 843-50.

Reynolds B.A. & Weiss S. (1992). Generation of neurons and astrocytes from isolated cells of the adult mammalian central nervous system. *Science* 255, 1707-10.

Ricci-Vitiani L., Lombardi D.G., Pilozzi E., Biffoni M., Todaro M., Peschle C. & De Maria R. (2007). Identification and expansion of human colon-cancer-initiating cells. *Nature* 445, 111–5.

Richardson G.D., Robson C.N., Lang S.H., Neal D.E., Maitland N.J. & Collins AT. (2004). CD133, a novel marker for human prostatic epithelial stem cells. *J Cell Sci* 117, 3539-45.

Robarge K.D., Brunton S.A., Castanedo G.M., Cui Y., Dina M.S., Goldsmith R., Gould S.E., Guichert O., Gunzner J.L., Halladay J., Jia W., Khojasteh C., Koehler M.F., Kotkow K., La H., Lalonde R.L., Lau K., Lee L., Marshall D., Marsters J.C. Jr, Murray L.J., Qian C., Rubin L.L., Salphati L., Stanley M.S., Stibbard J.H., Sutherlin D.P., Ubhayaker S., Wang S., Wong S. & Xie M. (2009). GDC-0449-a potent inhibitor of the Hedgehog pathway. *Bioorg Med Chem Lett* 19, 5576–81.

Salven P., Mustjoki S., Alitalo R., Alitalo K. & Rafii S. (2003). VEGFR-3 and CD133 identify a population of CD34+ lymphatic/vascular endothelial precursor cells. *Blood* 101, 168-72.

Sánchez-García I., Vicente-Dueñas C. & Cobaleda C. (2007). The theoretical basis of cancer-stem-cell based therapeutics of cancer: can it be put into practice? *Bioessays* 29, 1269-80.

Sarry J.E., Murphy K., Perry R., Sanchez P.V., Secreto A., Keefer C., Swider C.R., Strzelecki A.C., Cavelier C., Récher C., Mansat-De Mas V., Delabesse E., Danet-Desnoyers G., Carroll M. (2011). Human acute myelogenous leukemia stem cells are rare and heterogeneous when assayed in NOD/SCID/IL2Rγc-deficient mice. *J Clin Invest* 121, 384-95.

Schatton T., Murphy G.F., Frank N.Y., Yamaura K., Waaga-Gasser A.M., Gasser M., Zhan Q., Jordan S., Duncan L.M., Weishaupt C., Fuhlbrigge R.C., Kupper T.S., Sayegh M.H. & Frank, M.H. (2008). Identification of cells initiating human melanomas. *Nature* 451, 345-9.Stylianou S., Clarke R.B., Brennan K. (2006). Aberrant activation of notch signalling in human breast cancer. *Cancer Res* 66, 1517-25.

Shmelkov S.V., Meeus S., Moussazadeh N., Kermani P., Rashbaum W.K., Rabbany S.Y., Hanson M.A., Lane W.J., St Clair R., Walsh K.A., Dias S., Jacobson J.T., Hempstead B.L., Edelberg J.M. & Rafii S. (2005). Cytokine preconditioning promotes codifferentiation of human fetal liver $CD133^+$ stem cells into angiomyogenic tissue. *Circulation* 111, 1175-83.

Shmelkov S.V., Butler J.M., Hooper A.T., Hormigo A., Kushner J., Milde T., St Clair R., Baljevic M., White I., Jin D.K., Chadburn A., Murphy A.J., Valenzuela D.M., Gale N.W., Thurston G., Yancopoulos G.D., D'Angelica M., Kemeny N., Lyden D. & Rafii S. (2008). CD133 expression is not restricted to stem cells, and both $CD133^+$ and $CD133^-$ metastatic colon cancer cells initiate tumors. *J Clin Invest* 118, 2111-20.

Singh S.K., Clarke I.D., Terasaki M., Bonn V.E., Hawkins C., Squire J. & Dirks P.B. (2003). Identification of a cancer stem cell in human brain tumors. *Cancer Res* 63, 5821-8.

Singh S.K., Hawkins C., Clarke I.D., Squire J.A., Bayani J., Hide T., Henkelman R.M., Cusimano M.D. & Dirks P.B. (2004). Identification of human brain tumour initiating cells. *Nature* 432, 396-401.

Siu L.L., Papadopoulos K., Alberts S.R., Kirchoff-Ross R., Vakkalagadda B., Lang L., Ahlers C.M., Bennett K.L. & Van Tornout J.M. (2010). A first-in-human, phase I study of an oral hedgehog (HH) pathway antagonist, BMS-833923 (XL139), in subjects with advanced or metastatic solid tumors. *J Clin Oncol (ASCO)* abstract no. 2501.

Stingl J., Eirew P., Ricketson I., Shackleton M., Vaillant F., Choi D., Li H.I. & Eaves C.J. (2006). Purification and unique properties of mammary epithelial stem cells. *Nature* 439, 993-7.

Stylianou S., Clarke R.B., & Brennan K. (2006). Aberrant activation of Notch signalling occurs in human breast cancer. *Cancer Res* 66, 1517-25.

Triel C., Vestergaard M.E., Bolund L., Jensen T.G., Jensen U.B. (2004). Side population cells in human and mouse epidermis lack stem cell characteristics. *Exp Cell Res* 295, 79-90.

Ucar D., Cogle C.R., Zucali J.R., Ostmark B., Scott E.W., Zori R., Gray B.A. & Moreb J.S. (2009). Aldehyde dehydrogenase activity as a functional marker for lung cancer. *Chem Biol Interact* 178, 48-55.

Uchida N., Dykstra B., Lyons K., Leung F., Kristiansen M., Eaves C. (2004). ABC transporter activities of murine hematopoietic stem cells vary according to their developmental and activation status. *Blood* 103, 4487–95.

van de Wetering M., Sancho E., Verweij C., de Lau W., Oving I., Hurlstone A., van der Horn K., Batlle E., Coudreuse D., Haramis A.P., Tjon-Pon-Fong M., Moerer P., van den Born M., Soete G., Pals S., Eilers M., Medema R. & Clevers H. (2002). The beta-catenin/TCF-4 complex imposes a crypt progenitor phenotype on colorectal cancer cells. *Cell* 111, 241-50.

van Staveren W.C., Solís D.Y., Hébrant A., Detours V., Dumont J.E. & Maenhaut C. (2009). Human cancer cell lines: Experimental models for cancer cells in situ? For cancer stem cells? *Biochim Biophys Acta* 1795, 92-103.

Visvader J.E. & Lindeman G.J. (2008). Cancer stem cells in solid tumours: accumulating evidence and unresolved questions. *Nat Rev Cancer* 8, 755-68.

Von Hoff D.D., LoRusso P.M., Rudin C.M., Reddy J.C., Yauch R.L., Tibes R., Weiss G.J., Borad M.J., Hann C.L., Brahmer J.R., Mackey H.M., Lum B.L., Darbonne W.C., Marsters J.C. Jr, de Sauvage F.J. & Low J.A. (2009). Inhibition of the Hedgehog pathway in advanced basal-cell carcinoma. *N Engl J Med* 361, 1164–72.

Wang J., Sakariassen P.Ø., Tsinkalovsky O., Immervoll H., Boe S.O., Svendsen A., Prestegarden L., Rosland G., Thorsen F., Stuhr L., Molven A., Bjerkvig R. & Enger P.Ø. (2008). CD133 negative glioma cells form tumors in nude rats and give rise to CD133 positive cells. *Int J Cancer* 122, 761-8.

Weigmann A., Corbeil D., Hellwig A. & Huttner W.B. (1997). Prominin, a novel microvilli-specific polytopic membrane protein of the apical surface of epithelial cells, is targeted to plasmalemmal protrusions of non-epithelial cells. *Proc Natl Acad Sci USA* 94, 12425–30.

Weiss S., Dunne C., Hewson J., Wohl C., Wheatley M., Peterson A.C. & Reynolds B.A. (1996). Multipotent CNS stem cells are present in the adult mammalian spinal cord and ventricular neuroaxis. *J Neurosci* 16, 7599-609.

Wurdak H., Zhu S., Romero A., Lorger M., Watson .J, Chiang C.Y., Zhang J., Natu V.S., Lairson L.L., Walker J.R., Trussell C.M., Harsh G.R., Vogel H., Felding-Habermann B., Orth A.P., Miraglia L.J., Rines D.R., Skirboll S.L., Schultz P.G. (2010). An RNAi screen identifies TRRAP as a regulator of brain tumor-initiating cell differentiation. *Cell Stem Cell* 6,37-47.

Xu Q, Yuan X, Liu G, Black KL, Yu JS. (2008). Hedgehog signaling regulates brain tumor-initiating cell proliferation and portends shorter survival for patients with PTEN-coexpressing glioblastomas. *Stem Cells* 26, 3018-26.

Zhang L., Gao X., Wen J., Ning Y. & Chen Y.G. (2006). Dapper 1 antagonizes Wnt signaling by promoting dishevelled degradation. *J Biol Chem* 281, 8607-12.

Zhang S., Balch C., Chan M.W., Lai H.C., Matei D., Schilder J.M., Yan P.S., Huang T.H., Nephew K.P. (2008). Identification and characterization of ovarian cancer-initiating cells from primary human tumors. *Cancer Res* 68, 4311–20.

Zhao C., Chen A., Jamieson C.H., Fereshteh M., Abrahamsson A., Blum J., Kwon H.Y., Kim J., Chute J.P., Rizzieri D., Munchhof M., Vanarsdale T., Beachy P.A. & Reya T. (2009). Hedgehog signalling is essential for maintenance of cancer stem cells in myeloid leukaemia. *Nature* 458, 776–9.

Zhou B.B., Zhang H., Damelin M., Geles K.G., Grindley J.C. & Dirks P.B. (2009). Tumour-initiating cells: challenges and opportunities for anticancer drug discovery. *Nat Rev Drug Discov* 8, 806-23.

7

Flow Based Enumeration of Plasmablasts in Peripheral Blood After Vaccination as a Novel Diagnostic Marker for Assessing Antibody Responses in Patients with Hypogammaglobulinaemia

Vojtech Thon, Marcela Vlkova,
Zita Chovancova, Jiri Litzman and Jindrich Lokaj
Department of Clinical Immunology and Allergy, Medical Faculty of Masaryk University,
St. Anne's University Hospital, Brno
Czech Republic

1. Introduction

Hypogammaglobulinaemic patients are often started on immunoglobulin substitution therapy before antibody production is adequately evaluated. In such a situation, it is difficult to segregate transferred from antigen-induced specific antibody. Therefore we characterized changes in B-cell subpopulations in hypogammaglobulinaemic patients, including plasmablasts, in peripheral blood by flow cytometry after in vivo antigen challenge. We investigated the specificity of antibody production on the B-cell level by ELISPOT, which is independent of substitution therapy.

Common variable immunodeficiency (CVID) is characterized by low serum levels of IgG, IgA, normal or low levels of IgM and impaired antibody responses after vaccination (Conley et al. 1999). The clinical presentation of CVID includes recurrent respiratory tract infections by encapsulated bacteria, autoimmunity, granuloma formations, enteropathy and increased risk of malignancies. The diagnosis is established by exclusion and elimination of other disorders affecting B-cell differentiation. Although standard treatment include long-term immunoglobulin replacement and antimicrobial therapy, the mortality rate of CVID patients is higher than that of the general population (Chapel et al. 2008; Cunningham-Rundles & Bodian 1999).

Despite intensive research the immunopathogenesis of CVID has not yet been elucidated. It has been suggested that CVID is caused by defects in T cells, B cells, insufficient T-B cell interactions or impaired signaling required for B or T-cell maturation and function, but the characterization of the genetic defects remains unclear in the majority of patients. Molecular defects involving mutations in CD19 (van Zelm et al. 2006), ICOS (Grimbacher et al. 2003; Salzer et al. 2004), CD81 (van Zelm et al.), Msh5 (Sekine et al. 2007) and TACI (Castigli et al. 2005; Mohammadi et al. 2009; Salzer et al. 2005) were found in less than 10% of CVID patients (Cunningham-Rundles & Bodian 1999; Schaffer et al. 2007). CVID, therefore, is a heterogeneous group of patients expected to have multiple etiologies, all sharing similar immunologic and clinical characteristics.

Although the precise pathogenesis of CVID remains unknown, a number of common abnormalities involving peripheral blood lymphocytes were described including differences in the number of naïve B cells (follicular B cells), $CD21^{low}$ B cells, transitional B cells, non-class-switched IgM/IgD memory B cells (marginal zone-like B cells) (Klein et al. 1997; Shi et al. 2003; Tangye & Tarlinton 2009), class-switched memory B cells and plasmablasts (Carsetti et al. 2004; Sanchez-Ramon et al. 2008; Warnatz & Schlesier 2008; Weller et al. 2004). Specifically, CVID patients have reduced populations of $CD27^{+}$ memory B cells (class-switched memory B cells and marginal zone-like B cells) and increased percentages of undifferentiated B cells (immature $CD21^{low}$ B cells (Rakhmanov et al. 2009) and naïve $CD27^{-}$ B cells) associated with impaired class switching (Piqueras et al. 2003; Warnatz et al. 2002) and poor differentiation into plasma cells (Taubenheim et al. 2005) when compared to a control population (Ferry et al. 2005; Litzman et al. 2007).

In addition, a vast array of T-cell abnormalities has been described in CVID patients, including defects in TCR-dependent T-cell activation (Thon et al. 1997), reduced frequency of antigen-specific T cells, impaired IL-2 release in $CD4^{+}$ T cells (Funauchi et al. 1995), decreased lymphocyte proliferation to mitogens and antigens (Chapel et al. 2008), lack of generation of antigen-primed T cells after prophylactic vaccination (Bryant et al. 1990; Fischer et al. 1994; Giovannetti et al. 2007), impaired cytokine production (Fischer et al. 1994; Thon et al. 1997), reduced expression of CD40L on activated T cells (Farrington et al. 1994; Piqueras et al. 2003; Thon et al. 1997; Warnatz et al. 2002), significant decrease in Treg cells in CVID patients with granulomatous manifestations and immune cytopenias (Horn et al. 2009), significant reduction of frequency and absolute counts of $CD4^{+}$ T cells, percentage increase in $CD8^{+}$ T cells, decrease in distribution of $CD4^{+}$ and $CD8^{+}$ naïve T cells in comparison to healthy controls (Giovannetti et al. 2007; Mouillot et al. 2010). This complex list of T-cell abnormality likely plays a major role in determining the clinical course of CVID patients.

In spite all of these multiple T-cell defects proposed as possible cause of CVID, the classification schemes presently in use are based on functional or phenotypic characteristics of B cells (assessment of immunoglobulin synthesis in vitro and phenotypic subsets of peripheral blood B cells): Bryant British classification (Bryant et al. 1990), Freiburg classification (Warnatz et al. 2002), Paris classification (Piqueras et al. 2003) and the recent EUROclass classification (Wehr et al. 2008). A few authors, however, suggested T-cell phenotyping as an aditional parameter for classifying CVID, and current efforts aim at the definition of combined T and B-cell phenotyping for the classification of CVID (Mouillot et al. 2010; Warnatz & Schlesier 2008).

Although a lot is known about B cell subsets in of CVID patients, the way their B-cell subpopulations change in response to vaccination compared to normal individuals is largely unknown. Specifically, there are limited data as to antibody responses to protein or polysaccharide antigens and the quantity and quality of antibodies produced by patient from different groups of CVID patients.

We focused on (1) specific *in vitro* antibody production by individual B cells following vaccinations by T-dependent (protein) and T-independent (polysaccharide) antigens and (2) changes of B-cell subpopulation after vaccination in peripheral blood of CVID patients and healthy donors (Chovancova et al. 2011).

2. Methodological approach

2.1 Flow cytometry and assessment of plasmablasts

Blood samples from examine subjects were collected between 7 and 12 a.m. to exclude diurnal variation of lymphocyte subsets. Lymphocytes and B-cell subpopulations were analyzed directly from peripheral blood or from isolated PBMC (Litzman et al. 2007). The main B cell subpopulations identified in PBMCs were $CD21^{low}$ B cells characterized as $CD21^{low}CD38^{low}$, naïve B cells ($IgD^{+}CD27^{-}$), marginal zone-like B cells ($IgD^{+}CD27^{+}$), switched memory B cells ($IgD^{-}CD27^{+}$) and plasmablasts ($IgD^{-}CD27^{++}CD38^{++}$). Cells were identified using monoclonal antibodies (mAbs): FITC-conjugated anti-CD38, PE-conjugated anti-IgD, PE-conjugated anti-CD21, PC5-conjugated anti-IgM (all from *Pharmingen International, San Diego, CA, USA*) and PC5-conjugated anti-CD27 *(Beckman Coulter Miami, FL, USA)*. The B-cell subpopulations were analyzed by gating on $CD19^{+}$ cells (PC7-conjugated anti-CD19, *Beckman Coulter, Marseille, France*). Immunophenotyping of B lymphocytes was performed by five-colour cytometry Cytomix FC500 (*Beckman Coulter Miami, FL, USA*). The relative numbers of $CD19^{+}$ B cells are showed as mean ± SD.

2.2 Enzyme-linked immunosorbent spot assay (ELISPOT)

The ELISPOT assay provides both qualitative (type of immune protein) and quantitative (number of responding cells) information (Czerkinsky et al. 1983). We have modified the ELISPOT technique for the detection of specific antibody responses to TET and PPS.

96 wells microtitre plates (*MultiScreen™-HA, Millipore Corporation, Billerica, USA)* were coated with tetanus toxoid *(10 Lf/ml, ÚSOL, Prague, Czech Republic*) and PPS (*0.5 µg/ml, PNEUMO 23, Sanofi Pasteur, Lyon, France*) antigens in carbonate buffer (pH = 9.6) overnight at 4 °C. Plates were washed 3 times with PBS containing 0.05% Tween 20 and subsequently incubated for 30 minutes at 37 °C with 100 µl per well of blocking buffer (1% *solution of bovine serum albumin in PBS; Sigma Aldrich, Stenheim, Germany*). Plates were then stored at 4 °C until use. Peripheral blood mononuclear cells (PBMC), obtained from peripheral blood by gradient centrifugation (*Lymphoprep, Axis-Shields PoC AS, Oslo, Norway*) were added to the coated microtitre plates in RPMI 1640 medium (*Sigma Aldrich*) containing 10% heat-inactivated FCS (*LabMediaServis, Jaromer, Czech Republic*) at 4 different dilutions (1.25×10^5; 2.5×10^5; 5×10^5 and 1×10^6 in 100 µl/well for CVID patients and 0.625×10^5; 1.25×10^5; 2.5×10^5; 5×10^5 cells in 100 µl/well for controls and cultured overnight at 37 °C in 5% CO_2. After cells were washed off the plates 100 µl/well rabbit anti-human IgG, IgA or IgM conjugated to horseradish peroxidase (*Dako Cytomation, Glostrup, Denmark;* diluted 1:500 in PBS/Tween) were added to each well and incubated for 1h in the dark at room temperature. Plates were washed 3 times with PBS containing 0.05% Tween 20 followed by the addition of 100 µl/well of 3-amino-9-ethylcarbazole substrate solution (*AEC, Sigma Aldrich*) and incubated for 15 minutes at room temperature in the dark. Plates were rinsed with water and dried overnight at room temperature.

The red-coloured spots were counted with the AID ELISPOT reader (*AID, Autoimmun Diagnostika GmbH, Strassberg, Germany*). This provided accurate recognition and calculation of the spots and allowed objective differentiation between background and "real" spots. The results were expressed as a number of SFC per million B cells.

2.3 Immunization of subjects

Thirty-seven patients with established CVID (14 males, 23 females, age range 20 – 74 years) were examined. Twenty-six patients were treated with regular infusions of intravenous immunoglobulin (IVIG), six patients received regular subcutaneous immunoglobulin (SCIG) injections and one patient intramuscular immunoglobulin therapy (IMIG). Four patients were newly diagnosed and not yet on immunoglobulin replacement therapy at the time of the study.

All CVID patients were vaccinated simultaneously with tetanus toxoid (TET) vaccine (*ALTEANA, Sevapharma, Prague, Czech Republic*) and unconjugated pneumococcal polysaccharide (PPS) antigens (*PNEUMO 23, Sanofi Pasteur, Lyon, France*), except patient no. 34, who received PPS one year after TET. All patients on IVIG were vaccinated one week prior to administration of replacement therapy.

The control group consisted of 80 healthy individuals. Fifty (16 males, 34 females, age range 22 – 72 years) were vaccinated with TET; ten (4 males, 6 females, age range 15 – 46 years) were given PPS alone; twenty (8 males, 12 females, age range 14 – 50 years) received both TET and PPS. The study was approved by the Ethics Committee of Masaryk University, Brno and signed informed consent was obtained from each participant.

2.4 Enzyme-linked immunosorbent assay (ELISA) and immunoglobulin quantification

Commercially available kits were used for measuring specific IgG antibody levels against tetanus toxoid (*VaccZyme™ Human Anti Tetanus Toxoid IgG EIA Kit, The Binding Site Group Ltd, Birmingham, United Kingdom*) and IgG antibodies titers against IgA (*Human Anti-IgA isotype IgG ELISA, BioVendor, Brno, Czech Republic*) in serum.

Trough serum levels of immunoglobulins IgG, IgA and IgM were measured in CVID patients prior to the IVIG infusion by nephelometry using the BN2 Nephelometer *(Dade Behring, Marburg, Germany)* according to the manufacturer's instructions.

2.5 Statistical analysis

Data were analyzed using the STATISTICA software [*StatSoft, Inc. (2007), STATISTICA (data analysis software system), version 8.0.*; www.statsoft.com]. Mann-Whitney U-test and Wilcoxon matched pairs test were used for analyses of dependencies between particular parameters in studied groups; $p < 0.05$ was regarded as statistically significant.

3. Laboratory findings

3.1 Kinetics and optimal timing for detection of specific spot forming cells isolated from peripheral blood after vaccination

The kinetics of anti-TET (T-dependent) specific antibody production by peripheral blood B cells was tested by ELISPOT assay in healthy volunteers from day 5 to day 9 after antigenic challenge. The same strategy was used in the assessment of anti-PPS (T-independent) specific antibody production in healthy controls from day 1 to day 8 after antigen challenge. Day 7 was found to be optimal for the detection of specific antibody producing B-cells in peripheral blood for both antigens and all tested immunoglobulin isotypes (IgG, IgA, and IgM). Our findings are in agreement with previous studies (Kodo et al. 1984; Stevens et al. 1979; Thiele et al. 1982).

3.2 Kinetics and specific antibody responses against protein (T-dependent) and polysaccharide (T-independent) antigens in healthy individuals

The group of healthy controls was vaccinated with protein antigen (tetanus toxoid, TET), unconjugated PPS antigens (PNEUMO 23) either separately or in combination. We found no significant difference in the number of SFC (IgG, IgA, IgM) against vaccinated antigens whether they were administered separately or simultaneously (Mann-Whitney U-test, p with range between 0.56 to 0.98). The number of specific SFC against both types of vaccines in the cohort of healthy controls is shown in Table 1.

	SFC/10^6 B cells		
	MEDIAN	MINIMUM	MAXIMUM
IgG anti-TET	10 371	964	86 747
IgA anti-TET	532	24	9 707
IgM anti-TET	0	0	0
IgG anti-PPS	3 843	812	76 880
IgA anti-PPS	33 935	3 200	186 384
IgM anti-PPS	9 540	2 165	52 994

Table 1. The number of spot forming cells against protein (n=70) and polysaccharide (n= 30) antigens in a group of healthy controls. SFC/10^6 B cells (spot forming cells per million CD19+ B cells); IgG, IgA, IgM anti-TET (IgG, IgA, IgM antibodies specific spot forming cells against tetanus toxoid); IgG, IgA, IgM anti-PPS (IgG, IgA, IgM antibodies specific spot forming cells against pneumococcal polysaccharides)

3.3 Specific antibody response in subgroups of CVID patients

CVID patients (n = 37) were classified according to the Freiburg (Warnatz et al. 2002) and EUROclass classification (Wehr et al. 2008) (Table 2), allowing a comparative analysis of antibody production and clinical phenotype. As we had expected, the majority of our well-defined CVID patients did not mount a specific humoral immune response against the two vaccines but several patients produced low numbers of vaccine-specific SFC (see below).

As for EUROclass classification scheme, 3 patients of group smB+21^{norm} (n = 7, patient no. 18, 19, 20), 1 patient of group smB+21^{low} (n = 6, patient no. 13) and 1 patient of group smB-21^{low} (n = 12, no. 1) had detectable IgG antibody responses against tetanus toxoid. In group smB+21^{low} there was 1 patient (no. 14) who secreted IgM and another patient (no. 12) who formed IgA and IgM antibodies against PPS. The latter patient is the only one among the CVID group who formed specific antibodies of 2 different immunoglobulin isotypes. Regarding the group smB-21^{norm} (n = 12), no specific antibody production was detected. In the Freiburg classification all patients with detectable antibody responses (no. 12, 13, 14, 18, 19 and 20) were from group II the exception (no. 1) being a group Ia patient.

number	Freiburg classification	EURO classification	sex	age	replacement therapy	IgG	IgA	IgM	IgG anti-IgA	IgG anti-TET	IgA anti-TET	IgM anti-TET	IgG anti-PPS	IgA anti-PPS	IgM anti-PPS
						g/l			titer	SFC/10^6 B cells					
1	Ia	smB-21^{low}	F	40	IMIG	2.78	<0.01	< 0.04	neg	344	0	0	0	0	0
2	Ia	smB-21^{low}	F	74	IVIG	5.39	<0.01	< 0.05	neg	0	0	0	0	0	0
3	Ia	smB-21^{low}	M	47	SCIG	3.92	0.06	0.19	neg	0	0	0	0	0	0
4	Ia	smB-21^{low}	M	50	IVIG	3.37	<0.01	< 0.05	neg	0	0	0	0	0	0
5	Ia	smB-21^{low}	M	36	IVIG	7.35	<0.01	0.05	neg	0	0	0	0	0	0
6	Ib	smB-21^{norm}	F	66	IVIG	5.82	<0.01	0.10	n. d.	0	0	0	0	0	0
7	Ib	smB-21^{norm}	F	34	no	2.01	<0.01	< 0.05	neg	0	0	0	0	0	0
8	Ib	smB-21^{norm}	M	30	IVIG	5.77	<0.01	< 0.05	neg	0	0	0	0	0	0
9	Ib	smB-21^{norm}	F	20	no	0.66	<0.01	0.13	1:50	0	0	0	0	0	0
10	Ib	smB-21^{norm}	F	44	IVIG	3.16	<0.01	0.10	neg	0	0	0	0	0	0
11	Ib	smB-21^{norm}	M	55	IVIG	5.09	<0.01	0.32	neg	0	0	0	0	0	0
12	II	smB+21^{low}	F	71	IVIG	6.29	0.08	0.29	neg	0	0	0	0	2562	659
13	II	smB+21^{low}	M	19	IVIG	4.49	<0.01	0.07	neg	407	0	0	0	0	0
14	II	smB+21^{low}	M	24	no	4.99	<0.01	0.20	neg	0	0	0	0	0	104
15	II	smB+21^{low}	F	54	IVIG	6.95	<0.01	0.15	1:100	0	0	0	0	0	0
16	II	smB+21^{low}	F	41	SCIG	6.14	<0.01	0.05	neg	0	0	0	0	0	0
17	II	smB+21^{low}	M	57	SCIG	5.66	0.02	< 0.05	neg	0	0	0	0	0	0
18	II	smB+21^{norm}	F	19	SCIG	6.75	0.05	0.75	neg	185	0	0	0	0	0
19	II	smB+21^{norm}	M	44	IVIG	5.91	0.22	< 0.05	neg	713	0	0	0	0	0
20	II	smB+21^{norm}	M	44	IVIG	6.37	<0.01	0.10	neg	231	0	0	0	0	0
21	II	smB+21^{norm}	M	31	IVIG	3.80	0.02	0.07	n. d.	0	0	0	0	0	0
22	II	smB+21^{norm}	F	68	IVIG	6.35	<0.01	< 0.05	neg	0	0	0	0	0	0
23	II	smB+21^{norm}	M	59	IVIG	6.86	0.04	0.06	neg	0	0	0	0	0	0
24	II	smB+21^{norm}	F	41	IVIG	5.26	<0.01	0.08	neg	0	0	0	0	0	0

Table 2. Continues on next page

number	Freiburg classification	EURO classification	sex	age	replacement therapy	IgG	IgA	IgM	IgG anti-IgA	IgG anti-TET	IgA anti-TET	IgM anti-TET	IgG anti-PPS	IgA anti-PPS	IgM anti-PPS
						g/l			titer	SFC/10^6 B cells					
25	II	smB-21^{low}	F	42	IVIG	8.15	<0.01	0.50	neg	0	0	0	0	0	0
26	II	smB-21^{low}	F	58	IVIG	5.98	<0.01	< 0.05	neg	0	0	0	0	0	0
27	II	smB-21^{low}	F	57	IVIG	8.15	<0.01	< 0.05	neg	0	0	0	0	0	0
28	II	smB-21^{low}	M	34	IVIG	6.21	<0.01	0.05	neg	0	0	0	0	0	0
29	II	smB-21^{low}	F	43	IVIG	6.27	<0.01	< 0.05	neg	0	0	0	0	0	0
30	II	smB-21^{low}	F	50	SCIG	4.48	<0.01	< 0.05	neg	0	0	0	0	0	0
31	II	smB-21^{low}	F	28	IVIG	5.62	<0.01	< 0.05	neg	0	0	0	0	0	0
32	II	smB-21^{norm}	F	44	IVIG	6.75	<0.01	0.05	neg	0	0	0	0	0	0
33	II	smB-21^{norm}	F	61	IVIG	7.54	0.09	< 0.05	neg	0	0	0	0	0	0
34	II	smB-21^{norm}	F	27	no	2.35	<0.01	0.45	neg	0	0	0	0	0	0
35	II	smB-21^{norm}	F	40	IVIG	7.10	<0.01	0.09	neg	0	0	0	0	0	0
36	II	smB-21^{norm}	F	40	SCIG	8.51	<0.01	< 0.05	neg	0	0	0	0	0	0
37	II	smB-21^{norm}	M	19	IVIG	7.00	<0.01	< 0.05	neg	0	0	0	0	0	0

Table 2. (continued) Results of the ELISPOT assay in group of CVID patients. F (female); M (male); n.d. (not done); SFC/10^6 B cells (spot forming cells per million $CD19^+$ B cells); IgG, IgA, IgM anti-TET (IgG, IgA, IgM specific spot forming cells against tetanus toxoid); IgG, IgA, IgM anti-PPS (IgG, IgA, IgM specific spot forming cells against pneumococcal polysaccharides); IgG anti-IgA (IgG antibodies against IgA)

The decreased production of SFC in CVID patients was independent of replacement immunoglobulin treatment: four CVID patients without substitution therapy showed the same defect in the production of SFC and specific antibodies after vaccination as CVID patients on replacement therapy.

3.4 Changes of B-cell subpopulations in peripheral blood one week after vaccination

The mean percentage of $CD19^+$ B cells was 11 ± 4 % in healthy controls and 13 ± 7.6 % in CVID patients before vaccination. One week after vaccination the percentages were unchanged (12 ± 5 % in healthy controls and 13 ± 6.7 % in CVID patients).

We then examined the changes of absolute and relative numbers of plasmablasts and other B lymphocyte subpopulations in the peripheral blood one week after antigen challenge (Fig. 1, 2). In healthy controls no statistically significant changes in absolute and relative numbers of switched memory B cells were found between the two measurement time points, before

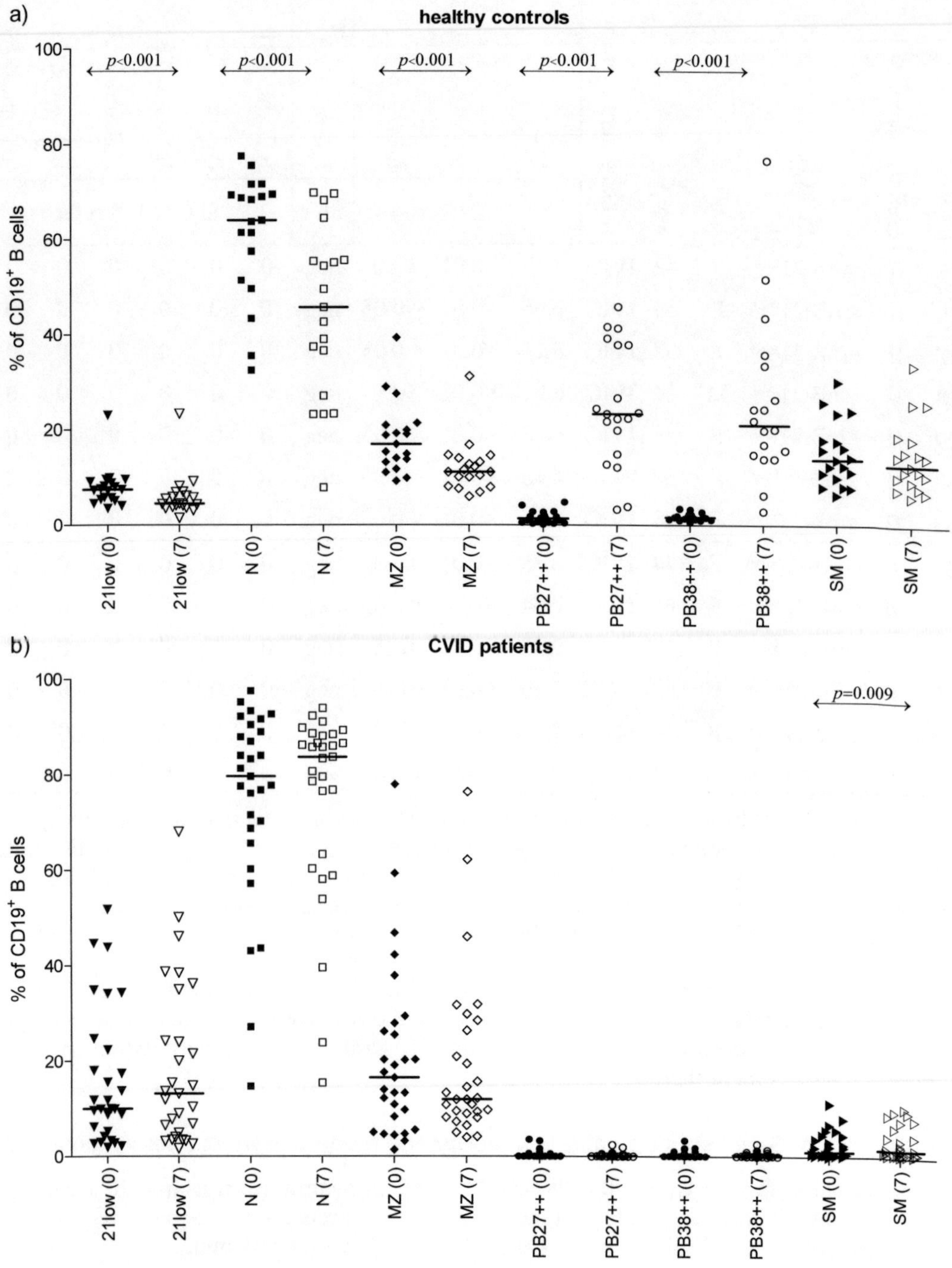

Fig. 1. Changes of relative numbers of B-cell subpopulations in healthy controls (HC; n = 19; a) and CVID patients (CVID; n = 29; b) before (0) and one week (7) after antigen challenge. 21^{low} ($CD21^{low}$ B cells), N (naïve B cells), MZ (marginal zone - like B cells), $PB27^{++}$ and $PB38^{++}$ (plasmablasts), SM (class-switched memory B cells)

and one week after vaccination. However, a highly significant increase in absolute as well as relative numbers of plasmablasts gated as IgD-CD27++ (PB CD27++) cells and IgM-CD38++ (PB CD38++) cells ($p<0.001$ in both cases) occurred (Fig. 3), while the absolute and relative numbers of CD21low B cells ($p<0.02$), naïve B cells ($p<0.001$) and MZ-like B cells ($p<0.001$) decreased. In contrast, among the cohort of CVID patients no statistically significant changes of examined cellular subpopulations, including plasmablasts (Fig. 1, 2 and 3) were observed except for a slight increase in smB cells to a level still well below the levels of healthy controls. This increase was statistically significant in Wilcoxon matched pairs test.

The fact that the number of plasmablasts corresponds with the number of SFC strongly suggest that the examination of peripheral blood plasmablasts on day 7 after vaccination can be used as a surrogate marker for specific antibody responses in normal controls and as a diagnostic procedure to identified CVID and other patients with defect in terminal B-cell differentiation (Chovancova et al. 2011).

4. Consequences

4.1 Hypogammaglobulinaemic patients and diagnostic vaccination

Poor vaccination responses to protein and polysaccharide antigens is essential for definition-based diagnosis of CVID (Conley et al. 1999). Quantitative assessment of specific antibody in serum is routinely performed by ELISA assay. However CVID patients are often started on immunoglobulin substitution therapy before antibody production is adequately evaluated. In such a situation, it is difficult to segregate transferred from antigen-induced specific antibody. We have designed a *in vitro* functional measurement of antibody production on the B-cell level using the ELISPOT technique, which is independent of substitution therapy (Chovancova et al. 2011). In addition, we monitored changes in B-cell subpopulations, including plasmablasts, in peripheral blood by flow cytometry after in vivo antigenic challenge.

The defect in the antibody production and SFC reduction observed in a cohort of CVID patients are not secondary to Ig substitution since the same defects were also seen in four CVID patients before starting Ig replacement therapy. IVIG treated CVID patients were vaccinated exactly one week before administration of immunoglobulin substitution. In this manner the theoretically possible influence of immunoglobulin replacement therapy on the generation of SFC was reduced.

Prior to this study, specific antibody production in substituted CVID patients following vaccination had been evaluated in serum. Goldacker et al. (Goldacker et al. 2007) measured specific antibodies in serum by ELISA assay. The contribution of parallel immunoglobulin substitution on antibody titers was difficult to correct and required a relatively complicated vaccination formula. Based on these calculations the authors reported a decrease in serum antibody levels against T-dependent and T-independent antigens in CVID patients between IVIG infusions. Using a meningococcal polysaccharide vaccine, Rezaei et al. described decreased vaccination response against meningococcal polysaccharide measured in serum of CVID patients while on IVIG (Rezaei et al. 2008; Rezaei et al. 2010). Immunization with a protein neoantigen, e.g. bacteriophage, and investigation of immune response with neutralization assay brought similar results (Ochs et al. 1971). Nevertheless, there is very little quantitative data correlating individual vaccination responses to proposed functional

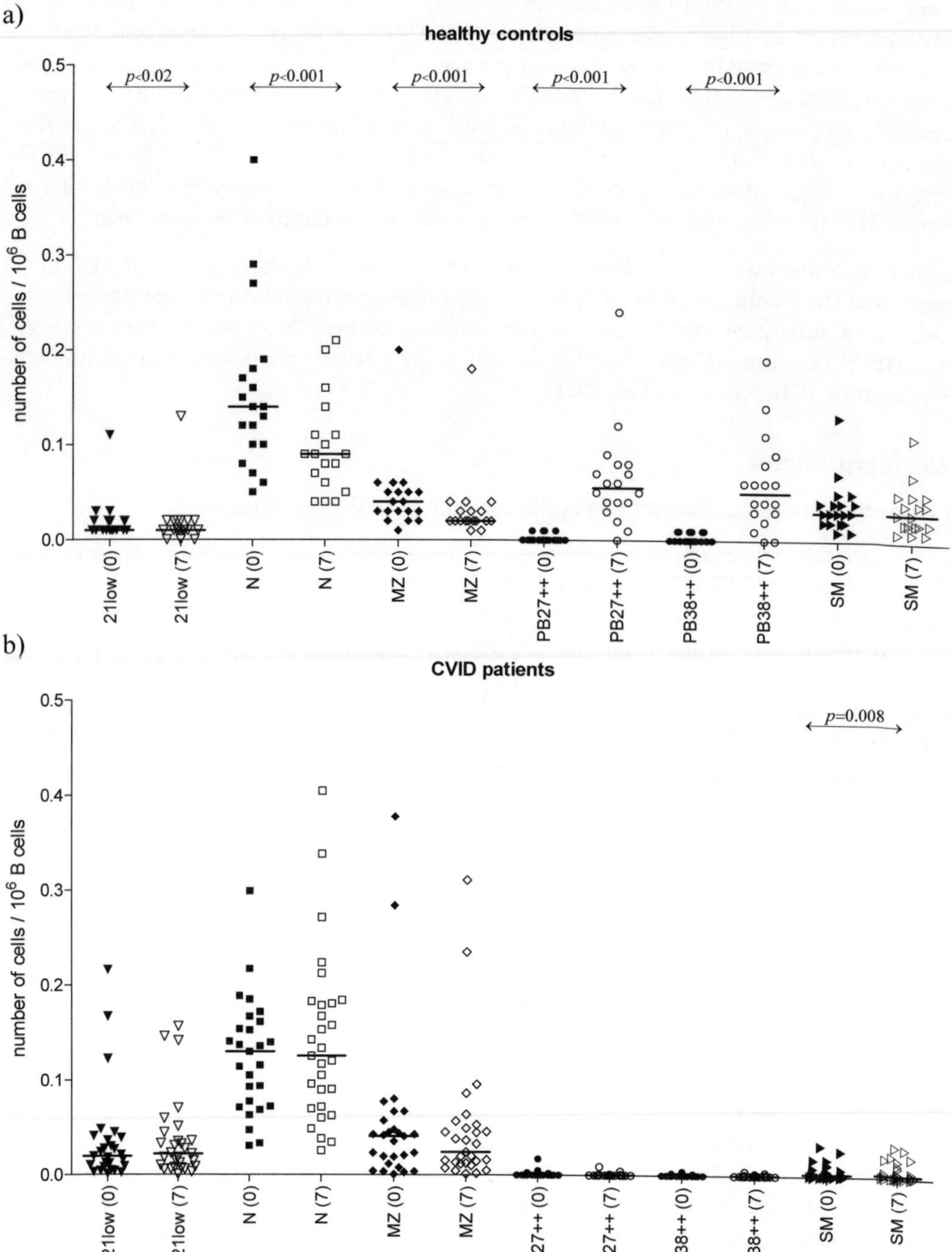

Fig. 2. Changes of absolute numbers of B-cell subpopulations in healthy controls (HC; n = 19; a) and CVID patients (CVID; n = 29; b) before (0) and one week (7) after antigen challenge. 21^{low} ($CD21^{low}$ B cells), N (naïve B cells), MZ (marginal zone - like B cells), $PB27^{++}$ and $PB38^{++}$ (plasmablasts), SM (class-switched memory B cells)

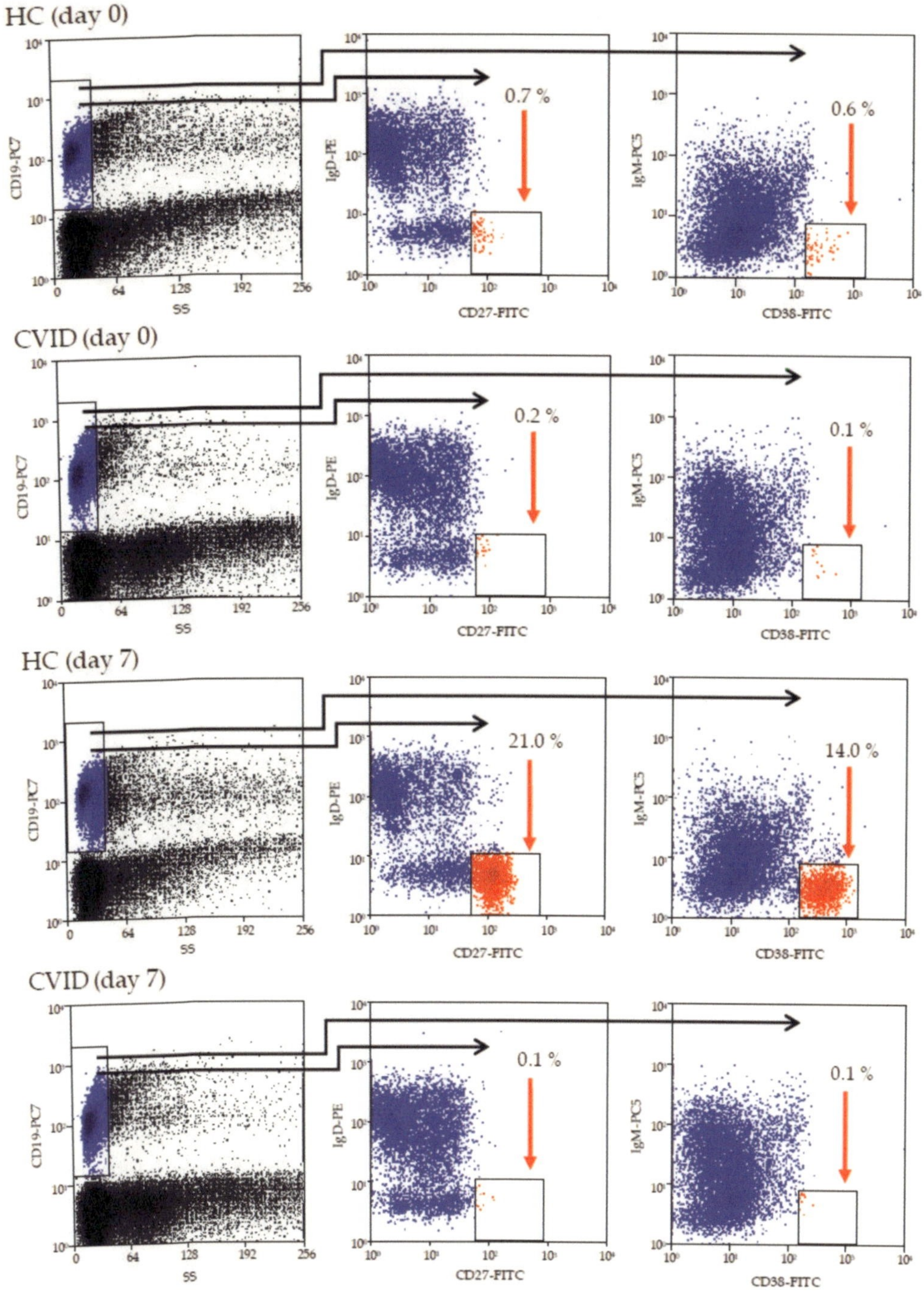

Fig. 3. Development of plasmablasts after vaccination. Plasmablasts (red arrows) were gated from CD19+ B cells (gate in column 1) as IgD-CD27++ (column 2) and IgM-CD38++ (column 3). The cells were investigated before (day 0) and on day 7 after vaccination. HC - healthy control; CVID - CVID patient, PB27++ and PB38++ - plasmablasts

classifications of CVID (Goldacker et al. 2007; Rezaei et al. 2008). Our group of CVID patients was arranged according to the Freiburg (Warnatz et al. 2002) and EUROclass classification (Wehr et al. 2008). As expected, the majority of our well-defined CVID patients (30/37) failed to mount a specific humoral immune response when analysed by SFCs collected from peripheral blood before and after immunization. The seven CVID patients who responded had much smaller quantities of specific SFC compared to healthy donors. All but one patient with measurable antibody responses belong to group II of the Freiburg classification or EUROclass group smB$^+$ which represent those CVID patients with nearly normal numbers of class-switched memory B cells. Patients in these groups are characterized by milder complications of the disease compared to other groups (Alachkar et al. 2006; Wehr et al. 2008).

4.2 Novel diagnostic tool using flow cytometry in hypogammaglobulinaemic patients with vaccination

During the last few years a number of studies described differences between B-cell subpopulations of CVID patients and those of healthy volunteers but the kinetics of these changes after encounter with an antigen in vivo (Pinna et al. 2009) has not previously been explored. We investigated the dynamic changes of CD21^{low} B cells, naïve B cells, marginal zone-like B cells, plasmablasts and switched memory B cells of CVID patients compared to healthy donors (Chovancova et al. 2011). Previous studies showed that memory B cells and plasmablasts have different kinetics in peripheral blood (Stevens et al. 1979). Plasmablasts reach their peak on day 7 after encounter with the antigen in peripheral blood while switched memory B cells showed a marked increase in number on day 14 after antigen challenge (Pinna et al. 2009). The absolute number of naïve B lymphocytes is determined by the generation of new naïve B cells from the bone marrow pool (a slow process) and by acute loss of naïve B lymphocytes via further maturation after antigen encounter (Agenes et al. 2000). Statistically significant up-regulation of naïve B cells and its continued accumulation after antigen challenge in CVID patients indicates disturbed conversion of undifferentiated B cells to more mature B-cell stages in germinal centers. Differentiation is crucially dependent on T-lymphocyte help, suggesting that the basic defects in the majority of CVID patients are not in B cells but in helper T-lymphocytes (Borte et al. 2009; Fischer et al. 1994; Fischer et al. 1996; Thon et al. 1997).

The reduced numbers of switched memory B cells which correlate with clinical complications (Ko et al. 2005; Viallard et al. 2006) and failure to increase the number of plasmablasts after antigen challenge may be explained by insufficient signals from helper T cells of CVID patients. In previous studies we and others have shown that B cells of CVID patients are able to produce antibodies if they are exposed *in vitro* to helper T-lymphocyte from healthy donors or to appropriate cytokines (Borte et al. 2009; Fischer et al. 1994; Fischer et al. 1996; Thon et al. 1997), [55]. Taubenheim et al. studied B-cell differentiation in lymph nodes from three CVID patients with splenomegaly and found distinct blocks in terminal plasma cell development but normal expression of a key regulator of terminal plasma cell differentiation, Blimp-1 (Taubenheim et al. 2005). Moreover, the clinically important observation that B cells from CVID patients may produce antibodies under certain circumstances correlates with the fact that CVID patients lacking IgA are able to generate IgG anti-IgA antibodies in vivo (Horn et al. 2007). Among our cohort of vaccinated CVID patients, two patients from subgroups Ib and II (Table 2) produced IgG anti-IgA antibodies in low titers although these two patients did not respond to vaccination.

Our observation that the majority of CVID patients lack antigen specific spot forming B cells and fail to increase circulating plasmablasts following *in vivo* antigen challenge provides a rapid screening test to demonstrate defective antibody responses in CVID patients, even when on replacement IVIG therapy (Chovancova et al. 2011).

5. Conclusion and clinical implications

Identification of circulating plasmablasts after vaccination is a new simple flow based test to assess antibody responses in hypogammaglobulinaemic patients, even if on immunoglobulin (IVIG or SCIG) replacement therapy.

6. Acknowledgement

We thank Prof. Dr. Hans D. Ochs for critical discussions. The research leading to these results has received funding from the Ministry of Health of the Czech Republic, Grant no. NR9035-4 and from the European Community's Seventh Framework Programme FP7/2007-2013 under grant agreement no. 201549 (EURO-PADnet HEALTH-F2-2008-201549).

7. References

Agenes, F., Rosado, M. M. & Freitas, A. A. (2000). Peripheral B cell survival. *Cell Mol Life Sci* Vol. 57, No. 8-9, (August 2000), pp. 1220-1228.

Alachkar, H., Taubenheim, N., Haeney, M. R., Durandy, A. & Arkwright, P. D. (2006). Memory switched B cell percentage and not serum immunoglobulin concentration is associated with clinical complications in children and adults with specific antibody deficiency and common variable immunodeficiency. *Clin Immunol* Vol. 120, No. 3, (September 2006), pp. 310-318.

Borte, S., Pan-Hammarstrom, Q., Liu, C., Sack, U., Borte, M., Wagner, U., Graf, D. & Hammarstrom, L. (2009). Interleukin-21 restores immunoglobulin production ex vivo in patients with common variable immunodeficiency and selective IgA deficiency. *Blood* Vol. 114, No. 19, (November 5 2009), pp. 4089-4098.

Bryant, A., Calver, N. C., Toubi, E., Webster, A. D. & Farrant, J. (1990). Classification of patients with common variable immunodeficiency by B cell secretion of IgM and IgG in response to anti-IgM and interleukin-2. *Clin Immunol Immunopathol* Vol. 56, No. 2, (August 1990), pp. 239-248.

Carsetti, R., Rosado, M. M. & Wardmann, H. (2004). Peripheral development of B cells in mouse and man. *Immunol Rev* Vol. 197, (February 2004), pp. 179-191.

Castigli, E., Wilson, S. A., Garibyan, L., Rachid, R., Bonilla, F., Schneider, L. & Geha, R. S. (2005). TACI is mutant in common variable immunodeficiency and IgA deficiency. *Nat Genet* Vol. 37, No. 8, (August 2005), pp. 829-834.

Chapel, H., Lucas, M., Lee, M., Bjorkander, J., Webster, D., Grimbacher, B., Fieschi, C., Thon, V., Abedi, M. R. & Hammarstrom, L. (2008). Common variable immunodeficiency disorders: division into distinct clinical phenotypes. *Blood* Vol. 112, No. 2, (July 2008), pp. 277-286.

Chovancova, Z., Vlkova, M., Litzman, J., Lokaj, J. & Thon, V. (2011). Antibody forming cells and plasmablasts in peripheral blood in CVID patients after vaccination. *Vaccine* Vol. 29, No. 24, (May 2011), pp. 4142-4150.

Conley, M. E., Notarangelo, L. D. & Etzioni, A. (1999). Diagnostic criteria for primary immunodeficiencies. Representing PAGID (Pan-American Group for Immunodeficiency) and ESID (European Society for Immunodeficiencies). *Clin Immunol* Vol. 93, No. 3, (December 1999), pp. 190-197.

Cunningham-Rundles, C. & Bodian, C. (1999). Common variable immunodeficiency: clinical and immunological features of 248 patients. *Clin Immunol* Vol. 92, No. 1, (July 1999), pp. 34-48.

Czerkinsky, C. C., Nilsson, L. A., Nygren, H., Ouchterlony, O. & Tarkowski, A. (1983). A solid-phase enzyme-linked immunospot (ELISPOT) assay for enumeration of specific antibody-secreting cells. *J Immunol Methods* Vol. 65, No. 1-2, (December 16 1983), pp. 109-121.

Farrington, M., Grosmaire, L. S., Nonoyama, S., Fischer, S. H., Hollenbaugh, D., Ledbetter, J. A., Noelle, R. J., Aruffo, A. & Ochs, H. D. (1994). CD40 ligand expression is defective in a subset of patients with common variable immunodeficiency. *Proc Natl Acad Sci U S A* Vol. 91, No. 3, (February 1994), pp. 1099-1103.

Ferry, B. L., Jones, J., Bateman, E. A., Woodham, N., Warnatz, K., Schlesier, M., Misbah, S. A., Peter, H. H. & Chapel, H. M. (2005). Measurement of peripheral B cell subpopulations in common variable immunodeficiency (CVID) using a whole blood method. *Clin Exp Immunol* Vol. 140, No. 3, (June 2005),pp. 532-539.

Fischer, M. B., Hauber, I., Eggenbauer, H., Thon, V., Vogel, E., Schaffer, E., Lokaj, J., Litzman, J., Wolf, H. M., Mannhalter, J. W. & et al. (1994). A defect in the early phase of T-cell receptor-mediated T-cell activation in patients with common variable immunodeficiency. *Blood* Vol. 84, No. 12, (December 15 1994), pp. 4234-4241.

Fischer, M. B., Hauber, I., Wolf, H. M., Vogel, E., Mannhalter, J. W. & Eibl, M. M. (1994). Impaired TCR signal transduction, but normal antigen presentation, in a patient with common variable immunodeficiency. *Br J Haematol* Vol. 88, No. 3, (November 1994), pp. 520-526.

Fischer, M. B., Wolf, H. M., Hauber, I., Eggenbauer, H., Thon, V., Sasgary, M. & Eibl, M. M. (1996). Activation via the antigen receptor is impaired in T cells, but not in B cells from patients with common variable immunodeficiency. *Eur J Immunol* Vol. 26, No. 1, (January 1996), pp. 231-237.

Funauchi, M., Farrant, J., Moreno, C. & Webster, A. D. (1995). Defects in antigen-driven lymphocyte responses in common variable immunodeficiency (CVID) are due to a reduction in the number of antigen-specific CD4+ T cells. *Clin Exp Immunol* Vol. 101, No. 1, (July 1995), pp. 82-88.

Giovannetti, A., Pierdominici, M., Mazzetta, F., Marziali, M., Renzi, C., Mileo, A. M., De Felice, M., Mora, B., Esposito, A., Carello, R., Pizzuti, A., Paggi, M. G., Paganelli, R., Malorni, W. & Aiuti, F. (2007). Unravelling the complexity of T cell abnormalities in common variable immunodeficiency. *J Immunol* Vol. 178, No. 6, (March 15 2007), pp. 3932-3943.

Goldacker, S., Draeger, R., Warnatz, K., Huzly, D., Salzer, U., Thiel, J., Eibel, H., Schlesier, M. & Peter, H. H. (2007). Active vaccination in patients with common variable immunodeficiency (CVID). *Clin Immunol* Vol. 124, No. 3, (September 2007), pp. 294-303.

Grimbacher, B., Hutloff, A., Schlesier, M., Glocker, E., Warnatz, K., Drager, R., Eibel, H., Fischer, B., Schaffer, A. A., Mages, H. W., Kroczek, R. A. & Peter, H. H. (2003). Homozygous loss of ICOS is associated with adult-onset common variable immunodeficiency. *Nat Immunol* Vol. 4, No. 3, (March 2003), pp. 261-268.

Horn, J., Manguiat, A., Berglund, L. J., Knerr, V., Tahami, F., Grimbacher, B. & Fulcher, D. A. (2009). Decrease in phenotypic regulatory T cells in subsets of patients with common variable immunodeficiency. *Clin Exp Immunol* Vol. 156, No. 3, (June 2009), pp. 446-454.

Horn, J., Thon, V., Bartonkova, D., Salzer, U., Warnatz, K., Schlesier, M., Peter, H. H. & Grimbacher, B. (2007). Anti-IgA antibodies in common variable immunodeficiency (CVID): diagnostic workup and therapeutic strategy. *Clin Immunol* Vol. 122, No. 2, (February 2007), pp. 156-162.

Klein, U., Kuppers, R. & Rajewsky, K. (1997). Evidence for a large compartment of IgM-expressing memory B cells in humans. *Blood* Vol. 89, No. 4, (February 1997), pp. 1288-1298.

Ko, J., Radigan, L. & Cunningham-Rundles, C. (2005). Immune competence and switched memory B cells in common variable immunodeficiency. *Clin Immunol* Vol. 116, No. 1, (July 2005), pp. 37-41.

Kodo, H., Gale, R. P. & Saxon, A. (1984). Antibody synthesis by bone marrow cells in vitro following primary and booster tetanus toxoid immunization in humans. *J Clin Invest* Vol. 73, No. 5, (May 1984), pp. 1377-1384.

Litzman, J., Vlkova, M., Pikulova, Z., Stikarovska, D. & Lokaj, J. (2007). T and B lymphocyte subpopulations and activation/differentiation markers in patients with selective IgA deficiency. *Clin Exp Immunol* Vol. 147, No. 2, (February 2007), pp. 249-254.

Mohammadi, J., Liu, C., Aghamohammadi, A., Bergbreiter, A., Du, L., Lu, J., Rezaei, N., Amirzargar, A. A., Moin, M., Salzer, U., Pan-Hammarstrom, Q. & Hammarstrom, L. (2009). Novel mutations in TACI (TNFRSF13B) causing common variable immunodeficiency. *J Clin Immunol* Vol. 29, No. 6, (November 2009), pp. 777-785.

Mouillot, G., Carmagnat, M., Gerard, L., Garnier, J. L., Fieschi, C., Vince, N., Karlin, L., Viallard, J. F., Jaussaud, R., Boileau, J., Donadieu, J., Gardembas, M., Schleinitz, N., Suarez, F., Hachulla, E., Delavigne, K., Morisset, M., Jacquot, S., Just, N., Galicier, L., Charron, D., Debre, P., Oksenhendler, E. & Rabian, C. B-Cell and T-Cell Phenotypes in CVID Patients Correlate with the Clinical Phenotype of the Disease. *J Clin Immunol* Vol. 30, No. 5, (May 2010), pp. 746-755.

Ochs, H. D., Davis, S. D. & Wedgwood, R. J. (1971). Immunologic responses to bacteriophage phi-X 174 in immunodeficiency diseases. *J Clin Invest* Vol. 50, No. 12, (Dec 1971) pp. 2559-2568.

Pinna, D., Corti, D., Jarrossay, D., Sallusto, F. & Lanzavecchia, A. (2009). Clonal dissection of the human memory B-cell repertoire following infection and vaccination. *Eur J Immunol* Vol. 39, No. 5, (May 2009), pp. 1260-1270.

Piqueras, B., Lavenu-Bombled, C., Galicier, L., Bergeron-van der Cruyssen, F., Mouthon, L., Chevret, S., Debre, P., Schmitt, C. & Oksenhendler, E. (2003). Common variable immunodeficiency patient classification based on impaired B cell memory differentiation correlates with clinical aspects. *J Clin Immunol* Vol. 23, No. 5, (September 2003), pp. 385-400.

Rakhmanov, M., Keller, B., Gutenberger, S., Foerster, C., Hoenig, M., Driessen, G., van der Burg, M., van Dongen, J. J., Wiech, E., Visentini, M., Quinti, I., Prasse, A., Voelxen, N., Salzer, U., Goldacker, S., Fisch, P., Eibel, H., Schwarz, K., Peter, H. H. & Warnatz, K. (2009). Circulating CD21low B cells in common variable immunodeficiency resemble tissue homing, innate-like B cells. *Proc Natl Acad Sci U S A* Vol. 106, No. 32, (August 2009), pp. 13451-13456.

Rezaei, N., Aghamohammadi, A. & Read, R. C. (2008). Response to polysaccharide vaccination amongst pediatric patients with common variable immunodeficiency correlates with clinical disease. *Iran J Allergy Asthma Immunol* Vol. 7, No. 4, (December 2008), pp. 231-234.

Rezaei, N., Aghamohammadi, A., Siadat, S. D., Moin, M., Pourpak, Z., Nejati, M., Ahmadi, H., Kamali, S., Norouzian, D., Tabaraei, B. & Read, R. C. (2008). Serum bactericidal antibody responses to meningococcal polysaccharide vaccination as a basis for clinical classification of common variable immunodeficiency. *Clin Vaccine Immunol* Vol. 15, No. 4, (April 2008), pp. 607-611.

Rezaei, N., Siadat, S. D., Aghamohammadi, A., Moin, M., Pourpak, Z., Norouzian, D., Mobarakeh, J. I., Aghasadeghi, M. R., Nejati, M. & Read, R. C. Serum bactericidal antibody response 1 year after meningococcal polysaccharide vaccination of patients with common variable immunodeficiency. *Clin Vaccine Immunol* Vol. 17, No. 4, (April 2010), pp. 524-528.

Salzer, U., Chapel, H. M., Webster, A. D., Pan-Hammarstrom, Q., Schmitt-Graeff, A., Schlesier, M., Peter, H. H., Rockstroh, J. K., Schneider, P., Schaffer, A. A., Hammarstrom, L. & Grimbacher, B. (2005). Mutations in TNFRSF13B encoding TACI are associated with common variable immunodeficiency in humans. *Nat Genet* Vol. 37, No. 8, (August 2005), pp. 820-828.

Salzer, U., Maul-Pavicic, A., Cunningham-Rundles, C., Urschel, S., Belohradsky, B. H., Litzman, J., Holm, A., Franco, J. L., Plebani, A., Hammarstrom, L., Skrabl, A., Schwinger, W. & Grimbacher, B. (2004). ICOS deficiency in patients with common variable immunodeficiency. *Clin Immunol* Vol. 113, No. 3, (December 2004), pp. 234-240.

Sanchez-Ramon, S., Radigan, L., Yu, J. E., Bard, S. & Cunningham-Rundles, C. (2008). Memory B cells in common variable immunodeficiency: clinical associations and sex differences. *Clin Immunol* Vol. 128, No. 3, (September 2008), pp. 314-321.

Sekine, H., Ferreira, R. C., Pan-Hammarstrom, Q., Graham, R. R., Ziemba, B., de Vries, S. S., Liu, J., Hippen, K., Koeuth, T., Ortmann, W., Iwahori, A., Elliott, M. K., Offer, S., Skon, C., Du, L., Novitzke, J., Lee, A. T., Zhao, N., Tompkins, J. D., Altshuler, D., Gregersen, P. K., Cunningham-Rundles, C., Harris, R. S., Her, C., Nelson, D. L., Hammarstrom, L., Gilkeson, G. S. & Behrens, T. W. (2007). Role for Msh5 in the regulation of Ig class switch recombination. *Proc Natl Acad Sci U S A* Vol. 104, No. 17, (April 2007), pp. 7193-7198.

Shi, Y., Agematsu, K., Ochs, H. D. & Sugane, K. (2003). Functional analysis of human memory B-cell subpopulations: IgD+CD27+ B cells are crucial in secondary immune response by producing high affinity IgM. *Clin Immunol* Vol. 108, No. 2, (August 2003), pp. 128-137.

Schaffer, A. A., Salzer, U., Hammarstrom, L. & Grimbacher, B. (2007). Deconstructing common variable immunodeficiency by genetic analysis. *Curr Opin Genet Dev* Vol. 17, No. 3, (June 2007), pp. 201-212.

Stevens, R. H., Macy, E., Morrow, C. & Saxon, A. (1979). Characterization of a circulating subpopulation of spontaneous antitetanus toxoid antibody producing B cells following in vivo booster immunization. *J Immunol* Vol. 122, No. 6, (June 1979), pp. 2498-2504.

Tangye, S. G. & Tarlinton, D. M. (2009). Memory B cells: effectors of long-lived immune responses. *Eur J Immunol* Vol. 39, No. 8, (Aug 2009) pp. 2065-2075.

Taubenheim, N., von Hornung, M., Durandy, A., Warnatz, K., Corcoran, L., Peter, H. H. & Eibel, H. (2005). Defined blocks in terminal plasma cell differentiation of common variable immunodeficiency patients. *J Immunol* Vol. 175, No. 8, (October 2005), pp. 5498-5503.

Thiele, C. J., Morrow, C. D. & Stevens, R. H. (1982). Human IgA antibody and immunoglobulin production after in vivo tetanus toxoid immunization: size and surface membrane phenotype analysis. *J Clin Immunol* Vol. 2, No. 4, (October 1982), pp. 327-334.

Thon, V., Wolf, H. M., Sasgary, M., Litzman, J., Samstag, A., Hauber, I., Lokaj, J. & Eibl, M. M. (1997). Defective integration of activating signals derived from the T cell receptor (TCR) and costimulatory molecules in both CD4+ and CD8+ T lymphocytes of common variable immunodeficiency (CVID) patients. *Clin Exp Immunol* Vol. 110, No. 2, (November 1997), pp. 174-181.

van Zelm, M. C., Reisli, I., van der Burg, M., Castano, D., van Noesel, C. J., van Tol, M. J., Woellner, C., Grimbacher, B., Patino, P. J., van Dongen, J. J. & Franco, J. L. (2006). An antibody-deficiency syndrome due to mutations in the CD19 gene. *N Engl J Med* Vol. 354, No. 18, (May 2006), pp. 1901-1912.

van Zelm, M. C., Smet, J., Adams, B., Mascart, F., Schandene, L., Janssen, F., Ferster, A., Kuo, C. C., Levy, S., van Dongen, J. J. & van der Burg, M. (2010). CD81 gene defect in humans disrupts CD19 complex formation and leads to antibody deficiency. *J Clin Invest* Vol. 2010, No. 120(4), (April 2010), pp. 1265-1274.

Viallard, J. F., Blanco, P., Andre, M., Etienne, G., Liferman, F., Neau, D., Vidal, E., Moreau, J. F. & Pellegrin, J. L. (2006). CD8+HLA-DR+ T lymphocytes are increased in common variable immunodeficiency patients with impaired memory B-cell differentiation. *Clin Immunol* Vol. 119, No. 1, (April 2006), pp. 51-58.

Warnatz, K., Denz, A., Drager, R., Braun, M., Groth, C., Wolff-Vorbeck, G., Eibel, H., Schlesier, M. & Peter, H. H. (2002). Severe deficiency of switched memory B cells (CD27(+)IgM(-)IgD(-)) in subgroups of patients with common variable immunodeficiency: a new approach to classify a heterogeneous disease. *Blood* Vol. 99, No. 5, (March 2002), pp. 1544-1551.

Warnatz, K. & Schlesier, M. (2008). Flowcytometric phenotyping of common variable immunodeficiency. *Cytometry B Clin Cytom* Vol. 74, No. 5, (September 2008), pp. 261-271.

Wehr, C., Kivioja, T., Schmitt, C., Ferry, B., Witte, T., Eren, E., Vlkova, M., Hernandez, M., Detkova, D., Bos, P. R., Poerksen, G., von Bernuth, H., Baumann, U., Goldacker, S., Gutenberger, S., Schlesier, M., Bergeron-van der Cruyssen, F., Le Garff, M., Debre, P., Jacobs, R., Jones, J., Bateman, E., Litzman, J., van Hagen, P. M., Plebani, A.,

Schmidt, R. E., Thon, V., Quinti, I., Espanol, T., Webster, A. D., Chapel, H., Vihinen, M., Oksenhendler, E., Peter, H. H. & Warnatz, K. (2008). The EUROclass trial: defining subgroups in common variable immunodeficiency. *Blood* Vol. 111, No. 1, (January 2008), pp. 77-85.

Weller, S., Braun, M. C., Tan, B. K., Rosenwald, A., Cordier, C., Conley, M. E., Plebani, A., Kumararatne, D. S., Bonnet, D., Tournilhac, O., Tchernia, G., Steiniger, B., Staudt, L. M., Casanova, J. L., Reynaud, C. A. & Weill, J. C. (2004). Human blood IgM "memory" B cells are circulating splenic marginal zone B cells harboring a prediversified immunoglobulin repertoire. *Blood* Vol. 104, No. 12, (December 2004), pp. 3647-3654.

8

Applications of Flow Cytometry in Solid Organ Allogeneic Transplantation

Dimitrios Kirmizis[1], Dimitrios Chatzidimitriou[2],
Fani Chatzopoulou[2], Lemonia Skoura[2] and Grigorios Miserlis[3]
[1]*Aristotle University, Thessaloniki,*
[2]*Laboratory of Microbiology, Aristotle University, Thessaloniki,*
[3]*Organ Transplant Unit, Hippokration General Hospital, Thessaloniki,*
Greece

1. Introduction

The implementation of flow cytometry assays in evaluation of transplant recipients began in 1983 when Garavoy et. al. applied this technology to study the in vitro production of HLA antibodies and observed that flow cytometric technology identified serum HLA antibody levels so low that the complement dependent cytotoxicity assays could not detect them. Since even low levels of antibodies have been associated with early rejection episodes and graft loss, antibody detection by flow cytometry has become a routine technique for the study of donor and recipient compatibility, especially for renal allograft candidates and patients submitted to desensitizing pre-emptive therapies. Nowadays, flow cytometric based assays have become some of the most valuable tools to monitor allograft recipients both pre and post transplantation, with the detection and characterization of HLA-specific alloantibody being the principal application in organ transplantation.

2. Flow cytometry crossmatch

Flow cytometry crossmatch (FCXM), in contrast to standard complement-dependent cytotoxicity (CDC), measures alloantibody levels by quantifying the fluorescence intensity staining of anti-immunoglobulin (anti-Ig) reagents following the incubation of donor lymphocytes with patient serum, which is a more demanding and less well-defined application. The FCXM is typically performed by first incubating donor lymphocytes from peripheral blood, lymph node, or spleen with the recipient's serum, followed by a second incubation with a fluorescein-conjugated, anti-human- IgG (or anti-human-IgM) antibody. Phycoerythrin conjugated anti-CD3 antibody is also added to measure the anti-Ig-fluorescence on both T and non-T cells. Staining intensity produced by the patient's serum compared against that of a normal control serum provides the FCXM score. More recently, pretreatment of target cells with the proteolytic enzyme Pronase, a method which eliminates nonspecific binding of IgG to Fc receptors on B-cells, has been reported to further increase the sensitivity of the assay (Vaida et al, 2001).

Target cells

Although B lymphocytes also express HLA Class I antigens, FCXM refers to T lymphocytes, which are the target of choice to measure cytotoxic alloantibodies directed against donor's HLA Class I antigens. T cells abundantly express HLA Class I antigens, but not Class II (T lymphocytes from organ donors are in general not activated), and produce very low levels of nonspecific fluorescence. IgG antibodies against other surface components are rarely found, so that a positive reaction is, as a rule, a good indicator for HLA Class I antibodies. However, the expression of individual HLA specificities is variable (Kao et al, 1988) and the signal-to-noise ratio is less favorable (Cook et al, 1985). As mentioned above, alloantibodies against Class I antigens, HLA-DR or DQ can be detected on B cells as well. However, the B-cell FCXM is not as reliable as the T-cell FCXM, and it remains difficult to interpret. The low sensitivity of the test in this case is attributed to the fact that B cells are in general less reliable than T cells as antibody targets, despite the use of a B-cell-specific marker (such as CD19 or CD20) when testing donor peripheral blood lymphocytes, whereas the background fluorescence of B cells is considerably higher than that of T cells (Scornik et al, 1985). In addition, a positive test may or may not be due to antibodies, because aggregated IgG or immune complexes can also bind to B cells.

The T-cell FCXM: Because of the higher sensitivity of FCXM, often in cases where the standard complement-dependent cytotoxicity (CDC) is negative, antidonor antibodies are detected by the FCXM. Although the concentration of these antibodies is probably not sufficiently high to produce a hyperacute rejection of the graft, it has been shown that patients with a positive T-cell FCXM and a negative CDC, especially those who lost a previous graft or had broadly reactive HLA antibodies before the transplant, have a higher risk for graft loss (Garavoy et al, 1983; Talbot et al, 1992; Barteli et al, 1992; Kerman et al, 1990; Ogura et al, 1993, 1994; Mahoney, 1990; Cook, 1987), which is attributed to the fact that previous transplants induce greatly expanded memory clones that may mediate graft rejection if they recognize antigens in the new transplant (Scornik et al, 1992). On the contrary, it seems that in nonsensitized, first renal transplant candidates, graft survival is as good as with negative FCXM results (Talbot et al, 1992; Scornik et al, 1994). Thus, the greatest value of the FCXM is in the pretransplant evaluation of patients at high immunological risk (retransplant and sensitized patients); a negative result puts them in the same outcome probability bracket as first transplant candidates, whereas a positive result makes the decision to transplant rather risky.

The B-Cell FCXM: The role of anti-HLA Class I antibodies in transplantation has been controversial (Braun, 1989). There is growing evidence that in the absence of Class I antibodies low-titer DR or DQ antibodies, as measured by cytotoxicity, are not detrimental for graft survival (Karuppan et al, 1990), albeit high-titer antibodies can produce hyperacute graft rejection (Scornik et al, 1992), although they do not always do so (Taylor et al, 1987; Panajotopoulos et al, 1992). A published report concluded that the mere presence of B-cell antibodies is not a risk factor, but that when the antibody concentration was above an arbitrary level, there was a decreased graft survival. The majority, but not all, of these cases were also positive by cytotoxicity (Lazda, 1994). Thus, it is not clear whether the B-cell FCXM contributes additional information to the cytotoxicity technique and, given the technical problems in using B-cell FCXM and its poor correlation with cytotoxicity, its clinical relevance remains to be proven.

Result evaluation

The variance between patient and control sera staining intensity can be expressed either as a difference or shift (patient's serum minus control serum) or as a ratio (patient's serum divided by control serum). To account for the variability of the test, the distinction between a positive and a negative FCXM result is usually performed by testing a number of normal sera, with cutoff point the mean of all normal results plus 2 or 3 standard deviations (Garavoy et al, 1983; Talbot et al, 1992; Berteli et al, 1992; Scornik et al, 1989). This cutoff, however, may not be sufficient to account for the variability of the test and, to avoid false-positive results, it is often nescessary to use a relatively high cutoff and sacrifice some sensitivity to gain specificity. Current literature lacks unanimity on FCXM, with several publications not providing their cutoff points and others reporting various shifts above normal control staining intensity (Cicciarelli et al, 1992; Kerman et al, 1990; Ogura et al, 1993; 1994; Mahoney et al, 1990). The distinction between weakly positive and negative results is also particularly problematic with the FCXM (Scornik, 1995).

Clinical application

The choice of one or the other is usually based on the individual preference of a laboratory as it considers the relative advantages and disadvantages of the assays for clinical use. The FCXM is more sensitive, quantitative, and objective than CDC. On the other hand, CDC benefits from an experience of over 30 years of use and, being a microtechnique, is better suited for testing multiple specimens. In practice, whereas many centers consider FCXM as a sine qua non in order to proceed to transplant, other centers consider the FCXM to be "too sensitive" and the exclusion of a patient from being transplanted based on a positive result too conservative. In essence, even though the sensitivity of FCXM is significantly better compared to CDC based assays, its specificity (especially that of the B-cell FCXM) for HLA antibodies is low. Indeed, it is now well known that except for donor directed HLA antibodies, clinically irrelevant autoantibodies, non-HLA antibodies and even non-HLA specific immunoglobulins that bind to surface Fc receptors can also lead to positive crossmatches. In these cases, positive crossmatches not due to HLA antibodies are not actually false positive reactions, but they are clinically inconsequential. Nonetheless, a positive T lymphocyte FCXM in many centers was formerly always ascribed to HLA class I antibodies and a positive B cell crossmatch was considered due to class II HLA antibodies. The development of solid-phase antibody detection assays, particularly those utilizing flow cytometry or a Luminex platform, in the last years permitted the clinical determination of the cause of a positive FCXM, ie whether the positive FCXM was in fact due to clinically relevant (HLA class I and/or class II) antibodies. The implementation of these assays revolutionarized allogeneic transplantation, in regard to interpretion of a positive FCXM. In solid phase antibody detection assays, clusters of class I or class II molecules (specifically, the entire class I or class II set of proteins expressed by a single individual) or, as of recently, individual HLA alleles, are adhered to microparticles that bind only to HLA specific antibodies. Thus, when a FCXM is positive but flow based solid phase antibody detection documents absence of HLA antibodies in the same serum, the positive crossmatch should be interpreted as clinically irrelevant.

In kidney transplantation, in parallel with donor HLA typing, the initial screening of potential recipients' sera with donor cells to exclude patients who have clear reactivity against that donor can only be done by CDC, unless the number of potential recipients is significantly reduced by some other selection criteria. Once the recipient is identified, the final crossmatch is generally performed in most laboratories by CDC, whereas FCXM is done as an additional test in presensitized or retransplant candidates, although some programs perform it routinely in all patients. As long as the turn-around time of the FCXM is faster than CDC, the decision whether to transplant or not can be made based on the FCXM alone when the FCXM results are negative as well as when FCXM is positive in sensitized patients. In the remaining cases where FCXM is positive in patients who are not clearly sensitized, it is prudent to base the final decision on the results of all tests (FCXM, T-cell CDC, and B-cell CDC) (Scornik, 1995). Indeed, over the last two decades a positive FCXM has been shown to be a test conveying patients a higher risk not only for early antibody-mediated rejection and graft loss (Nelson et al., 1996; Talbot et al., 1992, Graff et al, 2010), but also for increased late renal allograft loss (Graff et al, 2009) as well as decreased survival (Ilham et al., 2008; Lindemann et al., 2010).

FCXM is a practical alternative to CDC in heart and liver transplantation because of its faster turnaround time, a lower incidence of ambiguous results due to poor cell viability, and the direct detection of IgG antibodies, which avoids the false-positive reactions caused by IgM autoantibodies. Although preformed anti-donor antibodies can cause early heart transplant rejection and compromise patient survival (Singh et al, 1983; Ratkovec et al, 1992), pretransplant crossmatch is performed only occasionally in heart transplantation. The liver is less susceptible to antibody induced damage (Fung et al, 1987), although recent reports indicate that preformed antibodies do represent a higher risk for rejection (Takaya et al, 1992; Nikaein et al, 1994). A positive crossmatch during or after the transplantation alert the clinicians for suspected early rejection episode. Antibodies detected by the FCXM but not by CDC also appear to be of significance in heart (Shenton et al, 1991) and liver (Ogura et al, 1994) transplantations. The procedures outlined for heart and liver are likely to apply to other solid organ transplants, such as lung and pancreas, as well albeit there is little information about the effect of anti-donor antibodies in these clinical settings.

Future prospectives

Due to its superior performance characteristics, an increasing number of transplant programs perform the FCXM prospectively as a test complementary to CDC. Yet, a systematic evaluation of its capabilities and limitations is still missing. The main weak points of the technique that still warrant further elucidation are the variability of the background fluorescence for T and, especially, B cells, the changing behaviour of target cells according to their source or integrity, and the possibility of using standards or positive controls that can serve as reliable references for antibody binding are factors that still need to be studied in detail. In all cases, a complete understanding by the laboratory personnel of the technical principles and the clinical implications of the test is a prerequisite in order to provide a meaningful result and consult to the clinicians.

3. Flow cytometry HLA specificity

Flow cytometry is used before and after transplantation to assess the specificity of anti-HLA antibodies. Single HLA antigen beads are used to determine specific HLA antibodies in high Panel Reactive Antibody (PRA) containing sera. In this technique, nucleated leucocytes are added to monoclonal antibodies that are labelled with a molecule that fluoresces. Cells with surface antigens that bind to the antibody become fluorescent. The flow cytometer detects the fluorescent cells by detecting the light emitted from them as they pass through a laser beam. The antibody screen consists of testing the serum of the patient with a panel of 30 or more cells. The objective is to detect alloantibodies and to determine their HLA specificity so that donors carrying the target HLA antigens can be excluded beforehand. Flow cytometry has been used to screen for antibodies by using cell panels from 5-10 individuals (Scornik et al, 1984). This panel size is not sufficient to identify individual HLA antigen specificities but it is a sensitive way to determine the presence or absence of alloantibodies. The flow cytometry screen has been simplified by mixing several target cells in one tube (Cicciarelli et al, 1992), although this procedure has not become widely accepted. Given the increasing use of the FCXM at the time of transplantation, there is a growing need to perform antibody screens with the same degree of sensitivity. Some laboratories test larger cell panels, which is obviously an option for selected cases but not for routine use. Flow cytometry antibody screening with fewer (ex. 10) panel cells permits its application in all organ transplant candidates when first evaluated, whereas further testing is then decided according to the initial results. The later approach provides highly accurate and fast information and substantially reduces repeat or duplicate testing. With the use of the flow cytometry antibody detection assays described above donors expressing any of those antigens would be avoided, increasing the likelihood that, when a donor is crossmatched with the particular candidate recipient, the final result (predicted by "virtual crossmatching") will be negative.

4. Posttransplant monitoring

Antibodies produced after transplantation can mediate acute rejection, although not all rejection episodes involve detectable antibodies. After the organ transplant, detection of antidonor antibodies can confirm a suspected diagnosis of rejection and the need for immediate antirejection therapy, indicate bone marrow toxicity during immunosuppressive therapies, and help in the differentiation of infections from transplant rejection (Shanahan, 1997). A variety of cell surface markers and activation antigens can be used depending on the clinical condition and the organ transplanted. Posttransplant antibody monitoring is not routinely necessary but it may be helpful in some cases of heart (Suciu-Foca et al, 1991; Smith et al, 1991) or kidney (Scornik et al, 1989; Martin et al, 1987; Zhang et al, 2005, Reed et al, 2006) transplantation. Flow cytometry is very useful because results with frozen donor cells are more consistent than when using the CDC technique and because differences between the pretransplant and posttransplant specimens can be detected with higher sensitivity. Results are usually not affected when patients have already been treated with OKT3 (OKT3 in the patient's serum kills T lymphocytes in the CDC test). In the presence of OKT3, the fluorescent CD3 reagent for flow cytometry staining should be replaced by another T-cell marker for satisfactory T-cell cluster separation. Finally, immunophenotyping of lymphocyte subsets with the use of flow cytometry, i.e. the analysis of cell surface markers using fluorochrome-conjugated monoclonal antibodies (ex., CD3+, CD4+, CD8+ T cells, CD19+ B cells, and CD3-, CD56+ NK cells) can be used for assessing the immune status of the patient and monitor effectiveness of immunotherapies.

5. ATG/ALG therapy monitoring

One of the mainstays of therapy against the rejection process in transplantation, either as a prophylaxis or as treatment, is the use of anti-lymphocyte globulin (ALG) and anti-thymocyte globulin (ATG). Polyclonal heterologous products act principally by reducing the level of peripheral blood T-lymphocytes. The majority of transplant centres administer

ATG/ALG in an empirical fashion according to a fixed dose regimen. Due to the idiosyncratic respone of individual patients, a fixed dose regimen may undersuppress some patients or result in oversuppression, which may, in turn, lead to acute renal allograft rejection or opportunistic infections.

The standard methods for monitoring the efficacy of ATG therapy are the determination of serum IgG levels (McAlack et al, 1979) and the detection of circulating T-cell levels with the use of E-rosettes employing sheep erythrocytes (Cosimi et al, 1976). The reproducibility of the E-rosette assay system was questioned when flow cytometric measurement of monoclonal antibody-labelled T lymphocytes was introduced (Cosimi et al, 1981). Flow cytometric analysis of monoclonal antibody-labelled T lymphocytes proved to be more accurate, more reproducible, and easier to perform (No authors listed, 1985) than the E-rosette assay, with the optimal threshold T-cell count for such treatment being approximately 50 T cells/μL (Shenton et al, 1994). Flow cytometry with the use of three fluorescent markers provides an excellent, rapid and reproducible way of measuring such cells. The lymphocytes are identified using right-angle light side scatter (RALS) vs anti-CD45 (PerCP) plots, with the use of anti-CD3-FITC markers for the determination of the percentage of T cells and the inclusion of Leu-M3-PE (anti-CD14) for the removal of monocytes from the gate. By spiking the labelled sample with fluorescent beads the number of T cells/μL can be calculated.

6. Conclusion

Flow cytometric based assays have become amongst the most valuable tools to monitor allograft recipients both pre and post transplantation nowadays. Their principal applications in solid organ transplantation are the FCXM and the detection and characterization of HLA-specific alloantibodies. Whereas they have been in clinical use for more than a decade, the accumulating experience of the laboratories and the clinicians have generated expectations for even more exciting applications in the years to come.

7. References

Bell A, Shenton B.K, Garner S. Proc R Soc Med, 33, 219, 1998.

Berteli AJ, Daniel V, Mohring K, et al.: Association of kidney graft failure with a positive flow cytometry crossmatch. Clin Transplant 6:31-34, 1992.

Braun WE: Laboratory and clinical management of the highly sensitized organ transplant recipient. Hum Immunol 26:245-460, 1989.

Cicciarelli J, Helstab K, Mendez R: Flow cytometry PRA, a new test that is highly correlated with graft survival. Clin Transplant 6:159-164, 1992.

Cook DJ. Scornik JC: Purified HLA antigens to probe human alloantibody specificity. Hum Immunol 14:234-244, 1985.

Cook DJ, Terasaki PI, Iwaki Y, et al.: An approach to reducing early kidney transplant failure by flow cytometry crossmatching. Clin Transplant 1:253-256, 1987.

Cosimi AB, Wortis HH, Delmonico FL, Russell PS. Randomized clinical trial of antithymocyte globulin in cadaver renal allograft recipients: importance of T cell monitoring. Surgery. 1976; 80: 155-63.

Cosimi AB, Colvin RB, Burton RC, et al.: Use of monoclonal antibodies to T-cell subsets for immunologic monitoring and treatment in recipients of renal allografts. N Engl J Med. 1981;305:308-14.

Fung JJ, Makowka L, Griffin M, et al.: Successful sequential liver kidney transplantation in patients with preformed lymphocytotoxic antibodies. Clin Transplant 1:187-194, 1987.

Garovoy MR, Rheinschmidt M, Bigos M, et al.: Flow cytometry analysis: a high technology crossmatch technique facilitating transplantation. Transplant Proc 15:1939-1944, 1983.

Graff RJ, Xiao H, Schnitzler MA, et al. The role of positive flow cytometry crossmatch in late renal allograft loss. Hum Immunol 70, 502-505, 2009.

Graff RJ, Buchannan PM, Dzebisashvili N, et al. The Clinical Importance of Flow Cytometry Crossmatch in the Context of CDC Crossmatch Results. Transplant Proc 42, 3471-3474, 2010.

Ilham, M. A., Winkler, S., Coates, E., Rizzello, A., Rees, T. J., Asderakis, A. Clinical significance of a positive flow crossmatch on the outcomes of cadaveric renal transplants. Transplant Proc. 40, 1839–1843, 2008.

Kao KJ, ScornikJC, Riley WJ, McQueen C: Association between HLA phenotypes and HLA concentration in plasma or platelets. Hum Immunol 21:115-124, 1988.

Karuppan SS, Lindholm A, Moller E: Characterization and significance of donor-reactive B cell antibodies in current sera of kidney transplant patients. Transplantation 49:510-515, 1990.

Kerman RH, Van Buren CY, Lewis RM, et al.: Improved graft survival for flow cytometry and antihuman globulin crossmatch-negative retransplant recipients. Transplantation 4952-56, 1990.

Lazda VA. Identification of patients at risk for inferior renal allograft outcome by a strongly positive B cell flow cytometry crossmatch. Transplantation 57964-969, 1994.

Lindemann, M., Nyadu, B., Heinemann, F. M., m Kribben, A., Paul, A., Horn, P. A., Witzke, O. High negative predicative value of an amplified flow cytometry crossmatch in living donor kidney transplantation. Hum. Immunol. 71, 771–776, 2010.

Mahoney R, Ault KA, Given SR, et al.: The flow cytometric crossmatch and early renal transplant loss. Transplantation 49:527-535, 1990.

Martin S, Dyer PA, Mallick NP, et al.: Posttransplant antidonor lymphocytotoxic antibody production in relation to graft outcome. Transplantation 44:50-53, 1987.

McAlack RF, Stern S, Beizer R, et al.: Immunologic monitoring parameters in ALG- versus non-ALG-treated renal transplant patients. Transplant Proc., 11, 1431-2, 1979

Nelson, P. W., Eschliman, P., Shield, C. F., Aeder, M. I., Luger, A. M., Pierce, G. A., Bryan, C. F. Improved graft survival in cadaveric renal transplantation by flow cytometry crossmatching. Arch. Surg. 131, 599–603, 1996.

Nikaein A, Backman L, Jennings L, et al.: HLA compatibility and liver transplant outcome. Improved patient survival by HLA and crossmatching. Transplantation 58:786-792, 1994.

No authors listed. Transplantation immunology and monitoring. Transplant Proc. 1985;17: 547-677.

Ogura K, Terasaki PI, Johnson C, et al.: The significance of a positive flow cytometry crossmatch test in primary kidney transplantation. Transplantation 56:294-298, 1993.

Ogura K, Terasaki PI, Koyama H, et al.: High one-month liver failure rates in flow cytometry crossmatch-positive recipients. Clin Transplant 8111-115, 1994.

Panajotopoulos N, lanhez LE, Neumann J, et al.: A successful second renal allograft across positive B cell crossmatch due to IgG anti-HLA DR5 antibody. Clin Transplant 6:196-198, 1992.

Ratkovec RM, Hammond EH, OConnell JB, et al.: Outcome of cardiac transplant recipients with a positive donor-specific crossmatch. Preliminary results with plasmapheresis. Transplantation 54:65 1-655, 1992.

Reed EF, Demetris AJ, Hammond E, et al. Acute antibody-mediated rejection of cardiac transplants. J Heart Lung Transplant 2006; 25:153-9.

Scornik JC, Ireland JE, Howard RJ, Pfaff WW: Assessment of the risk for broad sensitization by blood transfusions. Transplantation 37: 249-253, 1984.

Scornik JC, Brunson ME, Howard RJ, Pfaff WW: Alloimmunization, memory, and the interpretation of crossmatch results for renal transplantation. Transplantation 54:389-394, 1992.

Scornik JC, LeFor WM, Cicciarelli JC, et al.: Hyperacute and acute kidney graft rejection due to antibodies against B cells. Transplantation 54:61-64, 1992.

Scornik JC, Brunson ME, Schaub B, et al.: The crossmatch in renal transplantation. Evaluation of flow cytometry as a replacement for standard cytotoxicity. Transplantation 57:62 1-625, 1994

Scornik J.C. (1995). Detection of Alloantibodies by Flow Cytometry: Relevance to Clinical Transplanation. Cytometry, 22, 259-263.

Shanahan T. Application of flow cytometry in transplantation medicine. Immunol Invest. 1997;26:91-101.

Shenton BK, Glenville BE, Mitchenson AE, et al.: Use of flow cytometric crossmatching in cardiac transplantation. Transplant Proc 23: 1153-1154, 1991.

Shenton BK, White MD, Bell AE, Clark K, Rigg KM, Forsythe JL, Proud G, Taylor RM. The paradox of ATG monitoring in renal transplantation. Transplant Proc. 1994; 26:3177-80.

Singh G, Thompson M, Griffith B, et al.: Histocompatibility in cardiac transplantation with particular reference to immunopathology of positive serologic crossmatch. Clin Immunol Immunopathol 28: 56-66, 1983.

Smith JD, Danskine AJ, Rose ML, Yacoub MH: Specificity of lymphocytotoxic antibodies formed after cardiac transplantation and correlation with rejection episodes. Transplantation 53:1358-1362, 1992.

Suciu-Foca N, Reed E, Marboe C, et al.: The role of anti-HLA antibodies in heart transplantation. Transplantation 5 1:716-724, 1991.

Takaya S, Bronsther O, Iwaki Y, et al.: The adverse impact on liver transplantation of using positive cytotoxic crossmatch donors. Transplantation 53; 400-406, 1992.

Talbot D, Cavanagh G, Coates E, et al,: Improved graft outcome and reduced complications due to flow cytometric crossmatching and DR matching in renal transplantation. Transplantation 53:925-928, 1992.

Taylor CJ, Chapman JR, Fuggle SV, et al.: A positive B cell crossmatch due to IgG anti-HLA-DQ antibody present at the time of transplantation in a successful renal allograft. Tiss Antigens 30:104-112, 1987.

Vaidya, S., Cooper, T., Avandsalehi, J., Titus, B., Brooks, K., Hymel, P., Noor, M., Sellers, R., Thomas, A., Stewart, D., Daller, J., Fish, J. C., Gugliuzza, K. K., Bray, R. A.. Improved flow cytometric detection of HLA alloantibodies using pronase: potential clinical impact. Transplantation 71, 422–428, 2001.

Zhang Q, Liang LW, Gjertson DW, Lassman C, Wilkinson AI, Kendrick E, Pham TP, Danovitch G, Gritsch A, Reed EF. Development of post transplant anti-donor HLA antibodies is associated with acute humoral rejection and early graft dysfunction. Transplantation; 79: 591-8, 2005.

9

The Use of Flow Cytometry to Monitor T Cell Responses in Experimental Models of Graft-Versus-Host Disease

Bryan A. Anthony and Gregg A. Hadley
The Ohio State University
USA

1. Introduction

1.1 Introduction to the immune system and flow cytometry

The immune system is a collection of dynamic cells that work together and interact to perform a variety of bodily functions. The immune system is involved in many disease states and changes to the immune system can be very impactful in progression or amelioration of a disease. The ability to monitor immune responses during disease progression and resolution can help to elucidate the underlying mechanisms of immune-mediated diseases

Flow cytometry is a method of monitoring immune responses using antibodies labeled with fluorochromes either directly or indirectly through a fluoresceinated secondary reagent. Antibodies are proteins that can bind to a particular epitope with very high affinity. To monitor immune responses via flow cytometry, immune cells must be isolated and incubated with antibodies to markers of choice. During co-incubation, antibodies randomly encounter cells in suspension and bind to the epitopes for which they are specific for. Following co-incubation, excess antibody is washed off and the cell suspension can either be passed through a flow cytometer immediately or the cell suspension can be fixed and passed through a flow cytometer at a later time. The resulting data are then analyzed and interpreted.

1.2 Introduction to applications of flow cytometry in graft-versus-host disease

Graft-versus-host disease (GVHD) is an immune mediated disease that results following bone marrow transplant. GVHD is caused by donor T cells that react to alloantigens expressed on host tissues. GVHD pathology is generally confined to the epithelia of the skin, liver, and intestinal tract. Following transplantation, T cell responses go through several phases with each phase characterized by various T cell activities. Flow cytometry provides a powerful tool to determine the disease state at any given time, characterize T cell responses, and examine the effectiveness of therapeutic intervention.

In this chapter, we will discuss the application of flow cytometry to characterizing T cell responses during GVHD. We will discuss isolating T cells from relevant immune compartments, applying flow cytometry to identifying disease states over time, defining the roles of T cell subsets during GVHD, identifying the effectiveness of specific T cell depletion in vivo during GVHD, and the use of bioluminescent imaging to integrate flow cytometric data with T cell trafficking properties.

To monitor T cell responses during GVHD, T cells can be isolated from several locations. In this section of the chapter, we will describe methods for isolating and purifying T cell subsets from the intestinal tract, peripheral blood, mesenteric lymph node, and spleen. By examining these specific locations, researchers can gain insight into pathogenic T cell development and maintenance. We will provide data regarding T cell yield and expected ratios of various T cell subsets in each location.

Flow cytometry can be a valuable asset in identifying disease progression. Flow cytometry allows for both cell surface and intracellular identification of T cells. This section of the chapter will focus on how to identify disease states during GVHD based on cell surface staining as well as identify intracellular cytokine production characteristic of pathogenic T cells. We will discuss typical surface staining of T cells during various phases of GVHD.

The roles of T cell subsets in GVHD can be explored using data that characterizes T cell responses during GVHD. In this section of the chapter, we will discuss how flow cytometric analysis can be used to generate hypotheses about the roles of T cell subsets during GVHD. We will instruct the reader how to analyze flow cytometry data, draw subsequent conclusions, and generate hypotheses to confirm their conclusions. We will provide examples of this practice in the context of GVHD.

The final section of this chapter will focus on using flow cytometry to determine the effectiveness of therapeutic interventions. Our lab has used immunotoxins and depleting antibodies as potential therapies for GVHD. Flow cytometry plays a large role in determining the mechanism of action of our therapies as well as determining if the therapy was successful. In this section, we will include data showing how flow cytometry can be used to determine the effectiveness of immunotherapies.

2. Graft-versus-host disease

2.1 Introduction to bone marrow transplantation

Bone marrow transplantation represents a curative therapy for a variety of hematopoietic deficiencies including blood cancers. Because of the potentially fatal side effects, transplants are often only used when standard therapies are ineffective. Immediately prior to the transplant, the host is given a conditioning regimen of radiation and/or chemotherapy to suppress or ablate the host immune system. In doing so, the host is cured of their blood disorder; however, they are also severely immunocompromised and will not survive without a bone marrow transplant to restore immune function. Donor bone marrow can be isolated by injecting a syringe into a marrow containing bone and extracting marrow. This is a very laborious and painful process for the donor. Alternatively, a less invasive method of extracting hematopoietic stem cells involves treating the donor with granulocyte colony-stimulating factor (G-CSF) and pheresing stem cells out of the blood. Treatment with G-CSF mobilizes stem cells from the bone marrow into circulation, and stem cells can then be isolated from peripheral blood. Donor stem cells are isolated and injected into the immunosuppressed host.

2.2 Graft-versus-host disease

Acute Graft-versus-host disease is the most common detrimental outcome following bone marrow or hematopoietic stem cell transplants. In 1966, Billingham described three criteria for GVHD: 1) the graft must contain a sufficient number of immunologically competent cells, 2) the host must contain important isoantigens lacking in the graft, and 3) the host must be incapable of mounting an immune response against the graft (Billingham, 1966). There are four stages of GVHD that classify the severity of the disease with stage I being the least severe and stage IV being the most severe. Various stages are defined by the degree of pathology associated with each target organ (Table 1). There are several genetic risk factors that can negatively impact a recipient's probability of getting severe GVHD. These risk factors include, but are not limited to polymorphisms in proinflammatory cytokines such as TNFα and INFγ as well as polymorphisms in anti-inflammatory cytokines such as IL-10 and TGFβ (Ball & Egeler, 2008). Other risk factors include age/sex of the donor and recipient, donor stem cell source, and degree of HLA mismatch (Koreth & Antin, 2008). It is of great importance to match the donor and recipient as closely as possible. The degree of HLA mismatch between the donor and recipient positively correlates with the severity of GVHD (Park et al., 2011). GVHD is caused by mature lymphocytes that are unintentionally isolated during graft procurement that generate an immune response to host antigens. It is not uncommon for the number of mature lymphocytes to vastly outnumber the stem cells in the transplant inoculum (Korbling & Anderlini, 2001). T cells represent the highest single cell type population (Korbling & Anderlini, 2001), and are the primary mediators of GVHD. Mature donor antigen presenting cells (APCs) and B cells contribute to the pathogenesis of GVHD by priming T cells against host tissue. However, donor T cells alone are sufficient to cause GVHD (Shlomchik et al. 1999). Interestingly, depletion of donor CD4+ T cells is ineffective in reducing GVHD severity, but selective depletion of CD8+ T cells ameliorates GVHD severity (Nagler et al., 1998; Nimer et al., 1994). These data suggest that CD8+ T cells play a dominant role in promoting GVHD pathology. Patients that develop acute GVHD often develop chronic GVHD. Chronic GVHD is characterized by the delay in onset as well as the breadth of target organ involvement. Acute GVHD is diagnosed if onset occurs within 100 days of transplant; whereas, clinical manifestations occurring after 100 days post

Stage	*Skin*	*Liver*	*GI Tract*
0	No rash due to GVHD	Normal serum bilirubin	None
I	Mild maculopapular rash over less than 25% of the body	Bilirubin from 2 to <3 mg/dl	Diarrhea >500-1000 ml/day
II	Moderate maculopapular rash over 25%-50% of the body	Bilirubin from 3 to <6 mg/dl	Diarrhea >1000-1500 ml/day
III	Severe maculopapular rash covering greater than 50% of the body	Bilirubin from 6 to < 15mg/dl	Diarrhea >1500 ml/day
IV	Severe maculopapular rash covering greater than 50% of the body.	Bilirubin > 15mg/dl	Diarrhea >1500 ml/day; abdominal pain or ileus

Adapted from Ball & Egeler, 2008, Bone Marrow Transplantation.

Table 1. Description of each clinical manifestation for each target organ at each stage of GVHD

transplant are characterized as chronic GVHD. Target organs affected by acute GVHD are largely limited to the skin, liver, and gut. In addition to the skin, liver, and gut, chronic GVHD can affect mucous membranes, lung, and musculoskeletal system (Koreth & Antin, 2008).

In addition to their ability to cause GVHD, donor T cells provide protective effects to transplant recipients. Donor T cells promote bone marrow engraftment, immunity to opportunistic infections, and eliminate residual malignant cells resistant to the host conditioning regimen. Elimination of residual tumor cells is seen in several solid tumors and a variety of hematological malignancies with chronic myeloid leukemia (CML) being the most sensitive (Morris et al., 2006). Immunity to residual tumor cells is termed the graft-versus tumor (GVT) effect and immunity to hematopoietic malignancy is termed the graft-versus-leukemia (GVL). Transplant recipients receive a variety of immunosuppressive drugs, many of which target T cells. Because T cells are a major defense against viral infections, reactivation and primary cytomegalovirus (CMV) infections are problematic post transplant (Bautista et al., 2008). Intense myeloablative condition regimens destroy host defense responsible for maintaining CMV latency. It has been established that total body irradiation (TBI) causes reactivation of latent murine CMV (mCMV) infections (Kurz et al. 1999). Virus-specific CTLs have been generated from *in vitro* expanded CD8+ T cells and adoptively transferred into recipients (Riddel et al., 1992). Identifying a target to reduce GVHD and maintain immunity to a broad spectrum of pathogens would be advantageous to advancing our understanding of the immune system after bone marrow transplantation.

In some transplants, T cells are depleted prior to transplant because the severity of GVHD can be predicted through analysis of the degree of mismatch between donor and host. Recipients of T cell depleted grafts do not develop GVHD, but they also do not benefit from the protective effects of T cells post transplant. It was shown that leukemic relapse and graft rejection were increased in patients who received T cell depleted grafts and concluded that global T cell depletion is not a viable treatment strategy (Horowitz et al., 1990). Therefore, GVHD research is focused on identifying a method to prevent GVHD while maintaining the beneficial T cell properties post transplant.

2.3 Animal models of GVHD

Animal GVHD models are often used in order to test hypotheses aimed to improve outcomes following bone marrow transplantation. GVHD is induced by irradiating recipient mice and adoptively transferring donor bone marrow cells. Unlike the clinical scenario, there are not enough donor T cells isolated during bone marrow procurement to induce GVHD, so exogenous T cells must be added to induce GVHD. The most common source of T cells used to induce GVHD is the spleen and/or lymph nodes. Whole splenocytes or various subsets of T cells can be purified and adoptively transferred with the bone marrow to induce GVHD.

Advances in clinical practice have been driven by breakthroughs discovered using small animal models of GVHD. Rat models of GVHD are widely used and provide researchers with a small animal model to test hypotheses to improve outcomes following bone marrow transplants. Given the additional size provided in rat models compared to murine models, transplant studies in which GVHD is a complication of solid organ allografts can be done (Wakely et al., 1990; Muramatsu et al., 2010). However, murine GVHD models remain the most prominent transplant models. The vast number of MHC combinations available and the array of transgenic mice create an ideal situation for testing hypotheses aimed to discover immunological mechanisms governing GVHD. Murine GVHD models can be divided into two main categories: MHC-matched and MHC disparate. The disease course following GVHD induction in MHC-disparate models is much more rapid than the disease course following GVHD induction in MHC-matched models, and can generally be induced by CD4+ or CD8+ T cells alone. Donor CD4+ and CD8+ T cells in an MHC-disparate model are directed against differences in major histocompatibility antigens; whereas, T cells in an MHC-matched model are directed against differences in the minor histocompatibility antigens (miHAs). miHAs are polymorphic proteins that vary between individuals. miHAs are sufficient to cause GVHD despite the lower frequency of donor T cells specific for miHA differences (Goulmy et al., 1996). An MHC-matched model that closely resembles the clinical scenario is the C57Bl/6 (B6) into BALB.B strain combination. Both strains are of the H-2b haplotype, but are disparate for multiple miHAs. This model was well characterized in the Korngold laboratory, and it was established that GVHD was principally caused by CD4-dependent CD8+ T cells (Berger et al., 1994; Friedman et al., 1998). Furthermore, the immunodominant hierarchy has been established and it is known that the H60 miHA is immunodominant (Choi et al., 2001). The delayed mortality in MHC-matched models allows for disease progression that is more consistent with clinical disease progressions. The similarity of the relative roles of T cell subsets between the clinical scenario and the B6 into BALB.B strain combination and the delayed disease course make this model useful to study underlying mechanisms of GVHD.

2.4 Effects of the conditioning regimen

GVHD is classified into three different phases. The first phase of GVHD comes as a result of the conditioning regimen the recipient receives to reduce or ablate the native immune system. The conditioning regimen is aimed to destroy rapidly dividing cells, so in addition to destroying lymphocytes, the conditioning regimen also attacks epithelial cells in the skin, the liver, and the gut. Destruction of epithelium in these compartments is thought to cause release of proinflammatory cytokines including, but not limited to IL-1 and TNFα. Increased cytokine production causes the upregulation of costimulatory molecules, adhesion molecules, and MHC antigens (Chang & See, 1986; Pober et al., 1996). This process is critical to the activation of host antigen presenting cells (APCs). Epithelial damage in the gut is particularly important in the initiation of GVHD. Damage to the intestinal epithelium causes systemic release of LPS, which further amplifies GVHD induction (Reddy, 2003). Released LPS is taken up by local APCs and an immune response is mounted against LPS, which, in turn further exacerbates GVHD progression and pathology.

2.5 Donor T cell activation

GVHD pathology is mediated by donor T cells directed against major and minor histocompatibility antigens in the host. Donor T cell trafficking to host secondary lymphoid tissue immediately following hematopoietic stem cell transplantation (HSCT) is a complex processes that displays extreme diversity between organs. Naïve T cells cause more severe

GVHD than memory T cells (Dutt et al., 2007); therefore, naïve T cell trafficking is an area of intense research. T cell priming in intestinal inductive sites (Peyer's patches, mesenteric lymph nodes) plays a major role in gut associated GVHD. In the gut, T cells enter secondary lymphoid tissue by T cell rolling initiated by the L-selectin (CD62L) expressed on all naïve T cells interacting with the peripheral node addressin (PNAd) on high endothelial venules (HEVs). Further tethering of the T cell to the HEV is achieved by the CCL21/CCR7 interaction. This interaction mediates upregulation of leukocyte function-associated antigen type 1 (LFA-1) on T cells, which firmly bind the T cell and HEV (Johansson-Lindbom & Agace, 2007). Peyer's patches and mesenteric lymph node HEVs express low levels of PNAd; however, mucosal addressin cell-adhesion molecule-1 (MAdCAM-1) serves as an additional ligand for CD62L in gut priming sites (Johansson-Lindbom & Agace, 2007). Another important ligand for MAdCAM-1 is the $\alpha4\beta7$ integrin. This integrin is expressed on naïve T cells and plays a critical role in directing naïve T cells to the gut, causing intestinal GVHD (Campbell & Butcher, 2002; Johansson-Lindbom & Agace, 2007; Mora et al., 2003; Stagg et al., 2002). Once in host lymphoid tissue, antigen presentation is primarily done by host APCs presenting self peptides. Donor derived dendritic cells can cross present host antigens; however, severe GVHD is dependent on host APCs presenting to alloreactive T cells (Shlomchik, 2007). Activated T cells leave through the efferent lymphatic system and return to circulation via the thorasic duct. When activated T cells return to sites of inflammation they migrate through blood vessel endothelium and into epithelial compartments.

2.6 Effector phase of GVHD

In the activation phase, donor T cells traffic to host secondary lymphoid tissue hours after transplant and expand within 2-3 days (Wysocki et al., 2005). In the lymphoid tissue, donor T cells are primarily primed by host antigen presenting cells (APCs) to mature into T helper 1 (Th1) CD4+ T cells or cytotoxic CD8+ T cells. Recently, it has been described that T helper 17 (Th17) cells can also mediate lethal GVHD in murine models (Carlson et al., 2009). Th17 cells are characterized by their ability to produce the cytokine IL-17, and have been shown to be proinflammatory (Gran et al., 2002; Gutcher et al., 2006; Krakowski & Owens, 1996; Zhang et al., 2003). Th1 CD4+ T cells are characterized by their production of proinflammatory cytokines such as IFNγ, TNFα, and IL-2. 3-7 days post transplant, activated T cells traffic to and expand in GVHD target organs (Wysocki et al., 2005). The effector phase of GVHD consists of activated T cells migrating to epithelial compartments of GVHD target organs and destroying host tissues. Th1 CD4+ T cells mediate GVHD primarily through Fas/FasL mediated apoptosis, but also mediate epithelial damage via IL-1 and TNFα (Teshima et al., 2002). CD8+ T cells kill target tissues by direct contact to target cell or by release of cytotoxic soluble mediators (Ferrara et al., 1999). Contact dependent CD8+ T cell killing mechanisms include the Fas/FasL interaction and perforin/granzyme mediated cytotoxicity (Ferrara et al., 1999). In murine models where appropriate genetic differences exist, CD4+ T cells can induce GVHD by responding to MHC Class II differences; whereas, MHC Class I differences will elicit CD8+ T cell driven GVHD responses (Sprent et al., 1990). However, differences in miHAs elicit GVHD reactions from either CD4+ or CD8+ T cells following HLA-matched bone marrow transplantation.

3. Characterization of T cells during GVHD

3.1 T cell phenotypes involved in GVHD

Initially upon transfer from donor to host, donor T cells are in a naive state. Naive T cells characteristically express the lymphocyte homing receptor CD62L (L-selectin). The ligands for CD62L are GlyCAM-1, CD34, MadCAM-1, and PSGL-1. Each of these ligands are expressed on endothelial cells or high endothelial venules in the lymph node. Naive T cells home to host secondary lymphoid compartments following transplant. Naive T cells can be activated directly by antigen presentation by host APCs or indirectly by antigen presentation by donor APCs (Shlomchik et al., 1999; Teshima et al., 2002). Following activation, donor T cells down regulate CD62L, thereby freeing them from lymphoid recirculation, and upregulate integrins such as LFA-1 (CD11a/CD18) and VLA-4 (CD49d/CD29) which enable extravasation into host tissues (Figure 1). Activated T cells also upregulate the C-Type lectin protein, CD69, and the high affinity alpha chain of the IL-2 receptor (CD25).

Effector memory T cells can be classified by their expression of the hyaluronic acid receptor, CD44. CD44 is expressed at low levels on naive cells, but is highly upregulated upon activation. Naive T cells can be isolated from donor mice and tested for the expression of naive or activation markers to predict the GVHD inducing potential of a given population of T cells. Furthermore, naive CD4+ T cells can be cultured to polarization to Th phenotype (Swain et al., 1991). Polarized CD4+ T cells can be transferred to irradiated recipients to induce GVHD (Fowler et al., 1996).

It is well documented that adoptive transfer of naive T cells causes lethal GVD across either major or minor histocompatibility differences (OKunewick et al., 1990; Sprent et al., 1990); however, T cells of effector or memory phenotype are not as effective as naïve T cells in inducing GVHD following adoptive transfer into allogeneic recipients (Anderson et al., 2003). Interestingly, central memory, effector memory, and effector CD8+ T cells have been shown to induce GVHD in a fully allogeneic strain combination (Zhang et al., 2005a); whereas, memory (characterized by the lack of CD62L expression) CD4+ T cells do not induce GVHD in either MHC-matched or MHC-disparate murine models (Anderson et al., 2003; Chen et al., 2004). The mechanisms governing the lack of GVHD induction by memory CD4+ T cells remains unclear. However, it has been hypothesized by Sondel and colleagues that the T cells transferred by Anderson et al., were of the terminally differentiated, CD4+CD44hiCD62L-CD25- effector memory variety (Sondel et al., 2003). Effector memory differ from activated memory cells by their lack of CD69L and CD25 expression and lack the ability to home to central lymphoid tissue (Figure 1) (Sondel et al., 2003). The inability to home to lymphoid compartments following transfer in to host circulation presumably prevents donor T cells from being effectively primed against host antigens, thus leaving them unable to induce GVHD. The specificity that exists in choosing the appropriate cell type to induce GVHD provides an opportunity to utilize flow cytometry to aid in the induction of GVHD. Flow cytometry can be used to confirm or test the purity of a cultured cell population that has been induced into a certain phenotype. Flow cytometry can also identify the composition of donor splenocytes or lymph node cells. Historical data from Jackson Laboratories shows that the spleen of female B6 mice is comprised of roughly 16% CD4+ T cells and 10% CD8+ T cells (Jackson Laboratories). When testing hypotheses, it is of great importance to optimize experiments in order to obtain the most accurate results. Using flow cytometry to understand the composition of a given cell population allows researchers to accurately perform and analyze experiments.

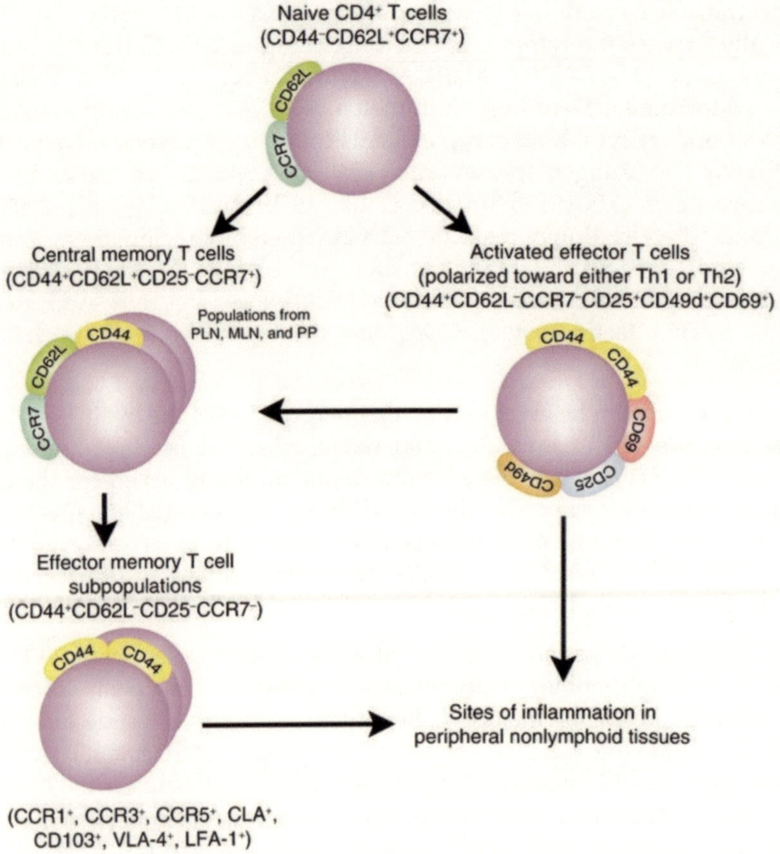

Fig. 1. Naïve CD4+ T cells develop into effector or memory CD4+ T cells. When naïve CD4+ T cells (initially CD44-CD62L+CCR7+) are activated they either develop into central memory CD4+ T cells (CD44+CD62L+CD25-CCR7+) or effector CD4+ T cells (CD44+CD62L-CCR7-CD25+CD49d+CD69+). Effector memory CD4+ T cells can extravasate into sites of inflammation or transition into central memory CD4+ T cells. Central memory CD4+ T cells can transition into effector memory CD4+ T cells (CCR1+CCR3+CCR5+CLA+CD103+VLA-4+LFA-1+). Adapted from Sondel et al., 2003, JCI

3.2 The role of regulatory T cells during GVHD

Regulatory T cells (Tregs) are a population of T cells that have been shown to suppress GVHD in murine models (Johnson et al., 2002). Tregs are characterized and controlled by several phenotypic markers with the most universal being expression of the transcription factor forkhead box P3 (Foxp3) (Hori et al., 2003). Despite being the universal Treg regulator, Foxp3 is also transiently upregulated following activation of CD4+ T cells (Esposito et al., 2010). Because of this, the function of Foxp3 expressing cells can be ambiguous. Transient Foxp3 expression by recently activated Th1 CD4 T cells is substantially lower than that in Foxp3 expressing Tregs (Esposito et al., 2010). Therefore, to accurately determine whether Foxp3 expression signifies a regulatory CD4+ T cell, protein quantification should be done. Protein quantification can be done through Western blotting and densitometry analysis. Moreover, CD25 is often used to classify CD4+ Tregs, but CD25 is also expressed on recently activated Th1, Th2, or Th17 T cells as well. Therefore, confirmation of a flow cytometric determination of a cellular phenotype may be supplemented using alternative methods.

CD4+ Tregs elicit several effector mechanisms, but they are widely regarded as immunosuppressive. Their immunosuppressive action can be carried out via cell-cell contact or secretion of anti-inflammatory cytokines including TGFβ and IL-10. Tregs can be further characterized by surface expression of several other proteins, including the αEβ7 integrin, CD103, which is broadly expressed by a variety of leukocyte subsets including activated CD8+ T cells, dendritic cells, and regulatory CD4+ and CD8+ T cells (Cepak et al., 1994; Cerf-Bensussan et al. 1987; Huehn et al. 2004). CD103+ Tregs have been shown to have immunosuppressive properties reaching or exceeding those of their CD103- counterparts (Lehman et al., 2002). There is a population of CD25-CD103+ Tregs that express CTLA-4, suppress T cell proliferation *in vitro*, and prevent severe colitis in the SCID mouse (Lehmann et al., 2002). CD25-CD103+ Tregs also produce a distinct cytokine profile. This subset of Tregs typically produces IL-4, IL-5, and IL-13 to a similar extent as Th2 CD4+ T cells; however, this cytokine profile is largely absent in their CD25+ counterparts (Lehmann et al., 2002).

CD4+CD25+CD103+ Tregs exhibit immunosuppressive properties *in vivo* as well as *in vitro*. Chronic GVHD frequently occurs in patients that develop acute GVHD, and *in vivo* transfer of CD4+CD25+CD103+ Tregs in mice has been shown to suppress ongoing chronic GVHD, and has been shown to reduce the number of alloantibody producing plasma cells and pathogenic T cells in GVHD target organs (Zhao et al., 2008). CD103 is also present on the surface of a population of CD8+ Tregs. CD8+ Tregs can acquire their antigen specificity peripherally and promote systemic tolerance. Antigen specific CD8+ Tregs can be induced by antigen injection into the anterior chamber of the eye. CD103 has been shown to be essential for the development and function of the CD8+ Tregs (Keino et al., 2006). Koch et al. characterized CD103+CD8+ Tregs as phenotypically different from other CD8+ suppressor T cell populations. CD103+CD8+ Tregs express CD28, but lack Foxp3, CD25, LAG-3, CTLA-4, and GITR (Koch et al., 2008).

3.3 Cell specific depletion during GVHD

Depletion of specific cell types can be an effective means to prevent GVHD. The most obvious clinical example of this is patients who receive T cell depleted grafts incur GVHD less frequently. However, this is not an effective treatment because globally depleting T cells results in increased rate of graft rejection, increased susceptibility to opportunistic infections, and increased rates of leukemic relapse. However, rare instances occur where the risk for severe GVHD is so great that the potential benefits outweigh the risks and T cells are selectively removed from the graft. In such instances, removal is done through the addition antibodies targeted to either CD4+ T cells, CD8+ T cells, or both. The antibodies are conjugated to magnetic beads and the graft-antibody mix is passed through a magnetic column. The magnetic beads bind to the magnetic column, so any CD4+ or CD8+ T cells bound by antibody are retained in the column while the remainder of the graft passes through freely. Flow cytometry can be used to confirm the presence or absence of T cells. Flow cytometric analysis can be done not only on the T cell depleted graft to confirm the absence of the pan T cell marker, CD3, but analysis can be done on the cells retained in the column to confirm a pure population of T cells. Despite the dogma regarding T cells as the central mediators of GVHD pathology, researchers are now focusing their efforts on the role of B cells during GVHD. Rituximab is a monoclonal antibody directed to CD20, a pan mature B cell marker, and causes B cell depletion by antibody dependent cellular cytotoxicity (ADCC), complement dependent cytotoxicity (CDC), and direct arrest of cellular growth. Studies have shown an amelioration of chronic GVHD in patients who received Rituximab suggesting a prominent role for B cells in the progression of chronic GVHD (Alousi et al., 2010).

4. Analyzing T cell responses during GVHD

4.1 Isolating T cells

To induce murine GVHD, T cells are infused via the tail vein and are immediately propelled into host circulation. Donor lymphocytes rapidly accumulate in host lymphoid tissue and expand within 2-3 days post transplant (Wysocki et al., 2005). At this point, donor lymphocytes can be isolated from either the secondary lymphoid tissue (spleen or lymph nodes) or peripheral blood. Peripheral blood is advantageous because it is not a terminal procedure; however, the lymphocyte yield is lower than that from the spleen or lymph nodes. Lymphocyte counts in the spleen of a naïve mouse can exceed 100 million cells. However, following lethal irradiation and GVHD induction, splenic lymphocyte counts may be limited to as low as 5 million total lymphocytes.

Peripheral blood should be collected using a submandibular bleed. This can be done using a lancet to stick the submandibular vein just before it opens to the jugular vein (Golde et al., 2005). The volume of blood collected should be less than 0.3 mL (Golde et al., 2005). Lymphocyte yield from peripheral blood will likely not exceed 1 million cells; however, yield will vary greatly with the strain combination used, disease state at which the blood was collected, and the volume of blood collected. Blood should be collected in a tube containing heparin (or any other anti-coagulation reagent) and the red blood cells should be lysed. Alternatively, the spleen can be removed following euthanization. The spleen should be minced and made into a single cell suspension and red blood cells should be lysed. Once the red blood cells are lysed, count the remaining lymphocytes and resuspend in FACS Buffer (10% FBS, 0.2% Sodium Azide in PBS).

4.2 Setting up a flow cytometry experiment

For each experiment that will be analyzed using flow cytometry, appropriate controls will need to be included. Those controls consist of a tube containing cells alone and a tube with each antibody alone. The cells alone control tube will allow the flow cytometer to calibrate the size and granularity of the cell population without antibody present. Additional tubes containing lymphocytes and each fluorochrome to be used in the experiment conjugated to an antibody that will positively bind the lymphocyte population (i.e. a positive control) should be added separately. The purpose of these tubes is to calibrate the cytometer to recognize each fluorochrome independently.

Lastly, isotype controls must be included and set up in individual tubes with lymphocytes. Isotypes are antibodies that are specific for an antigen that is not likely to be present on the cell population of interest. The isotype controls account for any non-specific binding of the antibodies of interest and can be helpful in accurately analyzing the data. If the experiment is designed to analyze cell populations of low frequency, it will be helpful to add each non-isotype antibody in addition to adding the isotype control (see example). It is preferable to use the lymphocytes to be used in the experimental tubes for all of the control tubes; however, if this is logistically impossible, alternative lymphocytes can be used.

For flow cytometry, incubate 1 million cells in separate test tubes that are compatible with the flow cytometer to be used with each antibody to be included in the experiment for 30 minutes in the dark at 4 degrees Celsius. During this incubation period, incubate lymphocytes with each positive control tube and isotype controls. After the incubation period, wash off excess antibody with 3 mL of FACS Buffer and resuspend with 300 uL of a fixative solution such as FACS Fix Solution (FACS Buffer with 10% Neutral Buffered Formalin). The cells should be analyzed on a flow cytometer as soon as possible, but can be delayed for up to several days.

Example Experiment: The goal in this example experiment is to identify the percent of naive CD8+ T cells in the spleen 7 days post transplant of 3 mice with GVHD.

- Each mouse is to be euthanized and the spleens are to be removed.
- Mince each spleen and create three single-celled suspensions by passing the spleen through a 40 uM nylon mesh filter.
- Collect each suspension, pellet the cells and lyse the red blood cells.
- Resuspend cells in FACS Buffer, count the cells, and transfer ~1 million cells (volume ~100 uL) into 3 tubes. These tubes will contain the antibodies to analyze the percent of naive CD8+ T cells.
- Combine all remaining cells and transfer ~1 million cells (volume ~100 uL) to 7 tubes. These tubes will make up the positive control and isotype tubes.
- Because we want to know the frequency of naive CD8+ T cells, we will need to stain the cells with 3 different antibodies: 1) CD3e (to identify T cells), 2) CD8a (to identify the CD8 population of T cells), and 3) CD62L (To identify the naive population of CD8+ T cells. Because these are three relatively common antigens, they should be available on a variety of fluorochromes. For this example, we will use CD3e-FITC, CD8a-PE, CD62L-APC. We will also need an isotype matched negative control for each antibody (Hamster IgG1-FITC, Rat IgG2a-PE, Rat IgG2a-APC respectively).
- See Table 2 for detailed experimental set up.
- Three mice were used (Tubes 5-7) so statistical analysis can be done to the flow cytometry data obtained.

4.3 Analyzing T cells from the gut during intestinal GVHD

During the conditioning regimen, the gut is heavily damaged and is a target organ of acute GVHD. Analyses of early T cell trafficking events indicate that T cells are primed against host antigens and migrate to the gut (Wysocki et al., 2005). The degree to which T cells are primed in the Peyer's patches is a controversial matter; however, it is clear that secondary lymphoid tissue in the gut contributes to the perpetuation of donor T cell pathology (Murai

	FITC	*PE*	*APC*
Tube 1	-	-	-
Tube 2	CD4		
Tube 3		CD4	
Tube 4			CD4
Tube 5	CD3e	CD8a	CD62L
Tube 6	CD3e	CD8a	CD62L
Tube 7	CD3e	CD8a	CD62L
Tube 8	Isotype CD3 (Hamp. IgG1)	CD8a	CD62L
Tube 9	CD3e	Isotype CD8a (Rat IgG2a)	CD62L
Tube 10	CD3e	CD8a	Isotype CD62L (Rat IgG2a)

Table 2. Sample of a table which describes the antibodies to be added to each tube

et al., 2003; Welniak et al., 2006). We and others have modified the protocol Isolation of Mouse Small Intestine Intraepithelial Lymphocytes, Peyer's Patch, and Lamina Propria Cells from the *Current Protocols in Immunology* series to isolate and analyze T cells that infiltrate the gut during GVHD. Briefly, the small intestine is removed and flushed with PBS. The Peyer's Patches are removed and the small intestine is cut longitudinally and into ~5 mm sections. Intraepithelial lymphocytes (IELs) and, during GVHD, gut infiltrating lymphocytes (GILs) are isolated from the intestinal sections.

Elegant flow cytometric experiments have been performed using GILs to test hypotheses regarding the role of T cell subsets during GVHD. El-Asady et al. used a competition based mixing experiment to show a role for CD103 in promoting CD8 T cell accumulation in the intestinal epithelium during GVHD. In this experiment, equal numbers of CD8+ T cells from CD90.1 (Thy1.1) congenic mice were mixed with CD8 T cells from a CD103-/- CD90.2 (Thy1.2) mouse and transferred into irradiated recipients. At various time points, GILs were isolated an analyzed for the proportion of CD103-/- CD8+ T cells in the gut compared to the spleen. Their data show that the proportion of CD103-/- CD8+ T cells is lower at day 28 than in earlier time points. This indicates that CD103-/- CD8+ T cells are less efficient in their ability to accumulate in the gut during GVHD suggesting that CD103 plays a significant role in promoting CD8+ T cell accumulation in the gut during GVHD (El-Asady et al., 2005). Furthermore, the T cell receptors on each set of CD8+ T cells is transgenic so that they only recognize an antigen expressed by host cells, thus adding a higher level of sophistication to the experiment and the conclusions that can be drawn from the results.

1. 1B2 is the antibody that binds to the transgenic T cell receptor. 1B2 positive cells indicate they are of donor origin and are specific for host antigens.
2. Thy1.1 (also known as CD90.1) positive cells represent the CD8 T cells that are able to express CD103.
3. The proportion of Thy1.1 cells increases compared to Thy1.1 negative (Thy1.2/CD90.2) cells indicating that CD103 deficient cells are unable to effectively accumulate in the gut during GVHD.
4. CD103-/- CD8 T cells are retained in the spleen with similar efficiency as wild type CD8 T cells.

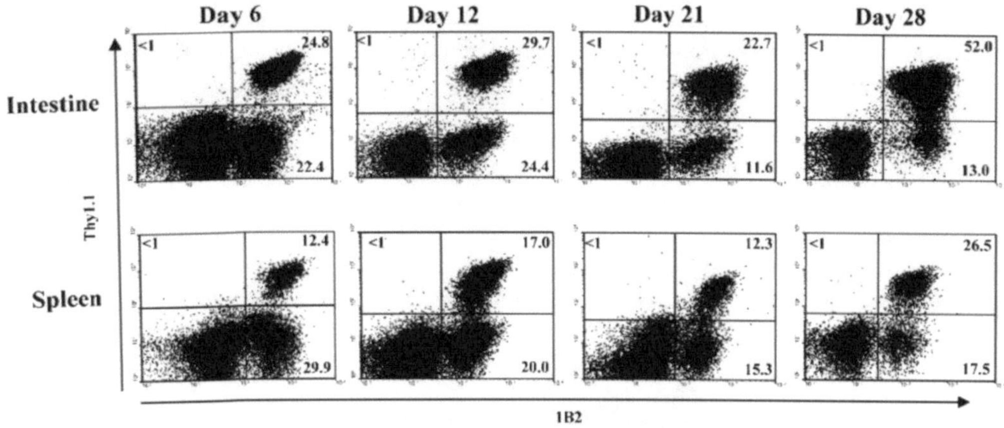

Fig. 2. CD103 promotes retention of CD8+ T cells in the gut during GVHD. Lethally irradiated BALB/c recipients were adoptively transferred with equal numbers ($0.5x10^6$) of donor (2C) CD103-/- (Thy1.2) or wild-type (Thy1.1) CD8+ T cells. Dot plots of 1B2 positive cells plotted against Thy1.1 positive cells show proportion of CD103-/- CD8+ T cells compared with wild-type CD8+ T cells at day 6, 12, 21, and 28. Adapted from El Asady et al., 2005, JEM

4.4 The use of intracellular flow cytometry to monitor T cell responses during GVHD

Intracellular staining for flow cytometry is a valuable technique for testing hypotheses regarding the function of various cell populations in that T cell function can be gleaned from the cytokines produced. To advance experiments in which surface markers are analyzed, cytokines can be probed for and analyzed via flow cytometry. Liu et al. exemplify the use of intracellular flow cytometry to help draw conclusions regarding the function of two T cell populations. In this study, intracellular flow cytometry was performed to compare the cytokine profile of wild type and CD103-/- CD8+ T cells. CD103-/- CD8+ T cells were shown to be equally effective in their ability to clear solid tumors as wild type CD8+ T cells following murine bone marrow transplantation. To confirm that CD103-/- CD8 T cells were mediating tumor clearance, those cells were isolated and the profile of cytokines produced queried (Liu et al., 2011). It was found that in fact CD103-/- CD8+ T cells produce the same levels of various proinflammatory cytokines as wild type CD8+ T cells. Coupling this finding with the finding that CD103-/- CD8 T cell recipients are able to clear tumor with similar efficacy as wild type CD8 T cell recipients leads to the logical conclusion that CD103-/- CD8+ T cells are functionally similar with regard to tumor fighting ability as compared to wild type CD8+ T cells.

4.5 Supplementing flow cytometry with bioluminescent imaging

Bioluminescent imaging (BLI) is a technique that utilizes the light as a product of the chemical reaction between the enzyme luciferase and its substrate luciferin. Luciferase is a gene naturally expressed by fireflies and is responsible for their characteristic green glow. The luciferase gene has been inserted into the murine genome on the B6 background generating a mouse that constitutively expresses luciferase (Cao et al., 2005). T cell populations have been purified and transferred with luciferase negative cell populations for induction of GVHD. Immediately following the administration of luciferin to GVHD recipients, recipients can be imaged in a charged coupled device (CCD) camera and a pseudo-colored image can be generated (Figure 3).

The non-invasive nature of BLI allows its use to supplement data generated via flow cytometry. Determining the cell source for lymphocyte isolation and analysis by flow cytometry is driven by hypothesis testing and historical results. By utilizing BLI, researchers can determine the anatomical location of T cell accumulation in real time and can isolate T cells based on their accumulation patterns rather than being restricted to analyzing experimental animals at specific time points and specific compartments.

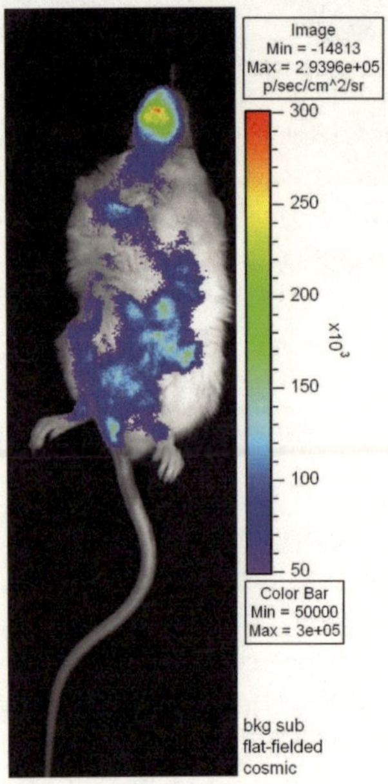

Fig. 3. Bioluminescent imaging as a supplement to flow cytometry: Lethally irradiated BALB/c recipients were adoptively transferred with 10^7 wild-type splenocytes and $2x10^6$ luciferase positive CD8+ T cells. A representative mouse is shown following 4 mg D-luciferin injection and imaging in Xenogen IVIS CCD camera for 5 minutes

5. GHVD treatments

5.1 Prophylactic treatment

In the absence of GVHD prophylaxis, the incidence of acute GVHD is nearly 100% (Sullivan et al., 1986). Prophylactic treatment with methotrexate results in a substantial decrease in the incidence of acute GVHD (Storb et al., 1974). Methotrexate - originally used as a chemotherapeutic agent - acts to inhibit folic acid metabolism and the cellular result is the inability to synthesize DNA; thus, resulting in inhibition of cellular proliferation. Treatments with calcineurin inhibitors (cyclosporine and tacrolimus) are more efficacious in preventing GVHD. Calcineurin inhibitors act to block the action of the transcription factor nuclear factor of activated T cells (NFAT) (Crabtree, 1989; Shaw et al.,1988). Prophylactic use of calcineurin inhibitors with low dose methotrexate results in as low as 20% GVHD incidence following bone marrow transplant (Nash et al., 1996; Storb et al., 1986). Flow cytometry can be used to monitor T cell responses following preventative treatment with methotrexate and/or calcineurin inhibitors. In murine models, carboxyfluorescein succinimidyl ester (CFSE) is used to monitor T cell proliferation by flow cytometry. CFSE is a fluorescent dye that is able to traverse cell membranes. CFSE is taken up by cells prior to adoptive transfer. As cells divide, CFSE is equally divided between daughter cells, so when cells are monitored by flow cytometry, cells that have gone through several rounds of divisions have markedly less CFSE than cells that have not proliferated.

5.2 Treatment of established GVHD

The primary treatment for established GVHD is the use of corticosteroids (Koreth & Antin, 2008). Binding of corticosteroids to their receptors on immune cells causes the upregulation of anti-inflammatory transcription factors and a suppression of the immune system. Although corticosteroids are ineffective prophylactically, their use for treatment of ongoing GVHD is widely established and effective (Chao et al., 2000). Intracellular flow cytometry can be used to track the production of pro- or anti-inflammatory cytokines following corticosteroid treatment. Other treatments for establish GVHD include mycophenolate mofetil (MMF) and sirolimus (also called rapamycin), but have yet to supplant corticosteroids as the gold standard for treatment of established GVHD. Patients with disease progression after three days of corticosteroid treatment or patients that do not show improvement after seven days of corticosteroid treatment are considered to be steroid-refractory and are treated with a more intense regimen. Such therapies include the use of monoclonal antibodies aimed to deplete T cell subsets. Monoclonal antibodies and/or fusion proteins can be used to block the action of proinflammatory cytokines. The efficacy of treatments for steroid-refractory GVHD is limited by lack of effectiveness or the high incidence of severe side effects.

5.3 Prospective therapeutic approach

Current prophylactic therapies of ongoing GVHD target a broad spectrum of cell types, and thus substantially inhibit post transplant immunity. Immunotherapies specifically targeted to GVHD-causing T cells are desirable. In mice, blockade of integrins expressed on T cells has been shown to be effective in preventing GVHD, while maintaining the beneficial properties of T cells post transplant (El-Asady et al., 2005; Liu et al., 2011). Waldman et al. has shown that the absence of the B7 integrin family on donor T cells results in reduced GVHD morbidity and mortality without compromising GVT effects (Waldman et al., 2006). Similarly, CD8+ T cells deficient in their ability to express CD103 are unable to induce GVHD, but maintain immunity to solid tumors (Lui et al., 2011). Flow cytometric sorting techniques can be used to selectively deplete T cells that express certain markers prior to transplantation. Cells are sorted based on fluorescence, so unbound cells are retained separately from cells bound by antibodies. This technique creates highly pure populations of cells of a given phenotype. Because proteins are expressed on T cell surfaces transiently and their expression is a dynamic process, cell sorting is limited to sorting cells based on their phenotype when analyzed. However, despite this limitation, the applications for flow cytometric sorting are vast due to the high throughput and accuracy with which cells are sorted.

Graft engineering is another therapeutic approach that has the potential to maintain post transplant immunity while preventing GVHD. Graft engineering is the idea of selectively depleting the mature donor T cell population of potentially pathogenic cells. The non-pathogenic cells are retained in the graft and are able to promote engraftment, post-transplant immunity, and GVT/GVL effects. Alternatively, T cells can be broadly depleted and repopulated with ex vivo expanded T cells that are specific for a particular tumor or microbial antigen. Several studies have demonstrated the ability to deplete alloreactive T cells or expand and adoptively transfer T cells specific for tumor (Verneris et al., 2001; Amrolia et al., 2004). Flow cytometry plays an important role in differentiating between tumor/pathogen reactive and alloreactive T cell populations. Because the sequences of many antigenic epitopes are known, synthetic peptides can be developed and conjugated to fluorochromes to be used for flow cytometry. T cells specific for the synthetic peptide bind their cognate antigen-fluorochrome complex and their frequency can be identified. Moreover, flow cytometric sorting techniques are able to remove these antigen-specific T cells from the graft. For ex vivo expansion of pathogen or tumor specific antigens, this application of flow cytometry is used to test the purity of the ex vivo expanded T cell population.

To broadly suppress GVHD, Tregs can be expanded ex vivo and adoptively transferred into bone marrow transplant recipients. Until recently, adoptive transfer of Tregs was confined to murine models; however, in 2011, Tregs were expanded ex vivo and adoptively transferred into bone marrow transplant recipients (Brunstein et al., 2011). Suppression of the ex vivo expanded Treg population was confirmed in vitro and following adoptive transfer the incidence rate of acute GVHD was significantly lower in patients who received Tregs (Brunstein et al., 2011). In mice, several groups have reported that adoptive transfer of Tregs can reduce GVHD incidence and severity (Edinger et al., 2003; Taylor et al., 2002). Tregs act to reduce GVHD by inhibiting proinflammatory effector responses by donor T cells, but interestingly, addition of exogenous Tregs does not inhibit GVL effects in mice (Edinger et al., 2003).

5.4 Concluding remarks

Current prophylactic and first-line therapies for GVHD are limited due to the breadth of immune suppression. Global immunosuppressive approaches limit the beneficial properties of T cells post transplant. The use of engineered grafts is an exciting therapeutic approach as it has the potential to separate GVHD from the beneficial GVL effects. Adoptive transfer of ex vivo expanded Tregs also has the potential to separate GVHD from GVL and has been shown to ameliorate GVHD in bone marrow transplant recipients. Innovative advances in the ability to modify T cell subsets have opened the door to novel therapeutic approaches to preventing GVHD without attenuating GVL effects.

In addition to facilitating the determination of efficacy of GVHD therapies, flow cytometry plays a central role in GVHD research. Flow cytometry aids researchers by allowing accurate identification of cellular phenotypes and cytokine profiles of cell populations involved in disease. GVHD remains the limiting factor to the broad use of bone marrow transplants as a curative therapy for hematological disorders. Flow cytometry is a valuable tool with a variety of applications to help separate GVHD from the beneficial properties of T cells post transplant.

6. References

Alousi AM, Uberti J, Ratanatharathorn V. The role of B cell depleting therapy in graft versus host disease after allogeneic hematopoietic cell transplant. *Leuk Lymphoma,* Vol. 51, No. 3, (2010/02/10), pp. 376-389, 1029-2403

Amrolia PJ, Muccioli-Casadei G, Huls H et al. (2006). Adoptive immunotherapy with allodepleted donor T-cells improves immune reconstitution after haploidentical stem cell transplantation. *Blood,* Vol. 108, No. 6, (2006/06/03), pp. 1797-1808, 0006-4971

Anderson BE, McNiff J, Yan J et al. (2003). Memory CD4+ T cells do not induce graft-versus-host disease. *J Clin Invest,* Vol. 112, No. 1, (2003/07/04), pp. 101-108, 0021-9738

Ball LM, Egeler RM. (2008). Acute GvHD: pathogenesis and classification. *Bone Marrow Transplant,* Vol. 41 Suppl 2, No. (2008/07/24), pp. S58-64, 0268-3369

Bautista G, Cabrera JR, Regidor C et al. (2009). Cord blood transplants supported by co-infusion of mobilized hematopoietic stem cells from a third-party donor. *Bone Marrow Transplant,* Vol. 43, No. 5, (2008/10/14), pp. 365-373, 1476-5365

Berger M, Wettstein PJ, Korngold R. (1994). T cell subsets involved in lethal graft-versus-host disease directed to immunodominant minor histocompatibility antigens. *Transplantation,* Vol. 57, No. 7, (1994/04/15), pp. 1095-1102, 0041-1337

Billingham RE. (1966). The biology of graft-versus-host reactions. *Harvey Lect,* Vol. 62, No. (1966/01/01), pp. 21-78, 0073-0874

Brunstein CG, Miller JS, Cao Q et al. Infusion of ex vivo expanded T regulatory cells in adults transplanted with umbilical cord blood: safety profile and detection kinetics. *Blood,* Vol. 117, No. 3, (2010/10/19), pp. 1061-1070, 1528-0020

Campbell DJ, Butcher EC. (2002). Rapid acquisition of tissue-specific homing phenotypes by CD4(+) T cells activated in cutaneous or mucosal lymphoid tissues. *J Exp Med,* Vol. 195, No. 1, (2002/01/10), pp. 135-141, 0022-1007

Cao YA, Bachmann MH, Beilhack A et al. (2005). Molecular imaging using labeled donor tissues reveals patterns of engraftment, rejection, and survival in transplantation. *Transplantation,* Vol. 80, No. 1, (2005/07/09), pp. 134-139, 0041-1337

Carlson MJ, West ML, Coghill JM, Panoskaltsis-Mortari A, Blazar BR, Serody JS. (2009). In vitro-differentiated TH17 cells mediate lethal acute graft-versus-host disease with severe cutaneous and pulmonary pathologic manifestations. *Blood,* Vol. 113, No. 6, (2008/10/30), pp. 1365-1374, 1528-0020

Cepek KL, Shaw SK, Parker CM et al. (1994). Adhesion between epithelial cells and T lymphocytes mediated by E-cadherin and the alpha E beta 7 integrin. *Nature,* Vol. 372, No. 6502, (1994/11/10), pp. 190-193, 0028-0836

Cerf-Bensussan N, Jarry A, Brousse N, Lisowska-Grospierre B, Guy-Grand D, Griscelli C. (1987). A monoclonal antibody (HML-1) defining a novel membrane molecule present on human intestinal lymphocytes. *Eur J Immunol,* Vol. 17, No. 9, (1987/09/01), pp. 1279-1285, 0014-2980

Chang RJ, Lee SH. (1986). Effects of interferon-gamma and tumor necrosis factor-alpha on the expression of an Ia antigen on a murine macrophage cell line. *J Immunol,* Vol. 137, No. 9, (1986/11/01), pp. 2853-2856, 0022-1767

Chao NJ, Snyder DS, Jain M et al. (2000). Equivalence of 2 effective graft-versus-host disease prophylaxis regimens: results of a prospective double-blind randomized trial. *Biol Blood Marrow Transplant,* Vol. 6, No. 3, (2000/06/28), pp. 254-261, 1083-8791

Chen BJ, Cui X, Sempowski GD, Liu C, Chao NJ. (2004). Transfer of allogeneic CD62L- memory T cells without graft-versus-host disease. *Blood,* Vol. 103, No. 4, (2003/10/11), pp. 1534-1541, 0006-4971

Choi EY, Yoshimura Y, Christianson GJ et al. (2001). Quantitative analysis of the immune response to mouse non-MHC transplantation antigens in vivo: the H60 histocompatibility antigen dominates over all others. *J Immunol,* Vol. 166, No. 7, (2001/03/20), pp. 4370-4379, 0022-1767

Crabtree GR. (1989). Contingent genetic regulatory events in T lymphocyte activation. *Science,* Vol. 243, No. 4889, (1989/01/20), pp. 355-361, 0036-8075

Dutt S, Tseng D, Ermann J et al. (2007). Naive and memory T cells induce different types of graft-versus-host disease. *J Immunol,* Vol. 179, No. 10, (2007/11/06), pp. 6547-6554, 0022-1767

Edinger M, Hoffmann P, Ermann J et al. (2003). CD4+CD25+ regulatory T cells preserve graft-versus-tumor activity while inhibiting graft-versus-host disease after bone marrow transplantation. *Nat Med,* Vol. 9, No. 9, (2003/08/20), pp. 1144-1150, 1078-8956

El-Asady R, Yuan R, Liu K et al. (2005). TGF-{beta}-dependent CD103 expression by CD8(+) T cells promotes selective destruction of the host intestinal epithelium during graft-versus-host disease. *J Exp Med,* Vol. 201, No. 10, (2005/05/18), pp. 1647-1657, 0022-1007

Esposito M, Ruffini F, Bergami A et al. IL-17- and IFN-gamma-secreting Foxp3+ T cells infiltrate the target tissue in experimental autoimmunity. *J Immunol,* Vol. 185, No. 12, (2010/11/26), pp. 7467-7473, 1550-6606

Ferrara JL, Levy R, Chao NJ. (1999). Pathophysiologic mechanisms of acute graft-vs.-host disease. *Biol Blood Marrow Transplant,* Vol. 5, No. 6, (1999/12/14), pp. 347-356, 1083-8791

Fowler DH, Breglio J, Nagel G, Hirose C, Gress RE. (1996). Allospecific CD4+, Th1/Th2 and CD8+, Tc1/Tc2 populations in murine GVL: type I cells generate GVL and type II cells abrogate GVL. *Biol Blood Marrow Transplant,* Vol. 2, No. 3, (1996/10/01), pp. 118-125, 1083-8791

Friedman TM, Gilbert M, Briggs C, Korngold R. (1998). Repertoire analysis of CD8+ T cell responses to minor histocompatibility antigens involved in graft-versus-host disease. *J Immunol,* Vol. 161, No. 1, (1998/07/01), pp. 41-48, 0022-1767

Golde WT, Gollobin P, Rodriguez LL. (2005). A rapid, simple, and humane method for submandibular bleeding of mice using a lancet. *Lab Anim (NY),* Vol. 34, No. 9, (2005/10/01), pp. 39-43, 0093-7355

Goulmy E, Schipper R, Pool J et al. (1996). Mismatches of minor histocompatibility antigens between HLA-identical donors and recipients and the development of graft-versus-host disease after bone marrow transplantation. *N Engl J Med,* Vol. 334, No. 5, (1996/02/01), pp. 281-285, 0028-4793

Gran B, Zhang GX, Yu S et al. (2002). IL-12p35-deficient mice are susceptible to experimental autoimmune encephalomyelitis: evidence for redundancy in the IL-12 system in the induction of central nervous system autoimmune demyelination. *J Immunol,* Vol. 169, No. 12, (2002/12/10), pp. 7104-7110, 0022-1767

Gunn D, Akuche C, Baryza J et al. (2005). 4,5-Disubstituted cis-pyrrolidinones as inhibitors of type II 17beta-hydroxysteroid dehydrogenase. Part 2. SAR. *Bioorg Med Chem Lett,* Vol. 15, No. 12, (2005/05/14), pp. 3053-3057, 0960-894X

Gutcher I, Urich E, Wolter K, Prinz M, Becher B. (2006). Interleukin 18-independent engagement of interleukin 18 receptor-alpha is required for autoimmune inflammation. *Nat Immunol,* Vol. 7, No. 9, (2006/08/15), pp. 946-953, 1529-2908

Hoffmann P, Ermann J, Edinger M, Fathman CG, Strober S. (2002). Donor-type CD4(+)CD25(+) regulatory T cells suppress lethal acute graft-versus-host disease after allogeneic bone marrow transplantation. *J Exp Med,* Vol. 196, No. 3, (2002/08/07), pp. 389-399, 0022-1007

Hori S, Nomura T, Sakaguchi S. (2003). Control of regulatory T cell development by the transcription factor Foxp3. *Science,* Vol. 299, No. 5609, (2003/01/11), pp. 1057-1061, 1095-9203

Horowitz MM, Gale RP, Sondel PM et al. (1990). Graft-versus-leukemia reactions after bone marrow transplantation. *Blood,* Vol. 75, No. 3, (1990/02/01), pp. 555-562, 0006-4971

Huehn J, Siegmund K, Lehmann JC et al. (2004). Developmental stage, phenotype, and migration distinguish naive- and effector/memory-like CD4+ regulatory T cells. *J Exp Med,* Vol. 199, No. 3, (2004/02/06), pp. 303-313, 0022-1007

Johansson-Lindbom B, Agace WW. (2007). Generation of gut-homing T cells and their localization to the small intestinal mucosa. *Immunol Rev,* Vol. 215, No. (2007/02/13), pp. 226-242, 0105-2896

Johansson-Lindbom B, Svensson M, Wurbel MA, Malissen B, Marquez G, Agace W. (2003). Selective generation of gut tropic T cells in gut-associated lymphoid tissue (GALT): requirement for GALT dendritic cells and adjuvant. *J Exp Med,* Vol. 198, No. 6, (2003/09/10), pp. 963-969, 0022-1007

Johnson BD, Konkol MC, Truitt RL. (2002). CD25+ immunoregulatory T-cells of donor origin suppress alloreactivity after BMT. *Biol Blood Marrow Transplant,* Vol. 8, No. 10, (2002/11/19), pp. 525-535, 1083-8791

JP OK, Kociban DL, Buffo MJ. (1990). Comparative effects of various T cell subtypes on GVHD in a murine model for MHC-matched unrelated donor transplant. *Bone Marrow Transplant,* Vol. 5, No. 3, (1990/03/01), pp. 145-152, 0268-3369

Keino H, Masli S, Sasaki S, Streilein JW, Stein-Streilein J. (2006). CD8+ T regulatory cells use a novel genetic program that includes CD103 to suppress Th1 immunity in eye-derived tolerance. *Invest Ophthalmol Vis Sci,* Vol. 47, No. 4, (2006/03/28), pp. 1533-1542, 0146-0404

Koch SD, Uss E, van Lier RA, ten Berge IJ. (2008). Alloantigen-induced regulatory CD8+CD103+ T cells. *Hum Immunol,* Vol. 69, No. 11, (2008/09/30), pp. 737-744, 0198-8859

Korbling M, Anderlini P. (2001). Peripheral blood stem cell versus bone marrow allotransplantation: does the source of hematopoietic stem cells matter? *Blood,* Vol. 98, No. 10, (2001/11/08), pp. 2900-2908, 0006-4971

Koreth J, Antin JH. (2008). Current and future approaches for control of graft-versus-host disease. *Expert Rev Hematol,* Vol. 1, No. 1, (2008/10/23), pp. 111, 1747-4094

Krakowski M, Owens T. (1996). Interferon-gamma confers resistance to experimental allergic encephalomyelitis. *Eur J Immunol,* Vol. 26, No. 7, (1996/07/01), pp. 1641-1646, 0014-2980

Kurz SK, Reddehase MJ. (1999). Patchwork pattern of transcriptional reactivation in the lungs indicates sequential checkpoints in the transition from murine cytomegalovirus latency to recurrence. *J Virol,* Vol. 73, No. 10, (1999/09/11), pp. 8612-8622, 0022-538X

Lehmann J, Huehn J, de la Rosa M et al. (2002). Expression of the integrin alpha Ebeta 7 identifies unique subsets of CD25+ as well as CD25- regulatory T cells. *Proc Natl Acad Sci U S A,* Vol. 99, No. 20, (2002/09/21), pp. 13031-13036, 0027-8424

Liu K, Anthony BA, Yearsly MM et al. CD103 deficiency prevents graft-versus-host disease but spares graft-versus-tumor effects mediated by alloreactive CD8 T cells. *PLoS One,* Vol. 6, No. 7, (2011/07/23), pp. e21968, 1932-6203

Mora JR, Bono MR, Manjunath N et al. (2003). Selective imprinting of gut-homing T cells by Peyer's patch dendritic cells. *Nature,* Vol. 424, No. 6944, (2003/07/04), pp. 88-93, 1476-4687

Morris ES, MacDonald KP, Hill GR. (2006). Stem cell mobilization with G-CSF analogs: a rational approach to separate GVHD and GVL? *Blood,* Vol. 107, No. 9, (2005/12/29), pp. 3430-3435, 0006-4971

Murai M, Yoneyama H, Ezaki T et al. (2003). Peyer's patch is the essential site in initiating murine acute and lethal graft-versus-host reaction. *Nat Immunol,* Vol. 4, No. 2, (2003/01/14), pp. 154-160, 1529-2908

Muramatsu K, Kuriyama R, Kato H, Yoshida Y, Taguchi T. Prolonged survival of experimental extremity allografts: a new protocol with total body irradiation, granulocyte-colony stimulation factor, and FK506. *J Orthop Res,* Vol. 28, No. 4, (2009/10/31), pp. 457-461, 1554-527X

Nagler A, Condiotti R, Nabet C et al. (1998). Selective CD4+ T-cell depletion does not prevent graft-versus-host disease. *Transplantation,* Vol. 66, No. 1, (1998/07/29), pp. 138-141, 0041-1337

Nash RA, Pineiro LA, Storb R et al. (1996). FK506 in combination with methotrexate for the prevention of graft-versus-host disease after marrow transplantation from matched unrelated donors. *Blood,* Vol. 88, No. 9, (1996/11/01), pp. 3634-3641, 0006-4971

Nimer SD, Giorgi J, Gajewski JL et al. (1994). Selective depletion of CD8+ cells for prevention of graft-versus-host disease after bone marrow transplantation. A randomized controlled trial. *Transplantation,* Vol. 57, No. 1, (1994/01/01), pp. 82-87, 0041-1337

Park M, Koh KN, Kim BE et al. The impact of HLA matching on unrelated donor hematopoietic stem cell transplantation in Korean children. *Korean J Hematol,* Vol. 46, No. 1, (2011/04/05), pp. 11-17, 2092-9129

Pober JS, Orosz CG, Rose ML, Savage CO. (1996). Can graft endothelial cells initiate a host anti-graft immune response? *Transplantation,* Vol. 61, No. 3, (1996/02/15), pp. 343-349, 0041-1337

Reddy P. (2003). Pathophysiology of acute graft-versus-host disease. *Hematol Oncol,* Vol. 21, No. 4, (2004/01/22), pp. 149-161, 0278-0232

Riddell SR, Watanabe KS, Goodrich JM, Li CR, Agha ME, Greenberg PD. (1992). Restoration of viral immunity in immunodeficient humans by the adoptive transfer of T cell clones. *Science,* Vol. 257, No. 5067, (1992/07/10), pp. 238-241, 0036-8075

Shaw JP, Utz PJ, Durand DB, Toole JJ, Emmel EA, Crabtree GR. (1988). Identification of a putative regulator of early T cell activation genes. *Science,* Vol. 241, No. 4862, (1988/07/08), pp. 202-205, 0036-8075

Shlomchik WD. (2007). Graft-versus-host disease. *Nat Rev Immunol,* Vol. 7, No. 5, (2007/04/18), pp. 340-352, 1474-1733

Shlomchik WD, Couzens MS, Tang CB et al. (1999). Prevention of graft versus host disease by inactivation of host antigen-presenting cells. *Science*, Vol. 285, No. 5426, (1999/07/20), pp. 412-415, 0036-8075

Sondel PM, Buhtoiarov IN, DeSantes K. (2003). Pleasant memories: remembering immune protection while forgetting about graft-versus-host disease. *J Clin Invest*, Vol. 112, No. 1, (2003/07/04), pp. 25-27, 0021-9738

Sprent J, Schaefer M, Korngold R. (1990). Role of T cell subsets in lethal graft-versus-host disease (GVHD) directed to class I versus class II H-2 differences. II. Protective effects of L3T4+ cells in anti-class II GVHD. *J Immunol*, Vol. 144, No. 8, (1990/04/15), pp. 2946-2954, 0022-1767

Stagg AJ, Kamm MA, Knight SC. (2002). Intestinal dendritic cells increase T cell expression of alpha4beta7 integrin. *Eur J Immunol*, Vol. 32, No. 5, (2002/05/01), pp. 1445-1454, 0014-2980

Storb R, Deeg HJ, Whitehead J et al. (1986). Methotrexate and cyclosporine compared with cyclosporine alone for prophylaxis of acute graft versus host disease after marrow transplantation for leukemia. *N Engl J Med*, Vol. 314, No. 12, (1986/03/20), pp. 729-735, 0028-4793

Storb R, Gluckman E, Thomas ED et al. (1974). Treatment of established human graft-versus-host disease by antithymocyte globulin. *Blood*, Vol. 44, No. 1, (1974/07/01), pp. 56-75, 0006-4971

Sullivan KM, Deeg HJ, Sanders J et al. (1986). Hyperacute graft-v-host disease in patients not given immunosuppression after allogeneic marrow transplantation. *Blood*, Vol. 67, No. 4, (1986/04/01), pp. 1172-1175, 0006-4971

Swain SL, Bradley LM, Croft M et al. (1991). Helper T-cell subsets: phenotype, function and the role of lymphokines in regulating their development. *Immunol Rev*, Vol. 123, No. (1991/10/01), pp. 115-144, 0105-2896

Taylor PA, Lees CJ, Blazar BR. (2002). The infusion of ex vivo activated and expanded CD4(+)CD25(+) immune regulatory cells inhibits graft-versus-host disease lethality. *Blood*, Vol. 99, No. 10, (2002/05/03), pp. 3493-3499, 0006-4971

Teshima T, Ordemann R, Reddy P et al. (2002). Acute graft-versus-host disease does not require alloantigen expression on host epithelium. *Nat Med*, Vol. 8, No. 6, (2002/06/04), pp. 575-581, 1078-8956

Verneris MR, Ito M, Baker J, Arshi A, Negrin RS, Shizuru JA. (2001). Engineering hematopoietic grafts: purified allogeneic hematopoietic stem cells plus expanded CD8+ NK-T cells in the treatment of lymphoma. *Biol Blood Marrow Transplant*, Vol. 7, No. 10, (2002/01/05), pp. 532-542, 1083-8791

Wakely E, Oberholser JH, Corry RJ. (1990). Elimination of acute GVHD and prolongation of rat pancreas allograft survival with DST cyclosporine, and spleen transplantation. *Transplantation*, Vol. 49, No. 2, (1990/02/01), pp. 241-245, 0041-1337

Waldman E, Lu SX, Hubbard VM et al. (2006). Absence of beta7 integrin results in less graft-versus-host disease because of decreased homing of alloreactive T cells to intestine. *Blood*, Vol. 107, No. 4, (2005/11/18), pp. 1703-1711, 0006-4971

Welniak LA, Kuprash DV, Tumanov AV et al. (2006). Peyer patches are not required for acute graft-versus-host disease after myeloablative conditioning and murine allogeneic bone marrow transplantation. *Blood*, Vol. 107, No. 1, (2005/09/15), pp. 410-412, 0006-4971

Wysocki CA, Panoskaltsis-Mortari A, Blazar BR, Serody JS. (2005). Leukocyte migration and graft-versus-host disease. *Blood,* Vol. 105, No. 11, (2005/02/11), pp. 4191-4199, 0006-4971

Zhang GX, Gran B, Yu S et al. (2003). Induction of experimental autoimmune encephalomyelitis in IL-12 receptor-beta 2-deficient mice: IL-12 responsiveness is not required in the pathogenesis of inflammatory demyelination in the central nervous system. *J Immunol,* Vol. 170, No. 4, (2003/02/08), pp. 2153-2160, 0022-1767

Zhang Y, Joe G, Hexner E, Zhu J, Emerson SG. (2005). Host-reactive CD8+ memory stem cells in graft-versus-host disease. *Nat Med,* Vol. 11, No. 12, (2005/11/17), pp. 1299-1305, 1078-8956

Zhang Y, Joe G, Hexner E, Zhu J, Emerson SG. (2005). Alloreactive memory T cells are responsible for the persistence of graft-versus-host disease. *J Immunol,* Vol. 174, No. 5, (2005/02/25), pp. 3051-3058, 0022-1767

Zhao D, Zhang C, Yi T et al. (2008). In vivo-activated CD103+CD4+ regulatory T cells ameliorate ongoing chronic graft-versus-host disease. *Blood,* Vol. 112, No. 5, (2008/06/14), pp. 2129-2138, 1528-0020

Zhu J, Zhang Y, Joe GJ, Pompetti R, Emerson SG. (2005). NF-Ya activates multiple hematopoietic stem cell (HSC) regulatory genes and promotes HSC self-renewal. *Proc Natl Acad Sci U S A,* Vol. 102, No. 33, (2005/08/06), pp. 11728-11733, 0027-8424

10

Lymphocyte Apoptosis, Proliferation and Cytokine Synthesis Pattern in Children with *Helicobacter pylori* Infection

Anna Helmin-Basa et al.*
Department of Immunology,
Collegium Medicum Nicolaus Copernicus University, Bydgoszcz,
Poland

1. Introduction

Helicobacter pylori (H. pylori) infection is usually acquired in early childhood. The majority of the infected children do not suffer from acute inflammatory complications and a few develop severe diseases such as peptic ulcer (Queiroz et al., 1991), mucosal atrophy, gastric carcinoma or MALT lymphoma (Guarner et al., 2003). The cellular basis for the mild gastric inflammatory changes in children with *H. pylori* infection is poorly understood. The few available studies in the *H. pylori*-infected children have revealed low expression of proinflammatory cytokines in the gastric mucosa (Bontems et al., 2003; Lopes et al., 2005), a rather low humoral systemic immune response manifested by *H. pylori*-specific IgG and IgA antibodies (Soares et al., 2005), and a high local Treg cell response (Harris et al., 2008).

In contrast to some studies on circulating T-lymphocyte distribution and activation in pediatric *H. pylori* infection (Helmin-Basa et al., 2011, Soares et al., 2005), estimation of apoptosis in different T lymphocyte subpopulations has not been evaluated separately in the peripheral blood of *H. pylori*-infected and non-infected children with gastritis. There is also the paucity of information regarding the *H. pylori*-specific peripheral cellular responses to live *H. pylori* carrying the cagA gene (*H. pylori cagA*+) which encodes an immunodominant 120-128 kD protein in the pediatric group.

As in the case of other intestinal microflora, *H. pylori* colonization of gastric mucosa results in a close and permanent bacterial contact with gut-associated lymphoid tissues (Acheson &

* Lidia Gackowska[1], Izabela Kubiszewska[1], Malgorzata Wyszomirska-Golda[1], Andrzej Eljaszewicz[1], Grazyna Mierzwa[2], Anna Szaflarska-Poplawska[3], Mieczyslawa Czerwionka-Szaflarska[2], Andrzej Marszalek[4] and Jacek Michalkiewicz[1,5]

[1]*Department of Immunology/ Collegium Medicum Nicolaus Copernicus University, Bydgoszcz, Poland*

[2]*Department of Pediatrics, Allergology and Gastroenterology/Collegium Medicum Nicolaus Copernicus University, Bydgoszcz, Poland*

[3]*Department of Pediatric Endoscopy and Gastrointestinal Function Testing/Collegium Medicum Nicolaus Copernicus University, Bydgoszcz, Poland*

[4]*Department of Clinical Pathomorphology/Collegium Medicum Nicolaus Copernicus University, Bydgoszcz, Poland*

[5]*Department of Clinical Microbiology and Immunology/Children's Memorial Hospital, Warsaw, Poland*

Luccioli, 2004). It leads to the stimulation of specific T cell responses induced by bacterial antigens, presented to the T cells by bacteria-loaded dendritic cells. This route of immunization leads to the generation of a T cell memory pool that is able to recognize a broad spectrum of bacterial antigens and that accumulates mainly in the lamina propria of the gastric mucosa (Hatz et al., 1996). However, because at least a part of this T cell population also enters the circulation the peripheral blood mononuclear cells (PBMCs) contain "memory" T cells which can respond by proliferation and cytokine expression to numerous bacterial microflora antigens, including entire *H. pylori* cells or their various products (Jacob et al., 2001; Windle et al., 2005). Since the presence of the *cagA* gene in *H. pylori* strains has commonly been associated with strong pro-inflammatory action (Peek et al., 1995), the *H. pylori cagA*+ strains were used here as PBMC inducers in order to stimulate lymphocyte apoptosis, proliferation, and cytokine expression. To the best of our knowledge this is the first report in which *H. pylori cagA*+ strains were used as PBMC stimulators in *H. pylori*-infected and noninfected children with gastritis. The PBMC model system has been used extensively for testing the immunomodulatory properties of a broad array of both Gram-positive and Gram-negative bacteria and their products, such as lipopolysaccharide (LPS), peptidoglycans and teichoic acid (Hessle et al., 1999, 2000; Karlsson et al., 2002). Using a PBMC model system, we studied live *H. pylori cagA*+-mediated acquired and innate cellular responses in children with gastritis. Innate responses included IL-12p40, IFN-gamma, TNF-alpha, IL-6 and IL-10 secretion levels, and the acquired response was assessed by *H. pylori*-induced lymphocyte proliferation. Since immune responses are strictly associated with lymphocyte apoptosis; therefore, the spontaneous and *H. pylori*-induced lymphocyte apoptosis were also tested.

The aim of this study was to assess the distribution and apoptosis of the most prevalent lymphocytes' subpopulations in the blood, and in addition to evaluate *H. pylori*-induced lymphocyte apoptosis, proliferation, and cytokine synthesis pattern (IL-12p40, IFN-gamma, TNF-alpha, IL-6 and IL-10) in *H. pylori*-infected and noninfected children with gastritis with the goal of comparing the results with those obtained from the control group formed by dyspeptic noninfected patients without gastritis.

2. Materials and methods

2.1 Patients

The study was undertaken according to Helsinki declaration with approval from the ethics committee of Collegium Medicum Nicolaus Copernicus University in Bydgoszcz, Poland. Informed consent was obtained from all the parents of patients and patients older than 16 years of age.

A total of 136 consecutive subjects older than 8 years of age with dyspeptic symptoms and residing in the Kuivia-Pomeranin district of Poland were included in this study. Exclusion criteria included: 1) previous diagnosis of other inflammatory disease, such as celiac disease, inflammatory bowel disease or allergy; 2) gastric perforation or hemorrhage, history of surgery, bleeding disorders, or evidence of other clinical conditions or intestinal parasites.

Each subject underwent an endoscopic examination of the upper part of the gastrointestinal tract as a result of reporting permanent abdominal pain. Three antral biopsies were taken from each patient. One biopsy specimen was subjected to a rapid urease test; the other two specimens were formalin-fixed and embedded in paraffin, sectioned and stained with hematoxylin and eosin for histological analysis, and Giemsa modified by Gray stain for *H. pylori* detection. Biopsy specimens were graded for gastritis by two independent pathologists according to the updated Sydney system. The histological variables (the presence and density of mononuclear and polymorphonuclear cells, glandular mucosa atrophy, intestinal metaplasia, and *H. pylori* colonization) were scored on a four-point scale: 0, none; 1, mild; 2, moderate; and 3, marked.

The urease test was performed in every patient. *H. pylori* infection was also excluded in every subject by performing the [^{13}C] urea breath test within one week of undergoing endoscopy. ^{13}C concentration was measured with an infra-red radiation analyzer (OLYMPUS Fanci 2) with 4‰ assumed as the cutoff point.

A patient was considered *H. pylori*-infected when the [^{13}C] urea breath test plus either the rapid urease test or microscopic evaluation were positive for *H. pylori*. When the results of all three tests were negative a patient was considered noninfected. Fifty-nine patients fulfilled the criteria for *H. pylori* positivity, while 77 patients fulfilled the criteria for *H. pylori* negativity. None of the patients had ulcer disease or macroscopic lesions of the duodenal mucosa in endoscopic examination.

Patients were divided into three groups:

1. Control group - 15 children (7 boys and 8 girls) aged 8-15 years (median age 14 years) without gastritis on histological examination and without *H. pylori* infection;
2. Noninfected children with gastritis (*Hp-*) - 62 children (20 boys and 42 girls) aged 8-18 years (median age 14 years) with recognized gastritis but without *H. pylori* infection;
3. *H. pylori*-infected children with gastritis (*Hp+*) - 59 children (28 boys and 31 girls) aged 8-18 years (median age 14 years) with recognized gastritis and *H. pylori* infection;

2.2 Bacteria

H. pylori strain 25A *cagA*-positive (*H. pylori cagA+*) was obtained from the Department of Microbiology and Clinical Immunology, Children's Memorial Hospital, Warsaw, Poland. Bacteria were washed twice with PBS pH 7.2 and adjusted to a density of 21 x 10^8 cells ml^{-1} in PBS.

2.3 Isolation of cells

At the time of endoscopy 10 ml of venous blood was obtained for immunologic testing from each patient. Peripheral blood mononuclear cells (PBMCs) were isolated from heparinized blood by Isopaque-Ficoll (Lymphoprep, Nycomed Pharma AS, Oslo, Norway) gradient centrifugation according to the procedure laid down by the manufacturer. Isolated PBMCs were resuspended in a PBS or culture medium made up of RPMI 1640 (Gibco, Paisley, UK) supplemented with 5% heat-inactivated human ABRh+ serum and gentamicin (40 µg ml^{-1}).

2.4 Phenotyping of cell surface antigens

Freshly isolated PBMCs were stained with fluorescein isothiocyanate (FITC)- and phycoerythrin (PE)-conjugated mouse anti-human monoclonal antibodies (BD Biosceinces,

New York, USA), specific for cell-surface markers with the following combinations: CD3/CD4, CD3/CD8, CD4/CD45RA, CD4/CD45RO, CD8/CD45RA, CD8/CD45RO. Simultest LeucoGate, (CD45-FITC/CD14-PE), and isotype control (IgG1-FITC/IgG2-PE) antibodies (BD Bioasceinces, San Diego, CA, USA) were included for each staining panel. Fluorescent staining was performed as described (Helmin-Basa et al., 2011). Briefly, 1 x 10^6 PBMCs in PBS were incubated with the indicated monoclonal antibodies for 20 min at RT in the dark. After one washing in PBS cell samples were submitted to the flow cytometric method for quantification of apoptosis using 7-Amino-Actinomycin D staining.

2.5 7-amino-actinomycin D (7-AAD) staining

After cell surface labeling, samples (1x10^6 cells) were incubated for 5-10 min at RT in the dark with 5 µl (0.25 µg) 7-AAD (BD Biosciences, San Diego, CA, USA). Then the samples (20 000 events per sample) were acquired on a FACScan flow cytometry (BD Biosciences, San Diego, CA, USA) equipped with a single 488 nm Argon laser, recorded in list mode and registered on logarithmic scales. 7-AAD emission was detected in the FL-3 channel (>650 nm). Analysis was performed with a Macintosh computer with the BD CellQuest Software (BD Biosciences).

2.6 Annexin V and propidum iodide staining in PBMC culture

After 72 hours culture of PBMCs (3 x 10^6 ml^{-1}) with *H. pylori cagA*+ (6.25 x 10^6 bacteria ml^{-1}), tetanus toxoid (TT, 5 UI ml^{-1}, Sigma-Aldrich) or without the stimulator, the percentage of live and dead lymphocytes were evaluated by flow cytometry (FACScan, BD Biosciences), using FITC Annexin V Apoptosis Detection Kit I (BD Biosciences, San Diego CA, USA). Briefly, 5 µl of Annexin V-FITC was added to 1 x 10^5 cells ml^{-1}, incubated for 20 minutes at RT in the dark, washed, and the cells were resuspended in 190 µl of binding buffer. Then 10 µl of propidium iodide was added 5-10 min before analysis by FACScan flow cytometry. The lymphocytes were gated and the live, apoptotic and dead cells were displayed on an FL-1 versus FL-3 fluorescence dot plot. Annexin V^-/PI^- cells represent live cells, the Annexin V^+/PI^- cells represent early apoptotic cells, the Annexin V^+/PI^+ cells are late apoptotic cells, and the Annexin V^-/PI^+ represent dead cells.

2.7 Proliferation assay in PBMC culture

The assay was made according to the procedure described previously (Gackowska et al., 2006, Michalkiewicz et al., 2003). Briefly, freshly isolated PBMCs were diluted in culture medium to a final concentration of 3 x 10^6 ml^{-1} and transferred in a volume of 100 µl (3 x 10^5) to flat-bottomed 96–well microplates (Costar, Cambridge, UK). Subsequently, 100 µl of culture medium alone (control) or containing live *H. pylori cells cagA*+ (6.25 x 10^6 cells ml^{-1}) or 20 µl of Concanavalin A (Con A 12.5 µg ml^{-1}, Sigma-Aldrich) or tetanus toxoid (TT 5 UI ml^{-1}, Sigma-Aldrich) was added. The cells were cultured in triplicates for seven (stimulation with *H. pylori cagA*+ and TT) or three (stimulation with Con A) days. Lymphocyte proliferation was assessed by pulsing the cells with 1 µCi ^3H thymidine (Amersham, Little Chalfont, UK) for the last 16 hours of the incubation period. The cultures were then harvested onto glass filter strips using an automated multisample harvester (Skatron, Lier, Norway) and analysed for ^3H-thymidine incorporation by liquid scintillation counting. Data is given as the stimulation index [SI], calculated by dividing the cpm obtained after stimulation by the cpm in corresponding cultures without a stimulator.

2.8 Cytokine assay in PBMC culture

Cytokine concentration (IL-12p40, IFN-gamma, TNF-alpha, IL-6 and IL-10) in cell culture supernatants was determined after 72 hours of *H. pylori cagA+* or Con A stimulation of PBMCs (3 x 10^6 ml^{-1}) using ELISA (Opt-EIA system, BD Biosciences, San Diego CA, USA), according to the manufacturer's procedure. Dose-response experiments performed for each cytokine indicated that the maximal secretion was obtained with 6.25 x 10^6 bacteria ml^{-1}, corresponding to a ratio of 2:1 (bacteria to PBMC) and 12.5 μg ml^{-1} of Con A that also induced the optimal proliferative response. For analysis of spontaneous cytokine secretion the cells were cultured alone in complete medium for 72 hours.

2.9 Statistical analyses

Data was expressed as means with standard deviation [SD] or medians with 95% confidence intervals (CI). The results were compared using the paired Student's *t* test or the Mann-Whitney's *U*-test as appropriate, depending on the normality of the data distribution, with STATISTICA for Windows release 5.0 (StatSoft, Tulusa, OK, USA) For normal distribution, variables were analyzed by the Kolmogorov-Smirnov test with Lilieforse correction. Statistical significance was considered as $p < 0.05$. The gastric inflammation was correlated with the percentage of positive cells using Spearman's coefficient of rank correlation. The level of significance was set at $p < 0.05$.

3. Results

3.1 Gastric mucosa histology

The intensity and activity of antral gastritis were greater in the *H. pylori*-infected children (*Hp+*) as compared to children with gastritis where *H. pylori* infection was excluded (*Hp-*) ($p < 0.05$), (Table 1). Neither atrophy nor intestinal metaplasia were seen in children's gastric mucosa.

Children	Antral mucosa				
	MN cells (intensity)	PMN cells (activity)	Atrophy	Intestinal metaplasia	*H. pylori*
Hp+	2 (1-3)	0 (0-2)	0	0	1 (0-3)
Hp-	2 (0-3)	0 (0-1)	0	0	0
Control group	0	0	0	0	0

Hp+, *H. pylori*-infected children; *Hp-*, noninfected children; MN: mononuclear cells;
PMN: polymorphonuclear cells.

Table 1. Gastric mucosa histology of *Hp+* and *Hp-* children, and control group (median score according to the update Sydney system: 0, none; 1, mild; 2, moderate; 3, marked)

3.2 The distribution of T-cell subsets in peripheral blood

There was an equal percentage of CD4+ and CD8+ T cell subsets in peripheral blood in the *Hp*+ and *Hp*- children and the control group (Table 2). However, the naive CD8+ T-cell subset (CD45RA+) was higher in the *Hp*+ children when compared to the control group ($p < 0.01$). In *Hp*- children, the proportion of memory CD8+ T-cell subset (CD45RO+) was increased ($p = 0.01$, *versus* control group). However, there was no correlation between the percentage of naive and memory T-cell subsets and the gastric inflammation scores in *Hp*+ and *Hp*- children.

T lymphocyte subsets		Means ± SD		
		Hp+ children (n = 13)	*Hp*- children (n = 15)	Control group (n = 12)
CD3+CD4+	%	39.95±4.78	36.96±6.76	38.98±5.92
CD3+CD8+	%	28.89±5.72	27.57±6.61	27.04±3.91
CD4+CD45RA+	%	29.51±8.62	26.31±6.15	22.95±0.65
CD4+CD45RO+	%	16.74±6.50	16.37±0.58	15.21±4.10
CD8+CD45RA+	%	34.95±1.72[a]	29.72±7.17	25.24±1.34
CD8+CD45RO+	%	10.44±2.78	9.91±0.52[a]	6.76±1.79

Hp+, *H. pylori*-infected children; *Hp*-, noninfected children; SD, standard deviation. Statistically significant differences (Student's *t* test): *versus* controls ([a]$p < 0.05$).

Table 2. The distribution of T-cell subsets in peripheral blood of *Hp*+ and *Hp*- children and the control group

3.3 Apoptosis of T-cell subsets in peripheral blood

Flow cytometric quantification of apoptotic T cell subsets in freshly isolated PBMCs showed significantly more apoptotic CD4+ and CD8+ T cells in both *Hp*+ ($p < 0.01$ and $p < 0.01$) and

T lymphocyte subsets		Means ± SD		
		Hp+ children (n = 13)	*Hp*- children (n = 15)	Control group (n = 12)
CD4+	%	10.48 ± 5.80[a,b]	4.50 ± 2.12[a]	2.13 ± 2.00
CD8+	%	8.46 ± 4.34[a,b]	5.01 ± 1.92[a]	1.48 ± 1.27
CD4+CD45RA+	%	5.24 ± 2.16[a]	4.62 ± 1.58[a]	0.36 ± 0.07
CD4+CD45RO+	%	5.11 ± 1.94[a]	7.37 ± 1.42[a]	0.55 ± 0.34
CD8+CD45RA+	%	4.69 ± 0.79[a]	5.45 ± 1.85[a]	0.68 ± 0.21
CD8+CD45RO+	%	6.12 ± 2.44	5.76 ± 1.51	4.17 ± 1.55

Hp+, *H. pylori*-infected children; *Hp*-, noninfected children; SD, standard deviation. Statistically significant differences (Student's *t* test): *versus* controls ([a]$p < 0.05$), *versus Hp*- children ([b]$p < 0.05$).

Table 3. Apoptosis in T-cell subsets in peripheral blood of *Hp*+ and *Hp*- children and the control group

Hp- (p = 0.01 and p < 0.01) children as compared with controls, but the percentages of apoptotic CD4+ and CD8+ T cells were higher in the former group (p < 0.01 and p = 0.02) (Table 3). Moreover, we found that the naive CD4+ and CD8+ T-cell subsets (CD45RA+) and memory CD4+ T-cell subset (CD45RO+) showed an increased apoptosis in both *Hp+* (p = 0.02, p < 0.01 and p = 0.01) and *Hp-* (p < 0.01, p = 0.02 and p < 0.01) children, but with no statistically significant differences between the groups.

3.4 The apoptosis of lymphocytes in *H. pylori*-induced PBMCs

The level of lymphocyte early apoptosis was unchanged in *H. pylori-* and TT-stimulated culture of PBMCs as compared with medium in both the *Hp+* and *Hp-* children. However, *Hp+* children had a higher level of spontaneous and TT-induced early apoptosis of lymphocytes than the *Hp-* ones (p = 0.02 and p < 0.01) (Fig. 1). Lymphocyte late apoptosis in *H. pylori-* and TT-induced PBMCs was equally high in both *Hp+* and *Hp-* children (*Hp+*: p = 0.01 and p = 0.09; *Hp-*: p = 0.01 and p = 0.01) when compared to the controls. Moreover, both *Hp+* and *Hp-* children had a low proportion of live lymphocytes in PBMC culture with *H. pylori* and TT (*Hp+*: p = 0.05 and p < 0.01; *Hp-*: p = 0.01 and p = 0.02), with no significant differences between the groups. However, only *Hp-* children have high percentage of dead (necrotic) cells in culture PBMC especially after TT stimulation (p < 0.01 *versus Hp+* children and controls).

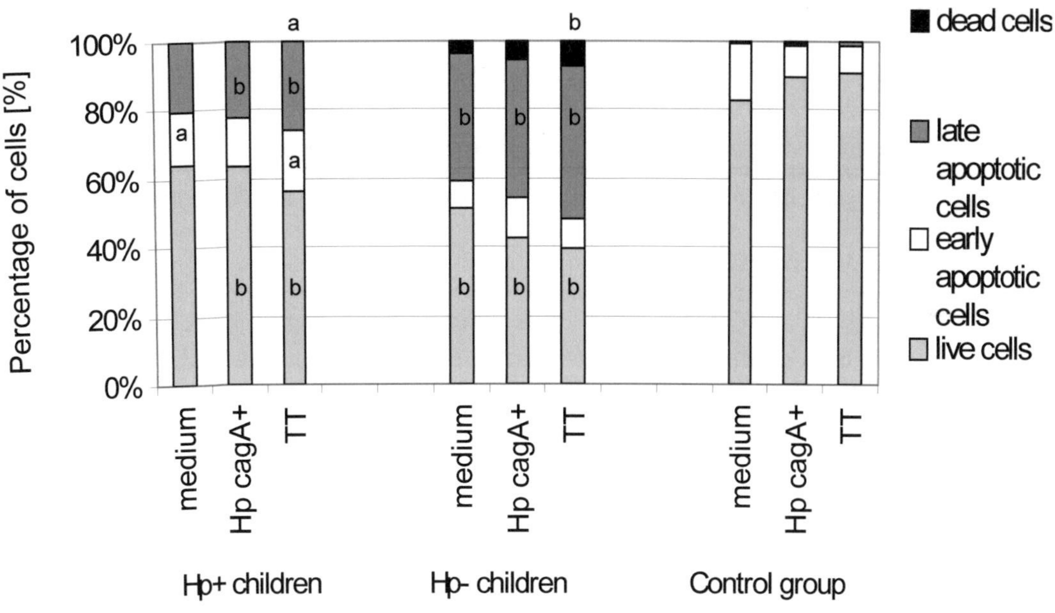

Hp+, *H. pylori*-infected children; *Hp-*, noninfected children; *Hp*, *H. pylori*; TT, tetanus toxoid. Results represent median values obtain from n independent experiments: *Hp+* children and controls: n = 6; *Hp-* children: n = 5. Statistically significant differences (Mann-Whitney's *U*-test): *versus Hp-* children (^{a}p < 0.05), *versus* controls (^{b}p < 0.05).

Fig. 1. The apoptosis of lymphocytes in PBMC culture in *Hp+* and *Hp-* children and the control group

3.5 The proliferative response in *H. pylori*-induced PBMCs

The changes in the mode of lymphocyte proliferation involved: a) lower lymphocyte response to *H. pylori* in the *Hp*+ children than in the *Hp*- ones ($p = 0.03$) and control group ($p < 0.01$); b) increased response to Con A in the *Hp*+ as compared to the *Hp*- children ($p = 0.02$) and control group ($p = 0.04$). However, lymphocytes of *Hp*+ and *Hp*- children and control group did not differ in their response to TT (Table 4).

Type of stimulator	Medians [CI]		
	Hp+ children (n = 46, 14 or 8)	*Hp*- children (n = 59, 21 or 13)	Control group (n = 13)
H. pylori cagA+	3.28[a,b] [1.55/26.09]	6.29 [3.50/45.68]	10.48 [8.26/24.16]
Concanavalin A	312.12[a,b] [190.63/513.91]	169.12 [111.44/199.25]	121.52 [90.60/181.82]
Tetanus toxoid	7.77 [0.45/18.02]	4.27 [3.06/25.68]	2.44 [0.71/5.01]

Hp+, *H. pylori*-infected children; *Hp*-, noninfected children; CI, confidence intervals. Statistically significant differences (Mann-Whitney's *U*-test): *versus* controls ($^{a}p < 0.05$), *versus Hp*- children ($^{b}p < 0.05$).

Table 4. PBMC proliferative response in *Hp*+ and *Hp*- children and the control group

3.6 The pattern of cytokine expression in *H. pylori*-induced PBMCs

The levels of *H. pylori*- or Con A-induced cytokines did not exceed the control values in both *Hp*+ and *Hp*- children. However, the profile of cytokine synthesis showed a different pattern: 1) IL-12p40 synthesis (Fig. 2): *H. pylori* was a poor IL-12p40 inducer both in the *Hp*+ and *Hp*- children ($p < 0.01$). However, in the *Hp*+ children production of IL-12p40 was higher than in the *Hp*- ones ($p = 0.02$). In contrast, Con A stimulation gave rise to a similar IL-12p40 level in both groups of children. Finally, the IL-12p40 synthesis profile in the *Hp*- children was similar to that of the control group with a better response to *H. pylori* than to Con A ($p = 0.04$ and $p < 0.01$). 2) IFN-gamma synthesis (Fig. 3): *H. pylori*-induced IFN-gamma synthesis remained unchanged in the *Hp*+ children, but it was slightly lower in the *Hp*- ones ($p = 0.01$) as compared with the control group. Con A was a significantly better IFN-gamma inducer than *H. pylori* in both *Hp*+ and *Hp*- children with no significant differences between the two groups. 3) TNF-alpha synthesis (Fig. 4): In the *Hp*- children, *H. pylori* and Con A-induced TNF-alpha levels were lower than in the control group ($p < 0.01$ and $p = 0.01$). However, Con A was a stronger inducer of TNF-alpha in the *Hp*+ children than in the *Hp*- ones ($p = 0.02$). 4) IL-6 synthesis (Fig. 5): *H. pylori* was a poorer IL-6 inducer in the *Hp*+ children than in the *Hp*- ones ($p = 0.03$) and control group ($p = 0.03$); this tendency was maintained with Con A being a worse stimulator of IL-6 in the *Hp*+ than in the *Hp*- children ($p < 0.01$). 5) IL-10 synthesis (Fig. 6): *H. pylori* was a better IL-10 inducer in the *Hp*+ than in *Hp*- children ($p = 0.03$). However, in both the *Hp*- children and control group Con A was a better IL-10 inducer than *H. pylori* ($p = 0.05$).

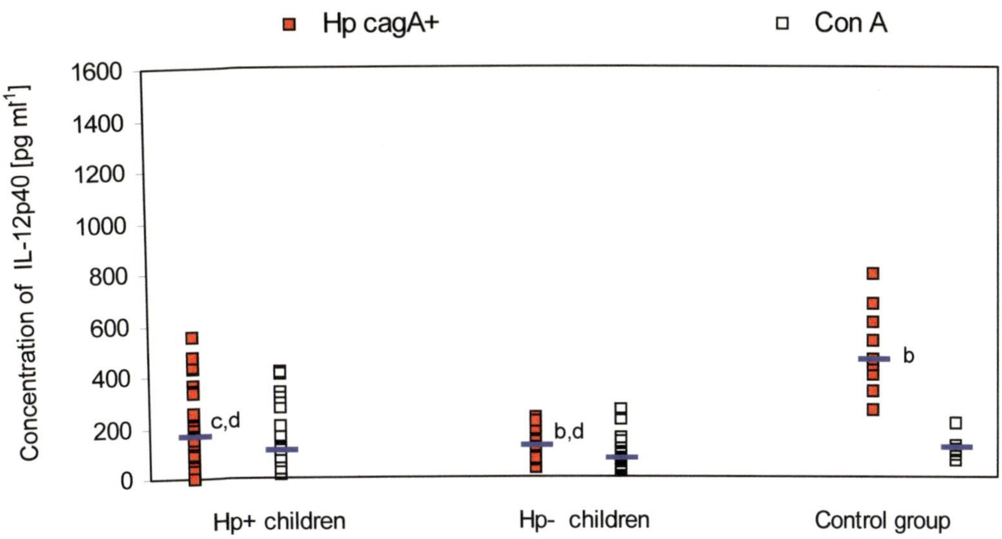

Hp, *H. pylori*; *Hp*+, Con A, Concanavalin A, *Hp*+, *H. pylori*-infected children; *Hp*-, noninfected children. Blue horizontal bars represent medians obtained from n independent experiments: *Hp*+ children: n = 29; *Hp*- children: n = 23; controls: n = 9. Statistically significant differences (Mann-Whitney's *U*-test): *versus* Con A stimulation. ($^{b}p < 0.05$), *versus Hp*- children ($^{c}p < 0.05$), *versus* controls ($^{d}p < 0.05$).

Fig. 2. Concentration of IL-12p40 in culture supernatants of PBMC in *Hp*+ and *Hp*- children and the control group

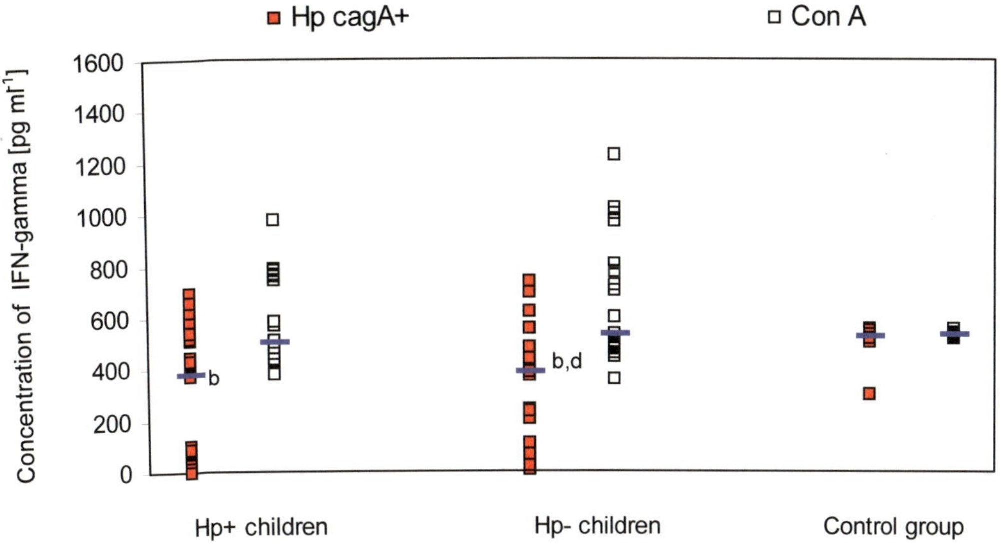

Hp, *H. pylori*; *Hp*+, Con A, Concanavalin A, *Hp*+, *H. pylori*-infected children; *Hp*-, noninfected children. Blue horizontal bars represent median values obtained from n independent experiments: *Hp*+ children: n = 27; *Hp*- children: n = 27; controls: n = 9. Statistically significant differences (Mann-Whitney's *U*-test): *versus* Con A stimulation. ($^{b}p < 0.05$), *versus Hp*- children ($^{c}p < 0.05$), *versus* controls ($^{d}p < 0.05$).

Fig. 3. Concentration of IFN-gamma in culture supernatants of PBMC in *Hp*+ and *Hp*- children and the control group

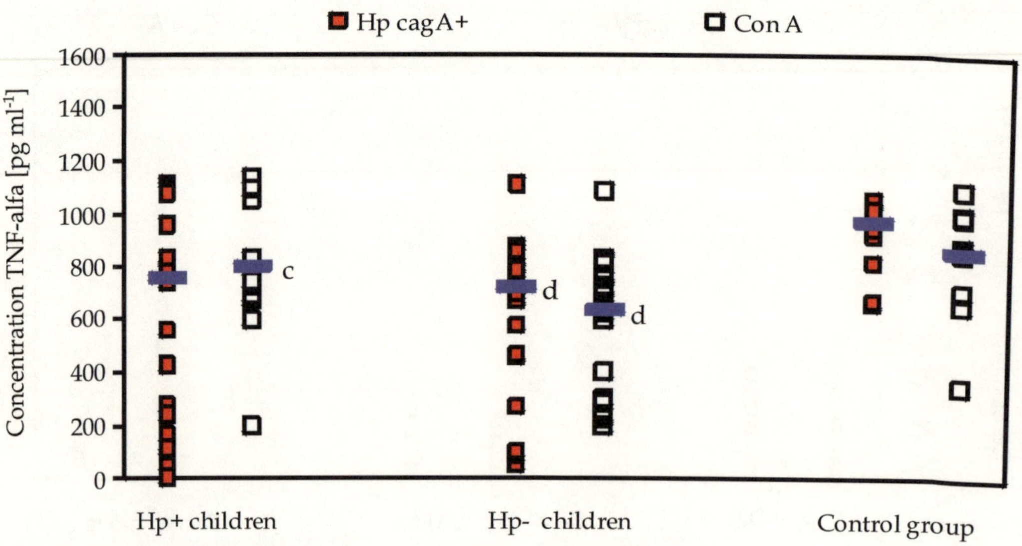

Hp, *H. pylori*; *Hp*+, Con A, Concanavalin A, *Hp*+, *H. pylori*-infected children; *Hp*-, noninfected children. Blue horizontal bars represent median values obtained from n independent experiments: *Hp*+ children: n = 19; *Hp*-children: n = 22; controls: n = 10. Statistically significant differences (Mann-Whitney's *U*-test): *versus Hp*- children ($^{c}p < 0.05$), *versus* controls ($^{d}p < 0.05$).

Fig. 4. Concentration of TNF-alfa in culture supernatants of PBMC in *Hp*+ and *Hp*- children and the control group

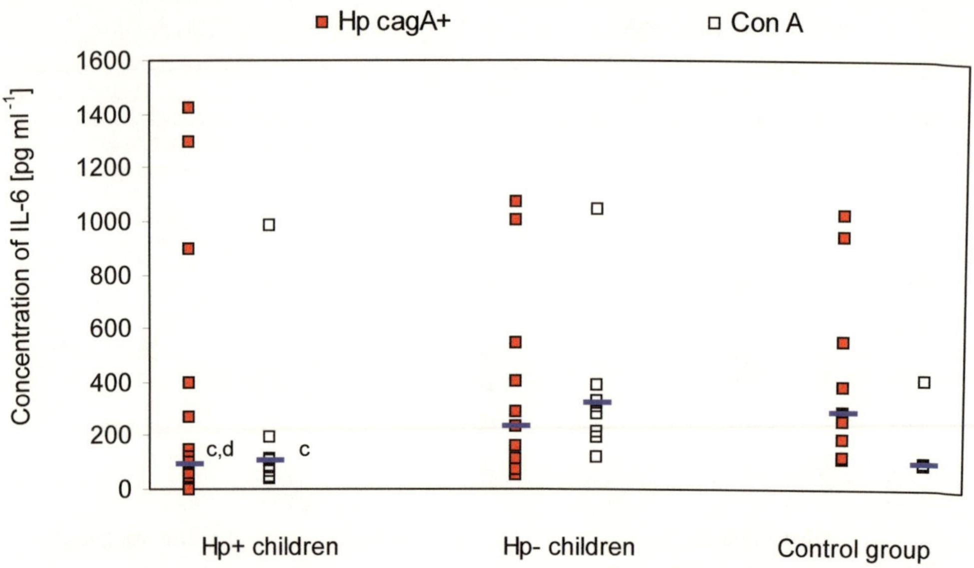

Hp, *H. pylori*; *Hp*+, Con A, Concanavalin A, *Hp*+, *H. pylori*-infected children; *Hp*-, noninfected children. Blue horizontal bars represent median values obtained from n independent experiments: *Hp*+ children: n = 21; *Hp* children: n = 12; controls: n = 11. Statistically significant differences (Mann-Whitney's *U*-test): *versus Hp*- children ($^{c}p < 0.05$), *versus* controls ($^{d}p < 0.05$).

Fig. 5. Concentration of IL-6 in culture supernatants of PBMC in *Hp*+ and *Hp*- children and the control group

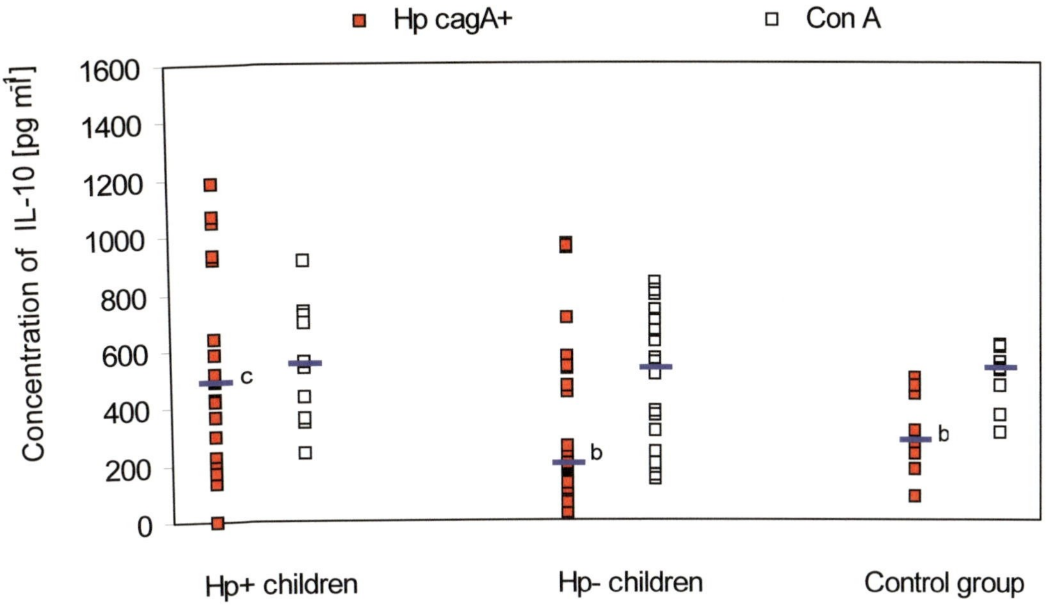

Hp, *H. pylori*; *Hp+*, Con A, Concanavalin A, *Hp+*, *H. pylori*-infected children; *Hp-*, noninfected children. Blue horizontal bars represent median values obtained from n independent experiments: *Hp+* and *Hp-* children: n = 23; controls: n = 8. Statistically significant differences (Mann-Whitney's *U*-test): *versus* Con A stimulation. ($^{b}p < 0.05$), *versus Hp-* children ($^{c}p < 0.05$).

Fig. 6. Concentration of IL-10 in culture supernatants of PBMC in *Hp+* and *Hp-* children and the control group

4. Discussion

In the present study *H. pylori*-infected and noninfected children with gastritis and the control group were compared with respect to 1) the distribution and apoptosis of T lymphocyte subsets in the blood, and 2) lymphocyte apoptosis, proliferation and cytokine synthesis pattern in the culture PBMCs. Additionally, the lymphocyte phenotypes of children with gastritis were correlated with gastric inflammation scores.

We report that the group of *H. pylori*-infected children have: 1) an elevated proportion of naive $CD8^{+}$ ($CD45RA^{+}$) T-cell population along with an increase in the percentage of apoptotic $CD4^{+}$ and $CD8^{+}$ T cells in the blood, 2) high spontaneous early lymphocyte apoptosis, low lymphocyte proliferation to *H. pylori* but a high response to Con A, and 3) slightly increased IL-10 expression along with decreased IL-6 expression in *H. pylori*-induced PBMC culture. Children with gastritis but without infection had a high percentage of memory $CD8^{+}$ T-cell subset ($CD45RO^{+}$) in the blood and a low INF-gamma and TNF-alpha in *H. pylori*-induced PBMC culture. Both *H. pylori*-infected and noninfected children with gastritis were characterized by 1) an increased percentage of apoptotic naive and memory $CD4^{+}$ and $CD8^{+}$ T-cell subsets in blood, 2) a high percentage of late apoptotic lymphocytes, along with a low proportion of live lymphocytes, and a low IL-12p40 expression in culture PBMCs.

An increase in the percentage of CD45RA-bearing $CD8^+$ T-cell subsets in the *H. pylori*-infected children may indicate that the infection with *H. pylori* induces the thymic T-cell renewal leading to the generation of T cells with high expression of CD45RA isoform. These results differ from those obtained in another study, also examining blood, which showed an unchanged proportion of circulating naive T cell subset ($CD45RA^+$) in a group of *H. pylori*-infected children [Helmin-Basa et al., 2011]. This discrepancy might result from a different number of examined children and the age of the children evaluated in previous study. However, similar changes have been observed in the gastric antral mucosa using quantitative immunohistochemistry [Maciorkowska et al., 2004].

Other differences that we have observed in *H. pylori*-infected children were the increase in the percentage of apoptotic $CD4^+$ and $CD8^+$ T lymphocytes in the blood and spontaneous early apoptosis of lymphocyte in PBMC culture. Similar changes have been observed in previous studies that evaluated the apoptosis of gastric mucosa inflammatory cells showing an increased apoptosis of $CD4^+$ T-cell subset using immunohistochemistry methods [Guarner et al., 2003, Kotłowska-Kmieć et al., 2009].

The noninfected children with gastritis had an elevated proportion of CD45RO-positive $CD8^+$ T-cell subset in the blood. These results are analogous to our previous study that also showed an increase in the percentage of circulating memory T cells with very high expression of CD45RO isoform in a group of noninfected children with gastritis [Helmin-Basa et al., 2011]. This suggests the activation of thymic–generated $CD45RA^+$ cells leading to the transition of the CD45RA isoform into CD45RO.

Additionally, our results have shown that circulating naive ($CD45RA^+$) and memory ($CD45RO^+$) T-cell subsets display high apoptosis in the *H. pylori*-infected and noninfected children with gastritis. $CD45RO^+$ cells may provide pro-inflammatory signals that contribute to the gastric inflammation. Hence, high apoptosis, especially of the memory T cells, can make the gastritis self-limited regardless of *H. pylori* infection.

We also found that the lymphocytes of the *H. pylori*-infected children had reduced proliferation in *H. pylori cagA*+-induced PBMC culture. These results essentially confirm some adult reports indicating that *H. pylori* infection is associated with a decreased peripheral lymphocyte response to live or killed *H. pylori* bacteria or their products (Fan et al., 1994; Malfitano et al., 2006; Lungren et al., 2003). Several mechanisms have been proposed as an explanation for this phenomenon, for example the active suppression of T and B lymphocyte proliferation potential, suppression of monocytes activation, inhibitory action of several virulent *H. pylori* products including CagA protein and VacA cytotoxin, and others (Boncristino et al., 2003; Wang et al., 2001). Profound low lymphocyte response to *H. pylori cagA*+ in infected children with high proliferation to antigen specific inducer (tetanus toxoid) and T -cell mitogen (Con A) in both the *H. pylori*-infected and noninfected children with gastritis, as well as in the controls leads to a number of conclusions. First-of-all, a low lymphocyte proliferation in response to *H. pylori* induction selectively found in the *H. pylori*-infected children is highly specific only for *H. pylori*. Secondly, the ongoing *H. pylori* infection creates conditions for *H. pylori* specific low T lymphocyte proliferation. This profile of response is also typical of gastric mucosa T cells in *H. pylori*-infected adults showing unresponsiveness to *H. pylori* antigens (Lungren et al., 2005; Ren et al., 2000) unless costimulatory cytokines are present (Ren et al., 2000).

We report here that lymphocytes of both *H. pylori*-infected and noninfected children with gastritis proved to be much more sensitive to *H. pylori* bacteria and tetanus toxoid-induced apoptosis than lymphocytes of the controls. These observations indicate that gastritis itself (independent of ongoing *H. pylori*-infection) makes peripheral lymphocytes sensitive to apoptosis. However, the higher early spontaneous lymphocyte apoptosis in *H. pylori*-infected children may suggest that ongoing *H. pylori* infection can make the lymphocyte apoptosis rate faster, possibly due to their prolonged contact with *H. pylori in vivo*. Our study of apoptotic lymphocytes in blood confirm that *H. pylori* infection increases apoptosis of circulating $CD4^+$ and $CD8^+$ T-cell subsets.

In general, our results concerning lymphocyte apoptosis are partly in agreement with other reports suggesting that *H. pylori*-induced apoptosis could be the reason for modest *H. pylori*-induced proliferation of T cells in *H. pylori*-infected subjects (Schmees et al., 2007). Some authors suggest that the apoptotic mechanism possibly involves Fas-bearing T cells through induction of FasL expression (Wang et al., 2000, 2001). Also, gastric T cells have been reported to express FasL and undergo apoptosis *in situ* following *H. pylori* infection as has also been shown previously (Galgani et al., 2004). The role of *cag* PAI in induction of T cell death through Fas/FasL interaction has also been strongly suggested on the basis that *cag* PAI-deficient strains of *H. pylori* were not able to induce apoptosis in T cells (Wang et al., 2001). In line with these results, Galgani e*t al.* (Galgani et al., 2007) have shown that *cagA*+ strains of *H. pylori* were highly effective inducers of apoptosis in human monocytes, but not in monocyte-derived dendritic cells. Our results also suggest that at least in the model of *H. pylori*-induced PBMCs *cagA* expression in the stimulating bacteria affected lymphocyte apoptosis levels.

Low *H. pylori*-induced IL-12p40 production found in the PBMCs of *H. pylori*-infected children may result either from limited number of IL-12 producing cells or from the defects in IL-12 regulation. Gastritis itself also limits the PBMC abilities in terms of IL-12p40 synthesis since *H. pylori*-activated PBMCs of noninfected children with gastritis also showed lower IL-12p40 production than controls; however, the values were higher than those of infected subjects. This observation may indicate that children gastritis itself, regardless of *H. pylori* infection, down-regulates IL-12p40 expression in *H. pylori*-induced PBMCs, and that *H. pylori*-infection makes this process more profound. Gram-negative bacteria have been found to induce rather low IL-12 synthesis in PBMCs but high IL-10 levels (Hessle et al., 1999, 2000). In this model system IL-12 is produced mainly by monocytes and is up-regulated by T cells, since their removal from PBMCs decreases the bacteria-induced IL-12 production (Hessle et al., 1999). Low IL-12p40 levels found in the *H. pylori cagA*+-induced PBMCs of the *H. pylori*-infected children and in a lesser degree also in the noninfected children with gastritis may result from two processes. Firstly, a high apoptosis of $CD4^+$ T cells participating in the up-regulation of IL-12 production by monocytes, and secondly, hypo-reactivity and/or apoptosis of monocytes directly induced either by *H. pylori* action (Galgani et al. 2004), or indirectly mediated by a relative excess of IL-10 (D'Andrea et al., 1993). Low IL-12 production may play a role in a complex and still poorly understood mechanism of rather limited *H. pylori*-mediated pro-inflammatory responses usually observed in children (Bontems at al. 2003, Lopes et al. 2005).

We have found that the production of INF-gamma decreased in noninfected children with gastritis but not in *H. pylori*-infected ones. This is in contrast with the IL-12p40 findings, and indirectly suggests that in the PBMC model system, *H. pylori cagA*+-induced IFN-gamma production essentially does not depend on IL-12p40. This observation confirms the results of other researchers showing that PBMC stimulation with Gram-negative bacteria results in a rather low and separately-independent IFN-gamma and IL-12 expression (Hessle et al., 2000).

In the *H. pylori*-infected children, but not in the noninfected ones, a relatively high *H. pylori cagA*+-mediated IFN-gamma synthesis was connected with relatively elevated IL-10 production (both responses were on the level of the controls). This observation may indicate a possible role of IL-10 in the down-regulation of IFN-gamma in the course of *H. pylori*-infection in children. This issue has been studied extensively by others (Holck et al., 2003). *H. pylori* bacteria (live or killed) and their antigens have been found to induce a higher IL-10 production in PBMCs of *H. pylori*-infected than noninfected adults (Haeberle et al., 1997; Jakob et al., 2001; Windle et al., 2005).

To the best of our knowledge, our report is the first showing a relative increase in IL-10 production in culture PBMCs of *H. pylori*-infected children. These results are consistent with previous findings, indicating that *H. pylori* infection is related to a high expression of IL-10 in the gastric mucosa both on mRNA and protein level (Bodger et al., 2001; Hida et al., 1999). IL-10 has long been considered a potent anti-inflammatory cytokine strongly implicated in *H. pylori* infection (Bodger et al., 2001). On the one hand it may protect from the harmful effects of potentially pro-inflammatory responses induced by *H. pylori,* but on the other, it may inhibit the protective mechanisms of immune responses directed against *H. pylori* antigens.

We also found that *H. pylori cagA*+ was a much lower IL-6 inducer in the culture PBMCs of *H. pylori*-infected than noninfected children with gastritis. Diminished IL-6 induction may play a role in the hypo-responsiveness of PBMCs to *H. pylori* stimulation in infected children. In our model system IL-6 is produced both by T cells and monocytes. IL-6 is a known strong co-stimulatory cytokine that plays a significant role in providing second signal to antigen-induced T cells (Shi et al., 1989).

In this study, *H. pylori* evoked a similar activity in stimulating TNF secretion in PBMCs of both *H. pylori*-infected and noninfected children. However, in the former group there was a tendency to a slightly lower TNF-alpha level. This partially confirms the findings of earlier studies in the stomach in which *H. pylori*-infected children and adults showed a similar concentration of this cytokine (Bontems et al., 2003). Unchanged or slightly decreased production of this cytokine in *H. pylori cagA*+-mediated PBMCs may also be contributing to the limited pro-inflammatory responses in children with gastritis.

5. Conclusion

In conclusion, *H. pylori* infection in children results in: a) increased percentage of peripheral blood memory $CD8^+$ T cells, b) high apoptosis of circulating $CD4^+$ and $CD8^+$ T-cell subsets, c) *H. pylori*-specific-peripheral hypo-responsiveness (low lymphocyte proliferation and IL-12p40 expression), and d) unchanged *H. pylori* dependent pro- inflammatory responses (IFN-gamma, TNF-alfa, respectively), associated with a high expression of IL-10 but low expression of IL-6. This response pattern, together with a high T-cell subsets apoptosis, may protect from more aggressive forms of *H. pylori*-induced inflammation, but on the other hand may also participate in the failure of eliminating the infection.

6. Acknowledgment

The study was supported by grant UMK 20/2010.

7. References

Acheson, D. W.& Luccioli S. (2004). Microbial-gut interactions in health and disease. Mucosal immune responses. *Best Pract Res Clin Gastroenterol,* Vol.18, No.2, (April 2004), pp, 387-404

Bodger, K., Bromelow, K., Wyatt, J. I. & Heatley, R. V. (2001). Interleukin 10 in *Helicobacter pylori* associated gastritis: immunohistochemical localisation and in vitro effects on cytokine secretion. *J Clin Pathol,* Vol.54, No.4, (April 2001), pp, 285-292

Boncristiano, M., Paccani, S. R., Barone, S., Ulivieri, C., Patrussi, L., Ilver, D., Amedei, A., D'Elios, M. M., Telford, J. L. & Baldari, C. T. (2003). The *Helicobacter pylori* vacuolating toxin inhibits T cell activation by two independent mechanisms. *J Exp Med,* Vol.198, No.12, (June 2003), pp, 1887-1897

Bontems, P.; Robert F.; Van Gossum A.; Cadranel S. &; Mascart F. (2003). *Helicobacter pylori* modulation of gastric and duodenal mucosal T cell cytokine secretions in children compared with adults. *Helicobacter,* Vol.8, No.3, (June 2003), pp, 216-226

D'Andrea, A., Aste-Amezaga, M., Valiante, N. M., Ma, X., Kubin, M. & Trinchieri, G. (1993). Interleukin 10 (IL-10) inhibits human lymphocyte interferon gamma-production by suppressing natural killer cell stimulatory factor/IL-12 synthesis in accessory cells. *J Exp Med,* Vol.178, No.3, (September 1993), pp, 1041-1048

Fan, X. J., Chua, A., Shahi, C.N., McDevitt. J, Keeling, P. W. & Kelleher, D. (1994). Gastric T lymphocyte responses to *Helicobacter pylori* in patients with *H pylori* colonisation. *Gut,* Vol.35, No.10, (October 1994), pp, 1379-1384

Gackowska, L., Michalkiewicz, J., Krotkiewski, M., Helmin-Basa, A., Kubiszewska, I., Dzierzanowska, D. (2006). Combined effect of different lactic acid bacteria strains on the mode of cytokines pattern expression in human peripheral blood mononuclear cells. *J Physiol Pharmacol.* Vol.57, No.9, (November 2006), pp, 13-21

Galgani, M., Busiello, I., Censini, S., Zappacosta, S., Racioppi, L. & Zarrilli, R. (2004). *Helicobacter pylori* induces apoptosis of human monocytes but not monocyte-derived dendritic cells: role of the cag pathogenicity island. *Infect Immun,* Vol.72, No.8, (August 2004), pp, 4480-4485

Guarner, J., Bartlett, J., Whistler, T., Pierce-Smith, D., Owens, M., Kreh, R., Czinn, S. & Gold, B. D. (2003). Can pre-neoplastic lesions be detected in gastric biopsies of children with *Helicobacter pylori* infection? *Pediatr Gastroenterol Nutr,* Vol. 37, No.3, (September 2003), pp, 309-314

Harris, P.R., Wright, S. W., Serrano, C., Riera, F., Duarte, I., Torres, J., Peña, A., Rollán, A., Viviani, P., Guiraldes, E., Schmitz, J. M., Lorenz, R. G., Novak, L., Smythies, L. E., Smith, P. D. (2008). *Helicobacter pylori* gastritis in children is associated with a regulatory T-cell response. *Gastroenterology*, Vol.134, No.2, (February 2008), pp, 491-499

Hatz, R. A., Meimarakis, G., Bayerdorffer, E., Stolte, M., Kirchner, T. & Enders, G. (1996). Characterization of lymphocytic infiltrates in *Helicobacter pylori*-associated gastritis. *Scand J Gastroenterol*, Vol.31, No.3, (March 1996), pp, :222-228

Helmin-Basa, A., Michalkiewicz, J., Gackowska, L., Kubiszewska, I., Eljaszewicz, A., Mierzwa, G., Bala, G., Czerwionka-Szaflarska, M., Prokurat, A. & Marszalek, A. (2011). Pediatric *Helicobacter pylori* infection and circulating T-lymphocyte activation and differentiation. *Helicobacter*, Vol. 16, No.1, (February 2011), pp, 27-35, ISSN

Hessle, C., Hanson, L. A., Wold & A. E. (1999). Lactobacilli from human gastrointestinal mucosa are strong stimulators of IL-12 production. *Clin Exp Immunol*, Vol.116, No.2, (May 1999), pp, 276-282

Hessle, C., Andersson, B. & Wold, A. E. (2000). Gram-positive bacteria are potent inducers of monocytic interleukin-12 (IL-12) while gram-negative bacteria preferentially stimulate IL-10 production. *Infect Immun, Vol.*68, No.6, (June 2000), pp, 3581-3586

Hida, N., Shimoyama, T. Jr., Neville, P., Dixon, M. F., Axon, A. T., Shimoyama, T. Sr. & Crabtree, J. E. (1999). Increased expression of IL-10 and IL-12 (p40) mRNA in *Helicobacter pylori* infected gastric mucosa: relation to bacterial *cag* status and peptic ulceration. *J Clin Pathol*, Vol. 52, No.9, (September 1999), pp, 658-664

Holck, S., Norgaard, A., Bennedsen, M., Permin, H., Norn, S. & Andersen, L. P. (2003). Gastric mucosal cytokine responses in *Helicobacter pylori*-infected patients with gastritis and peptic ulcers. Association with inflammatory parameters and bacteria load. *FEMS Immunol Med Microbiol*, Vol.36, No.3, (May 2003), pp, 175-180

Jakob, B., Birkholz, S., Schneider, T., Duchmann, R., Zeitz, M. & Stallmach, A. (2001). Immune response to autologous and heterologous *Helicobacter pylori* antigens in humans. *Microsc Res Tech*, Vol.53, No.15, (June 2001), pp, 419-424

Karlsson, H., Hessle, Ch. & Rudin, A. (2002). Innate immune response to human neonatal cells to bacteria from the normal gastrointestinal flora. *Infect Immun*, Vol.;70, No.12, (December 2002), pp, 6688-6696

Karttunen, R., Crowe, Haeberle, H. A., Kubin, M., Bamford, K. B., Garofalo, R., Graham, D. Y., El-Zaatari, F.,Karttunen, R., Crowe, S. E., Reyes, V. E. & Ernst, P. B. (1997). Differential stimulation of interleukin-12 (IL-12) and IL-10 by live and killed *Helicobacter pylori in vitro* and association of IL-12 production with gamma interferon-producing T cells in the human gastric mucosa. *Infect Immun*, Vol.65, No.10, (October 1997), pp, 4229-4235

Kotłowska-Kmieć, A., Bakowska, A., Wołowska, E., Łuczak, G. & Liberek, A. (2009). Periapoptotic markers in children with *Helicobacter pylori* infection. *Med Wieku Rozwoj*, Vol.13, No.4, (October-December 2009), pp, 231-236

Lopes, A. I.; Quiding-Jarbrink, M.; Palha, A.; Ruivo, J.; Monteiro, L.; Oleastro, M.; Santos, A. & Fernandes, A. (2005). Cytokine expression in pediatric *Helicobacter pylori* infection. *Clin Diagn Lab Immunol*, Vol.12, No.8, (August 2005), pp, 994-1002

Lungren, A., Suri Payer, E., Enarsson, K., Svennerholm, A. M. & Lundin, B .S. (2003). *Helicobacter pylori*-specific CD4+ CD25high regulatory T cells suppress memory T-cell responses to *H. pylori* in infected individuals. *Infect Immun*, Vol.71, No.4, (April 2003), pp, 1755-1762

Lundgren, A., Trollmo, C., Edebo, A., Svennerholm, A. M. & Lundin, B. S. (2005). *Helicobacter pylori*-specific CD4+ T cells home to and accumulate in the human *Helicobacter pylori*-infected gastric mucosa. *Infect Immun*, Vol.73, No.9, (September 2005), pp, 5612-5619

Maciorkowska, E., Kondej-Muszyńska, K., Kasacka, I., Kaczmarski, M., Kemona, A. (2004). Memory cells in the antral mucosa of children with Helicobacter pylori infection. *Rocz Akad Med Bialymst*, Vol.49, No.1, (2004), pp, 225-227

Malfitano, A. M. , Cahill, R., Mitchell, P., Frankel, G., Dougan, G., Bifulco, M., Lombardi, G., Lechler, R. I. & Bamford K. B. (2006). *Helicobacter pylori* has stimulatory effects on naive T cells. *Helicobacter*, Vol. 11, No.1, (February 2006), pp, 21-30

Michalkiewicz, J., Krotkiewski, M., Gackowska, L., Wyszomirska-Gołda, M., Helmin, A., Dzierzanowska, D.& Madaliński, K. (2003). Target cell for immunomodulatory action of lactic acid bacteria. *Microb Ecol Health Dis*, Vol. 15, No., (2003), pp, 185-192, ISSN

Peek, R. M. Jr., Miller, G. G., Tham, K. T., Perez-Perez, G. I., Zhao, X., Atherton, J. C. & Blaser, M. J. (1995). Heightened inflammatory response and cytokine expression in vivo to *cagA+ Helicobacter pylori* strains. *Lab Invest, Vol.*73, No.6, (December 1995), pp, 760-770

Queiroz, D. M., Rocha, G. A., Mendes, E. N., Carvalho, A. S., Barbosa, A. J., Oliveira, C. A. & Lima, G. F. Jr. (1991). Differences in distribution and severity of *Helicobacter pylori* gastritis in children and adults with duodenal ulcer disease. *J Pediatr Gastroenterol Nutr*, Vol.12, No.2, (February 1991), pp, 178-181

Ren, Z., Pang, G., Lee, R., Batey, R., Dunkley, M., Borody, T. & Clancy, R. (2000). Circulating T-cell response to *Helicobacter pylori* infection in chronic gastritis. *Helicobacter*, Vol.5, No.3, (September 2000), pp, 135-141

Schmees, C., Prinz, C., Treptau, T., Rad, R., Hengst, L., Voland, P., Bauer, S., Brenner, L., Schmid, R. M., Gerhard, M. (2007). Inhibition of T-cell proliferation by *Helicobacter pylori* gamma-glutamyl transpeptidase. Gastroenterology , Vol. 132, No.5, (May 2007), pp, 1820-1833

Shi, T., Liu, W. Z., Shi, G. Y.& Xiao, S. D. (1989). Synergistic interactions of IL-1 and IL-6 in T cell activation. Mitogen but not antigen receptor-induced proliferation of a cloned T helper cell line is enhanced by exogenous IL-6. J Immunol, Vol.143, No., (1989), pp, 896-901

Soares, T. F.; Rocha, G. A.; Rocha, A. M.; Correa-Oliveira, R.; Martins-Filho, O. A.; Carvalho, A. S.; Bittencourt, P.; Oliveira, C. A.; Faria, A. M. & Queiroz, D. M. (2005). Phenotypic study of peripheral blood lymphocytes and humoral immune response in *Helicobacter pylori* infection according to age. *Scand J. Immunol,* Vol.62, No.1, (July 2005), pp, 63-70

Wang, J., Fan, X., Lindholm, C., Bennett, M., O'Connoll, J., Shanahan, F., Brooks, E. G., Reyes, V. E & Ernst, P. B. (2000). *Helicobacter pylori* modulates lymphoepithelial cell interactions leading to epithelial cell damage through Fas/Fas ligand interactions. *Infect Immun,* Vol.68, No.7, (July 2000), pp, 4303-4311

Wang, J., Brooks, E. G., Bamford, K. B., Denning, T. L., Pappo, J.& Ernst, P. B. (2001). Negative selection of T cells by *Helicobacter pylori* as a model for bacterial strain selection by immune evasion. *J Immunol,* Vol.167, No.2, (July 2001), pp, 926-934

Windle, H. J., Ang, Y. S., Athie-Morales, V., McManus, R. & Kelleher, D. (2005). Human peripheral and gastric lymphocyte responses to *Helicobacter pylori* NapA and AphC differ in infected and uninfected individuals. Gut, Vol.54, No.1, (January 2005), pp, 25-32.

11

The Effect of Epigallocatechin Gallate (EGCG) and Metal Ions Corroded from Dental Casting Alloys on Cell Cycle Progression and Apoptosis in Cells from Oral Tissues

Jiansheng Su, Zhizen Quan, Wenfei Han, Lili Chen and Jiamei Gu
School of Stomatology, Tongji University,
Shanghai,
China

1. Introduction

1.1 The application of dental metallic materials

Metallic materials are the basis of dental materials science, which is an important part of dentistry. As a result of their good mechanical properties and some biological properties, metals are widely used in oral rehabilitation of dentition and mandibular defects, orthodontic and dental implants, as well as in the equipment for dental operations. Commonly used metals include nickel chromium, cobalt chromium, titanium, and silver palladium alloy; of these, nickel-chromium and cobalt-chromium alloys are in widespread clinical use in China because of their stable biological properties and moderate prices.

The oral environment is a very complex electrolyte environment with a large number of microorganisms, in which the metal prosthesis corrodes and releases metal ions. Microbial corrosion is a major contributor to this process. The products of bacterial metabolism (including organic and inorganic acids) can directly affect the pH on the surface or interface of a metal prosthesis, and thus affect the electrochemical reactivity, eventually promoting corrosion. Metal ions are increased in the saliva and oral soft tissue (e.g. gingiva & tongue smear) of patients who wear alloy prostheses. The metal ions released from dental casting alloys can potentially reduce the metabolism of cells, inhibit cell proliferation and have other toxic effects in vitro. Ions released from commonly used Ni-Cr alloys may induce adverse reactions, such as gingival inflammation and discoloration, oral cell mutation or cancer. Cobalt ions from Co-Cr alloy have been reported to stimulate allergic reaction. Another ion that may be released, molybdenum, though is not a main component of Co-Cr alloy, can potentially cause mutagenesis, inactive some important enzymes, such as alkaline phosphatase, and inhibit chromium absorption via leukocytes.

1.2 The biological effects of dental casting alloys

Microbial corrosion refers to electrochemical reactions aroused or catalyzed by microorganisms, rather than the metal specifically corroded by microorganisms. Microbial corrosion requires appropriate conditions for microbial reproduction, and is often the result of multi-microbial symbiosis and interaction. In the oral environment, dental casting alloys are sensitive to micro-organisms and tarnish, e.g. nickel, chromium, copper, aluminum, iron, palladium and zinc. It is reported that Actinomyces viscosus has a significant influence on the electrochemical corrosion of Ni-Cr alloy and Gold alloy; the existence of streptococcus mutans increases the corrosion of Ni-Cr alloy. On the other hand, oral bacteria can produce lactic acid and acetic acid. When fluoride ions, hydrogen peroxide and lactic acid exist simultaneously in the mouth, the corrosion of titanium would greatly increase. The biggest corrosion threat to iron is glucose, followed by acetic acid (Park et al., 2007). As mentioned above, the oral bacteria play an important role in material deterioration. Oral microorganisms should be considered when discussing biocompatibility of prostheses.

In conjunction with the corrosion process of dental casting alloys, many metal ions are absorbed within the digestive system. Per unit ion concentration, K^+, Cd^{2+}, V^{2+}, Ag^+, Hg^{2+}, Sb^{3+}, Be^{2+}, and In^{3+} have higher toxicity, while Sn^{4+}, Zr^{4+}, Nb^{5+}, and Mo^{6+} have lower toxicity. Cr^{6+} and Be^{2+} have the highest toxicity towards the cell membrane integrity and protein synthesis of human gingival fibroblasts; Ni^{2+} is moderately toxic to these cells, and Cr^{3+} and Mo^{6+} show the lowest toxicity. Ni^{2+}, Co^{2+}, Ti^{4+}, and V^{3+} could affect DNA synthesis, ALP (alkaline phosphatase) activity and calcification processes of osteoblast-like cells in vitro. Bone marrow cells can be significantly damaged when exposed to Cr^{6+} for 48h; Co^{2+}, Mo^{6+}, and Ni^{2+} also showed moderate toxicity; V^{5+} showed significant toxicity after 4 weeks.

The commonly used Ni-Cr alloy (which also contains Be) could cause gingival fibroblast morphology, viability and proliferation changes, increase the production of PCNA (Proliferating cell nuclear antigen) and Bcl-2 (B-cell lymphoma gene 2) proteins, and boost the production of IL-6, IL-8 and other cytokines involved in inflammation. These effects show positive correlations with concentration of Co, Cr and Cu ions. After wearing Ni-Cr alloy (with Be), animal experiments demonstrated apoptosis lymphocytes and DNA damage of buccal epithelial cells, which deteriorated further with increased wearing time; the gold alloy in contrast, produced no side effects. (Su et al., 2006a, 2006b, 2006c, 2008a, 2008b; Yu et al., 2007)

2. The tea application

Tea, which originated in China, and has spread over the world, has become a popular worldwide drink. Nowadays, over 34 countries produce tea, and there are more than 4 billion tea consumers in over 100 countries.

Tea is not only a refreshing drink, but also a healthy drink for the prevention of radiation sickness, cardiovascular diseases and cancer, with certain pharmacological effects. The main active ingredients in tea are tea polyphenols, which are strong antioxidants. These polyphenolic compounds mainly consist of catechins. They have a health benefits, including lowering blood cholesterol and blood pressure, and anti-cancer, anti-bacterial and anti-viral effects.

2.1 Biological effects of catechin

The green tea catechins make up approximately 60–80 wt.% of tea polyphenols. (-)-epigallocatechin gallate (EGCG) is the most abundant of the four major catechins which also include (-)-epicatechin gallate (ECG), (-)-epigallocatechin (EGC) and (-)-epicatechin (EC).

EGCG is also the most active component of green tea leaves. It has been shown to have biological effects, including antimutagenicity, antitumorigenesis, free radical scavenging, etc. Epidemiologic studies demonstrated that a low rate of tumorigenesis may be associated with the habit of drinking tea. Experiments in animal models and cells also suggested that green tea extract may contribute to the inhibition of the generation and development of tumors. In addition to the above-mentioned effect, EGCG, as reported, plays a critical role in inducing apoptosis of malignant cells, regulating key elements of signal pathway and inhibiting telomerase activity.

2.2 Biological effects of EGCG

EGCG is a potent antioxidant component that has demonstrated great antioxidant protection in experimental studies. It is also involved in protecting against free-radical DNA damage, and interferes with the binding of cancer-causing agents to cellular DNA. Besides, EGCG plays a role in inhibition of lipid peroxidation and inducement of apoptosis of malignant cells by regulating various signal pathways. For instance, EGCG may induce apoptosis of cells through binding to the antiapoptotic proteins Bcl-2 and Bcl-xL;

EGCG can negatively regulate protein serine/threonine phosphatase-2A (PP-2A) to positively regulate p53-dependent apoptosis. In addition: EGCG induces apoptosis of JB6 cells, which is associated with hyperphosphorylation of p53 and up-regulation of the proapoptotic gene, Bak (Qin et al., 2008); the interruption of the VEGF (vascular endothelial growth factor) signaling pathway by EGCG results in caspase activation and subsequent malignant cell death; EGCG induces stress signals by damaging mitochondria and ROS-mediated JNK activation in MIA PaCa-2 pancreatic carcinoma cells; EGCG-mediated caspase activation induces proteolytic cleavage of the NF-kappa B/p65 subunit, leading to the loss of transactivation domains, and driving the cells towards apoptosis; EGCG show its cytotoxicity to PC-3 cells by up-regulating the 67LR and the mitochondria-mediated apoptosis pathway (Zhang et al., 2008); and finally, EGCG treatment resulted in dose-dependent inhibition of TNF-α-induced production of MMP-1 and MMP-3 at the protein and mRNA levels in RA synovial fibroblasts (Yun et al., 2008).

The mechanism of the biological effects of EGCG may differ for different cell categories. Treatment of PC-3 cells with EGCG resulted in time and concentration-dependent activation of the extracellular signal-regulated kinase (ERK1/2) pathway. In contrast, EGCG treatment did not induce ERK1/2 activity in RWPE-1 cells (Albrecht et al., 2008). In HLE cells (hepatoma cell line), EGCG induced apoptosis, but not cell-cycle arrest, and appears to have down-regulated Bcl-2α and Bcl-xl by inactivation of NF-kappaB. Oral administration of EGCG showed similar effects in HLE xenograft tumors; in normal human primary epidermal keratinocytes (NHEK), one of the key mediators of EGCG action is p57/KIP2, a cyclin-dependent kinase (CDK) inhibitor. EGCG potently induces p57 in NHEK, but not in epithelial cancer cells. It is c-Jun N-terminal kinase (JNK) signaling that mediates EGCG-induced apoptosis, and exogenous expression of p57 suppresses EGCG-induced apoptosis via inhibition of JNK.

Research has indicated that the 67-kDa laminin receptor (67LR) mediates epigallocatechin gallate (EGCG)-induced cell growth inhibition and reduction of myosin regulatory light chain (MRLC) phosphorylation at Thr-18/Ser-19, which is important for cytokinesis through

67LR. EGCG at a physiological concentration can activate myosin phosphatase by reducing myosin phosphatase 1 (MYPT1) phosphorylation and that may be involved in EGCG-induced cell growth inhibition (Umeda et al., 2008). Matrix metalloproteinase (MMP-9) expression is linked with myeloid cell differentiation, as well as inflammation and angiogenesis processes related to cancer progression. EGCG inhibited MMP-9 secretion in a time- and dose-dependent manner. The gene and protein expression of MMP-9 and of the mRNA stabilizing factor HuR were also inhibited. In an invasion assay, EGCG repressed the invasion of lung carcinoma, and it down-regulated the expression of MMP-9. NF-kappa B localized in the nucleus of the 95-D cells was diminished in a dose-dependent manner in EGCG-treated cells. Thus, the inhibition of tumor invasion by EGCG was shown to be attributed to decreases in the expression of MMP-9 and NF-kappa B, which may result from decrease of intracellular oxidants (Annabi et al. 2007).

EGCG induced dose- and time-dependent apoptotic cell death accompanied by loss of mitochondrial transmembrane potential, release of cytochrome c into the cytosol, and cleavage of pro-caspase-9 to its active form; EGCG also enhanced production of intracellular reactive oxygen species (ROS) (Noda et al., 2007).

3. Tea and metal ions

3.1 The effect of tea polyphenols on the corrosion behavior of dental casting alloys

Ni-Cr alloy has become prevalent in oral prosthetic applications; although many instances of side effects caused by fixed nichrome dentures have been reported. Gingival inflammation and the appearance of marginal gingival blackening are both ascribed to release of metal ions from the denture. Thus, we wondered if the habit of drinking tea affected the corrosion behavior of dental casting alloys.

As reported, the recommended daily intake of tea is 6-16 g per person, and it differs with age. The major component of green tea, tea polyphenol, accounts for 20–30 wt.% of the dry weight of green leaves. The concentration of weak tea (4–6 g/L green tea) is equivalent to 1.25 g/L tea polyphenol solution, while strong tea (17–25 g/L green tea) is about 5 g/L. An average consumption of green tea (8-13g/L green tea) equates to 2.5g/L tea polyphenol solution.

Experiments showed that the effect of tea polyphenol on Ni-Cr alloy was the most obvious; it enhanced the corrosion rate of Ni-Cr alloy at low concentrations. Tea polyphenol at a concentration of 1.25 g/L had the lowest corrosion resistance compare to the other two groups (the alloy treated with 2.5g/L and 5g/L tea polyphenol).

With an increase in the concentration of tea polyphenol, the corrosion resistance of Ni-Cr alloy improved. A surface view of Ni-Cr alloy with a scanning electron microscope demonstrated that the surface of the alloy treated with 1.25 g/L tea polyphenol was the roughest, compared with the other samples. It was a very interesting result. Although the exact principle is unclear, the EGCG could formulate an insoluble chelate with Ni and/or Cr, thus precluding further corrosion.

Co-Cr alloy possesses good hardness and high strength, and more importantly does not contain adverse elements as Be and Ni. A great deal of scientific research has demonstrated that the corrosion of the alloy with Cr (>16%) is reduced because of the existence of a passive film on the surface. Treatment with a high concentration of tea polyphenol could further reduce the corrosion tendency of the Co-Cr alloy. Compared with in artificial saliva, the Co-Cr alloy in tea polyphenol has a lower corrosion tendency and corrosion rate.

Drinking tea at the recommended daily intake is helpful to enhance the corrosion resistance of Co-Cr alloy. Thus, it is advised that people with Co-Cr alloy prostheses increase their intake of tea polyphenol. This will give the prosthesis a long service life.

As titanium has good corrosion resistance, it is more and more widely used in clinical stomatology. In tea polyphenol solutions, with increasing concentration of polyphenols, the corrosion of titanium accelerates as its corrosion resistance decreases. Therefore, while lower concentrations of tea help to increase the corrosion resistance of titanium, if the concentration is much higher than the recommended amount for daily drinking the stability of titanium will be lower, as described above, with potentially harmful effects. So patients wearing titanium dentures should not drink concentrated tea solution.

We have studied both artificial saliva, and three different concentrations of polyphenol solutions. Among the three alloys studied, the corrosion rate of the titanium is slowest (i.e. its corrosion resistance is best); the corrosion rate of the nickel-chromium alloy is fastest (so its corrosion resistance is worst, and showed the most serious corrosion in the experiments) and the corrosion resistance of cobalt-chromium alloy is between that of titanium and nickel-chromium alloy.

3.2 Complexation reactions of tea polyphenols and metal ions

Polyphenols that are abundant in green tea contain multiple hydroxyl groups. As a result, green tea has a strong acid-base buffering capacity, and the polyphenols can complex with central ions such as Ni^{2+}, Bi^{3+}, Cr^{6+}, Fe^{3+}, Al^{3+}, Fe^{2+}, Mo^{6+}, Cu^{2+}, and Mn^{2+}, and form chelate rings. A number of studies show that flavonoids are strong chelating agents with Fe^{3+}. Catechins (flavonols) contain epigallocatechin gallate (EGCG), epigallocatechin (EGC), epicatechin gallate (ECG), and epicatechin (EC). All of them can form complexes with Fe^{3+}. A "B ring" catechol group is required for combination of polyphenols and Fe^{3+}; when the B ring of 3,4 o-hydroxy changes into a 3,4,5-trihydroxy gallic acyl group, the efficiency of the combination of polyphenol and Fe^{3+} is low. Although gallic acid (another phenolic acid) can form complexes with Fe^{3+}, the binding capacity of the polyphenols is weak because of the galloyl functional group. The functional groups and chemical characterization of polyphenols and metal ions have been studied for a long time. Chemical analysis and X-ray diffraction showed that catechin and Al^{3+} form a non-crystalline precipitate complex with a ratio of 1:1. Nuclear magnetic resonance spectroscopy shows the chemical shifts of catechins change upon complex formation; infrared absorption spectra show that the absorption bands of some functional groups of epicatechin disappeared

Some experiments show that catechins folded into a cavity-like structure around Zn^{2+} and Cu^{2+}, capturing Zn^{2+} and Cu^{2+} through the ring π-electron clouds of the aromatic compounds and forming complexes with 1:1 ratios. However, many studies suggest tea polyphenols and metal ions can coordinate in a wide variety of ways. The coordination modes of tea polyphenols and metal ions change with changing pH. Al different pH values, catechin and Fe^{3+} form complexes in different proportions: when $pH < 3$, Fe^{3+} and catechin combined at a molar ratio of 1:1; when $3 < pH < 7$, the molar ratio was 2:1; and when $pH > 7$, the molar ratio was 4:1. The stability constants of these complexes are in the range 10^5–10^{17} (Sungur & Uzar, 2007) . Electrospray mass spectrometry shows that catechins and iron ions form three different compounds (L^1Fe, L^1_2Fe and L^1_3Fe with one to three ligands) at different pH values (Elhabiri et al., 2007). Different kinds of polyphenols also have different coordination modes with metal ions. Studies show that EGC and EC combined with Mn^{2+} through the o-hydroxy of the B ring, while EGCG mainly combines with Mn^{2+} through the D ring (gallic ring), and then through the B ring (gallate catechin ring), as the coordination bond formed at the D-loop was stronger than that at the B ring. The same tea polyphenols and metal ions can form different complexes in different coordination modes. To form [Al (egcgH-2)]$^+$, two hydroxyl groups on the D-ring of epigallocatechin gallate become deprotonated, while to form [Al (egcgH-3)]^0, first one hydroxyl group on the B-ring and two on the D-ring are deprotonated, then Al^{3+} combines with two oxygen atoms on the D-ring and one on the B-ring to form a polymeric structure.

In addition, oxidation-reduction reaction can also take place between tea polyphenols and metal ions. The reduction potential of tea polyphenols is high, so it is easy for them to auto-oxidize under certain conditions. High valence metal ions can oxidize the polyphenols to their quinone or other derivatives, with the metal ions being reduced to their lower valent states. Catechins, the main components of tea polyphenols, have been shown experimentally to reduce Cu^{2+} and Fe^{3+} into Cu^+ and Fe^{2+}. Because the Cu^{2+}/Cu^+ redox potential is low, the Cu^{2+}/Cu^+ reaction is easier than the Fe^{3+}/Fe^{2+} reaction. When excess Fe^{3+} was added into gallic acid (GA), Fe^{3+} rapidly combined with the o-hydroxyl on the B-ring of gallic acid, and formed complexes at the ratio of 1:1, as indicated by the formation of a dark blue solution. Subsequently, other complexes can formed electron transfer reactions - Fe^{3+} was reduced to Fe^{2+}, and GA was oxidized to semiquinone, which then rapidly combined with the remaining Fe^{3+} to form benzoquinone.

4. Effects of interaction between EGCG and metal ions on cells

4.1 Effects of interaction between EGCG and metal ions on cell proliferation rate

We found that EGCG has a strong inhibitory effect on the growth of tongue squamous carcinoma cells; with significant inhibition beginning at 100 μM. In contrast, for gingival fibroblasts, a small inhibition of cell growth was noted at over 150 μM EGCG (Fig. 1). Some studies have shown that Ni^{2+} has carcinogenic effects, and some have shown that its toxicity and carcinogenic effects are related to its absorption, transport, distribution and retention in cells. Our studies show that when the concentration of EGCG is less than 150 μM, the growth of gingival fibroblasts remains almost unaffected (cell survival rate is more than 95%); when EGCG concentration ranges from 150 μM to 300 μM, a concentration- and time-dependent inhibition of growth of gingival fibroblasts is seen. These results indicated that EGCG may have little promotion on the growth of gingival fibroblasts at low concentrations, and strong inhibition at high concentrations (Fig. 1). Interestingly, we also found that the interactions between EGCG and Ni^{2+}/Co^{2+} enhanced the inhibition effect of EGCG on cell growth (Fig. 2, Fig. 4), as well as cell morphological changes. Cr^{3+}/Mo^{6+} have little effect on the growth of tongue squamous carcinoma cells and gingival fibroblast cells, and the interaction of EGCG and Cr^{3+}/Mo^{6+} produces no significant inhibition effects on tongue squamous carcinoma cells and gingival fibroblast cells (Fig. 3, Fig. 5).

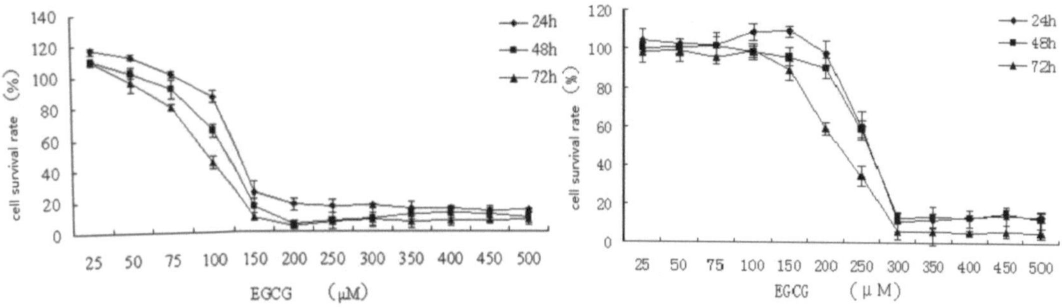

Fig. 1. Cell survival rates in tongue squamous cancer Cal-27 cells (left) and human gingival fibroblast cells (right) upon treatment with EGCG. The cell density was detected at 24, 48 and 72 h after cell seeding. Cell survival rate was calculated as the number of cells present at these time points compared with the initial cell seeding density. Data points represent the mean ± SD for each group

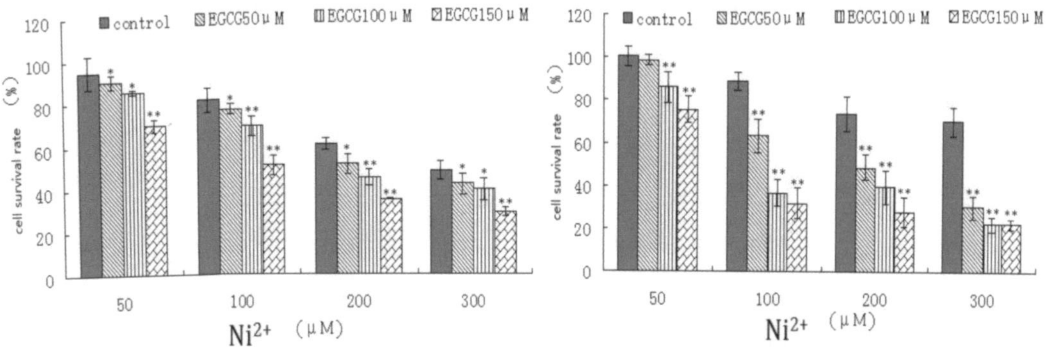

Fig. 2. Cell survival rates in tongue squamous cancer Cal-27 cells (left) and human gingival fibroblast cells (right) upon treatment with combinations of EGCG and Ni^{2+} for 48 hours compared with the control group (treatment with Ni^{2+} only). Data points represent the mean ± SD. n=6 (*, $p<0.05$; **, $p<0.01$)

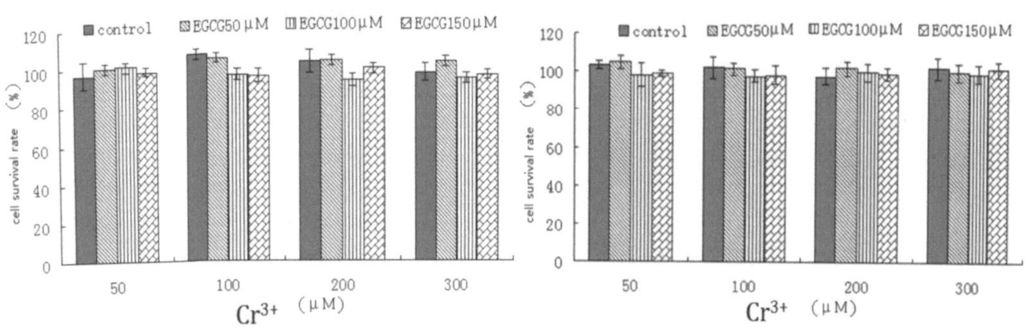

Fig. 3. Cell survival rates in tongue squamous cancer Cal-27 cells (left) and human gingival fibroblast cells (right) upon treatment with combinations of EGCG and Cr^{3+} for 48 hours compared with the control group (treatment with Cr^{3+} only). Data points represent the mean ± SD. n=6 (*, $p<0.05$; **, $p<0.01$)

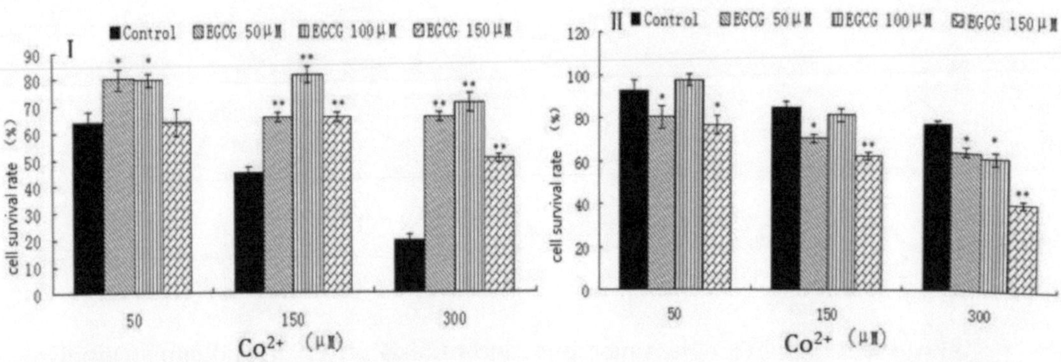

Fig. 4. Cell survival rates in tongue squamous cancer Cal-27 cells (left) and human gingival fibroblast cells (right) upon treatment with combinations of EGCG and Co^{2+} for 48 hours. The control group was treated with Co^{2+} only. Data points represent the mean ± SD. n=6 (*, $p<0.05$; **, $p<0.01$)

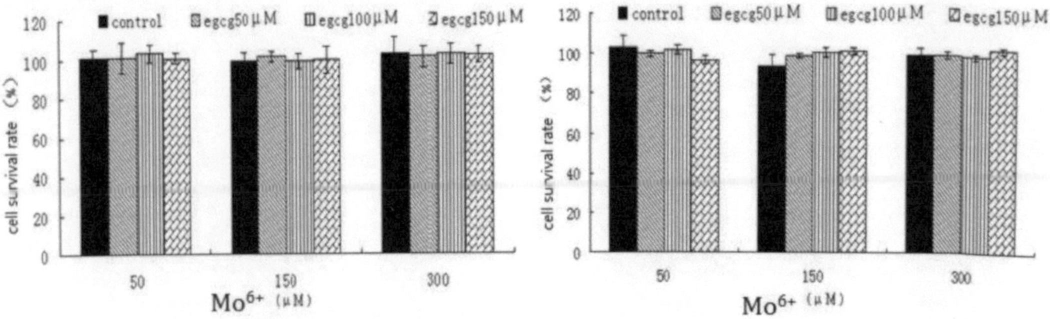

Fig. 5. Cell survival rates in tongue squamous cancer Cal-27 cells (left) and human gingival fibroblast cells (right) upon treatment with combinations of EGCG and Mo^{6+} for 48 hours compared with the control group (treatment with Mo^{6+} only). Data points represent the mean ± SD. n=6 (*, $p<0.05$; **, $p<0.01$)

4.2 The influence of the combination of metal ions and EGCG on cellular DNA

DNA is a biological macromolecule, which occupies a central and critical role in the cell as its genetic information. A variety of factors can cause DNA damage in cells, such as ionizing radiation, peroxides, thiols and certain metal ions. It has been reported that Ni^{2+} can decrease DNA synthesis, change the structure of DNA, reduce protein synthesis and inhibit DNA replication and transcription. It can also cause decrease of succinate dehydrogenase activity and total cellular protein. In addition, Ni^{2+} complexes with nitrogen compounds may damage DNA in breast cancer cells (Lü et al., 2009). However, Cr^{3+} is difficult to get into cells, and hence has no significant effect on the human gingival fibroblast cells (Elshahawy et al., 2009).

Single cell gel electrophoresis (SCGE), also called comet assay could detect the DNA damage on single cell level. The parameter of Olive Tail Moment reflects both intensity and extent of DNA damage. Ni^{2+} in combination with EGCG significantly increased the damage to human gingival fibroblast cells and tongue squamous cancer cells. The damage to tongue squamous cancer cells could also be increased by the combination of Cr^{3+} and EGCG. Furthermore, the damage to human gingival fibroblast cells and tongue squamous cancer cells caused by Cr^{3+} in combination with EGCG was significantly less than that produced by 100 μM EGCG alone (Figs. 6–7).

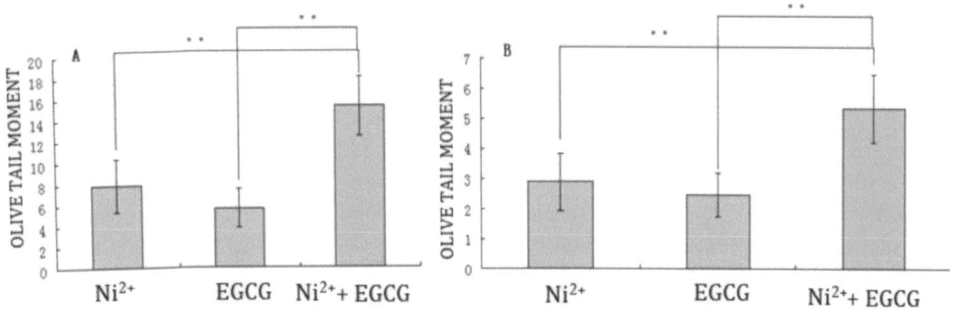

Fig. 6. Comet Assay: DNA damage in tongue squamous cancer Cal-27 cells (left) and human gingival fibroblast cells (right) after treatments with EGCG, Ni^{2+} and EGCG combined with Ni^{2+}. Cells were treated with 100 μM EGCG and/or 200 μM Ni^{2+} for 48 hours

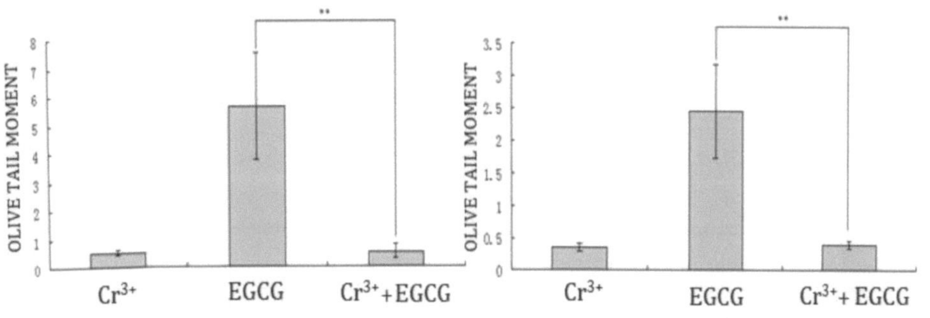

Fig. 7. Comet Assay: DNA damage in tongue squamous cancer Cal-27 cells (left) and human gingival fibroblast cells (right) after treatments with EGCG, Cr^{3+} and EGCG combined with Cr^{3+}. Cells were treated with 100 μM EGCG and/or 200 μM Cr^{3+} for 48 hours

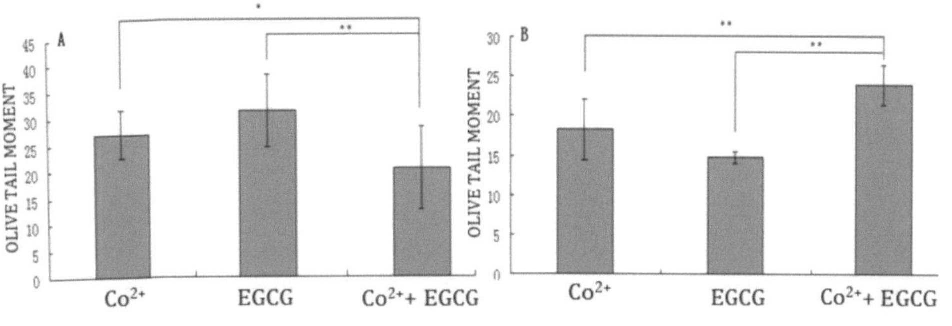

Fig. 8. Comet Assay: DNA damage in tongue squamous cancer Cal-27 cells (left) and human gingival fibroblast cells (right) after treatments with EGCG, Co^{2+} and EGCG combined with Co^{2+}. Cells were treated with 150 μM EGCG and/or 300 μM Co^{2+} for 48 hours

The combination of Co^{2+} and EGCG produced less DNA damage than either individual component on tongue squamous cancer cells, but increased the damage to human gingival fibroblast cell DNA. Mo^{6+} in combination with EGCG produced significantly less damage than EGCG alone to both human gingival fibroblast cells and tongue squamous cancer cells (Figs. 8–9).

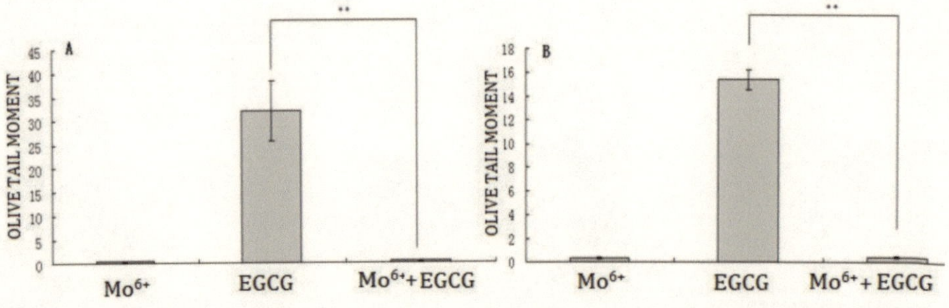

Fig. 9. Comet Assay: DNA damage in tongue squamous cancer Cal-27 cells (left) and human gingival fibroblast cells (right) after treatments with EGCG, Mo^{6+} and EGCG combined with Mo^{6+}. Cells were treated with 150 μM EGCG and/or 300 μM Mo^{6+} for 48 hours

4.3 The influence of interaction of metal ions and EGCG on cell cycle

Flow cytometry (FCM) is an efficient experimental method for cell cycle detection and estimation of apoptotic cells. Hence, we use FCM to measure the apoptosis. The result

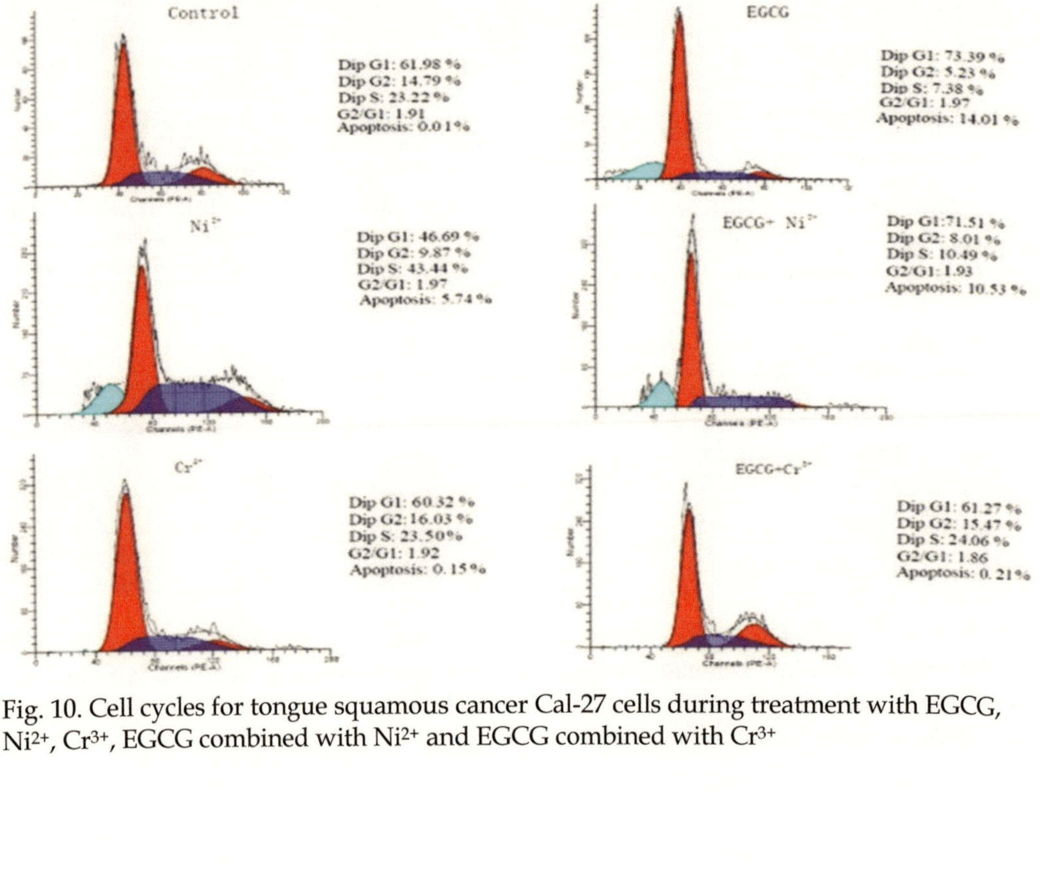

Fig. 10. Cell cycles for tongue squamous cancer Cal-27 cells during treatment with EGCG, Ni^{2+}, Cr^{3+}, EGCG combined with Ni^{2+} and EGCG combined with Cr^{3+}

showed that: EGCG induces G0/G1 cell cycle arrest and partial apoptosis in the tongue squamous cancer cells. Ni^{2+} arrests the cell cycle at S in the human gingival fibroblast cells and tongue squamous cancer cells. After exposure to the combination of EGCG and Ni^{2+}, the cell cycle is arrested at G0/G1 and apoptosis is increased. Compared with the Ni^{2+} induced effect, the effect of the combination of Ni^{2+} and EGCG is enhancement of the apoptosis of both human gingival fibroblast cells and tongue squamous cancer cells. This indicates that the cytotoxicity of Ni^{2+} enhanced after co-treatment with Ni^{2+} and EGCG. In contrast, Cr^{3+} has no obvious influence on the cell cycle of the human gingival fibroblast cells and tongue squamous cancer cells. The effect on the cell cycle of human gingival fibroblast cells and tongue squamous cancer cells induced by EGCG could be reduced by combination of Cr^{3+} and EGCG. (Figs. 10–11)

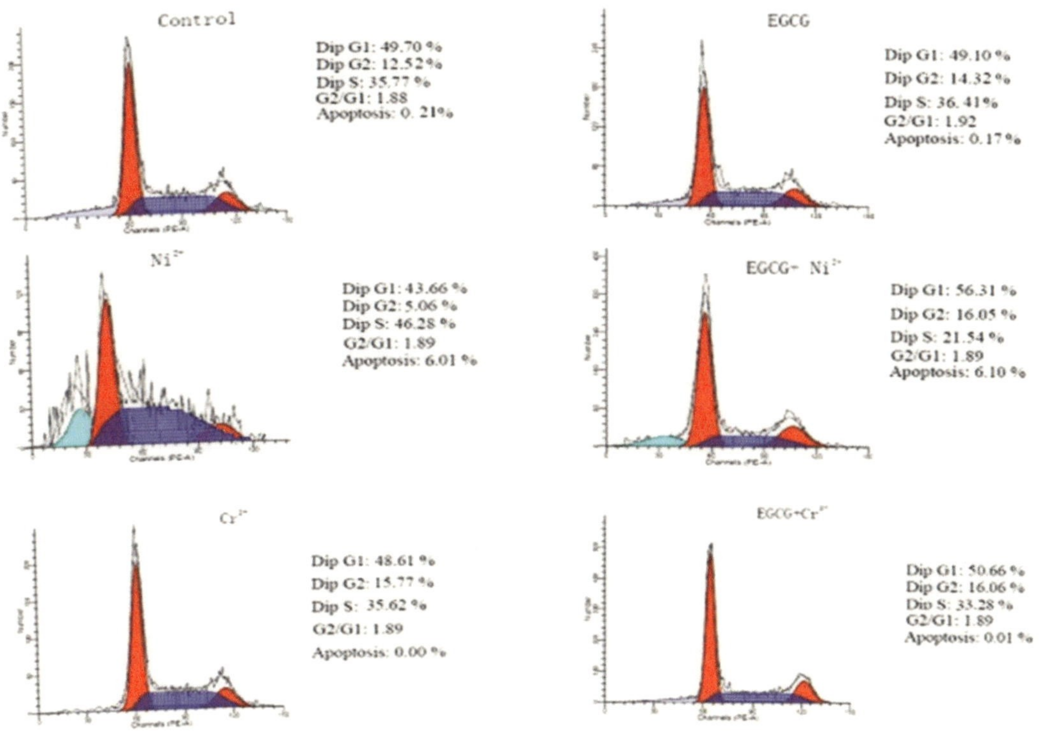

Fig. 11. Cell cycles for human gingival fibroblast cells during treatment with EGCG, Ni^{2+}, Cr^{3+}, EGCG combined with Ni^{2+} and EGCG combined with Cr^{3+}

Both EGCG and Co^{2+} inhibited the cell cycle of tongue squamous cancer cells, block the DNA synthesis and arrest the cell cycle at G0/G1. However, the combination of EGCG and Co^{2+} significantly reduced the inhibition effect caused by EGCG or Co^{2+} individually, and increased the percentage of cells in the G2/M phase. There was no significant change in the cell cycle between the group of Cal-27 cells treated with Mo^{6+} and the control group, and the cell cycle arrest of Cal-27 cells induced by EGCG could be reduced combination with Mo^{6+} to the extent that no significant difference was seen compared with the control group. (Figs. 12–13)

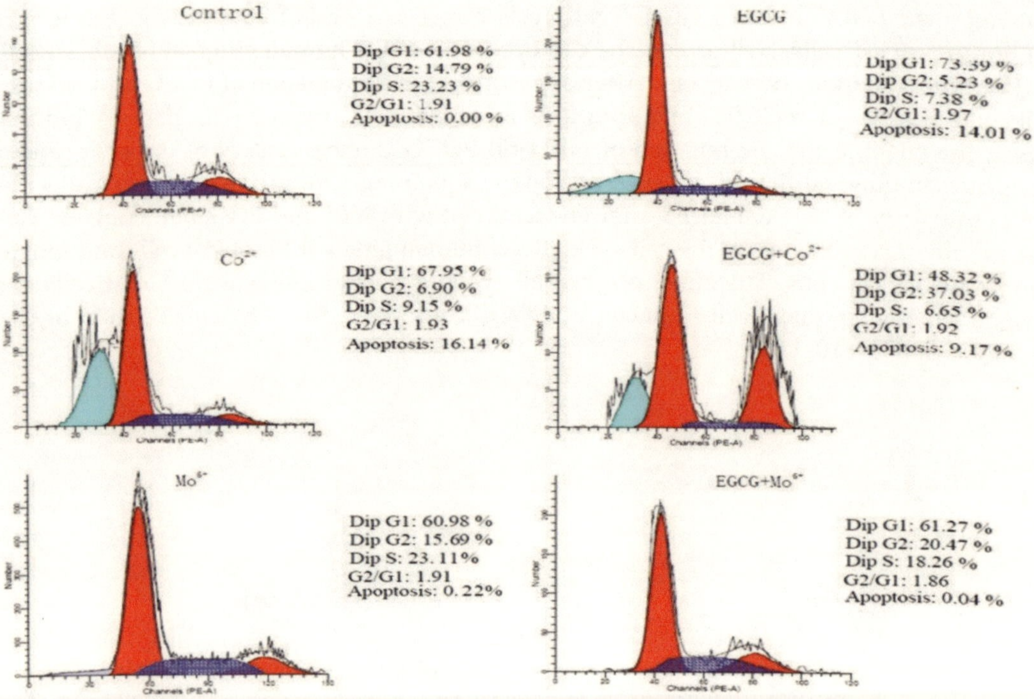

Fig. 12. Cell cycles for tongue squamous cancer Cal-27 cells during treatment with EGCG, Co^{2+}, Mo^{6+}, EGCG combined with Co^{2+} and EGCG combined with Mo^{6+}

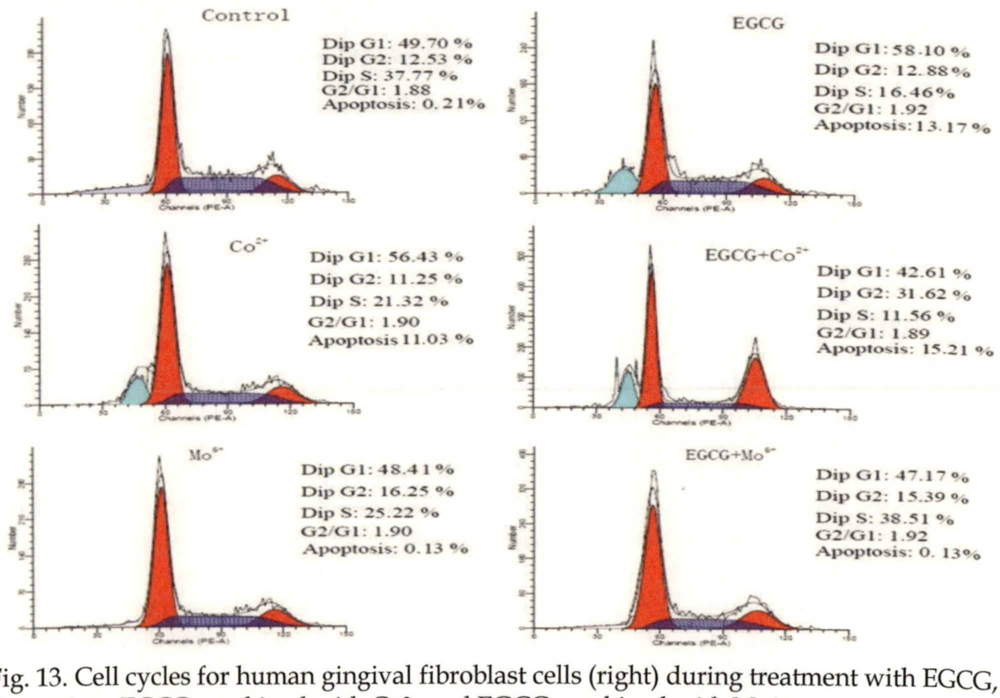

Fig. 13. Cell cycles for human gingival fibroblast cells (right) during treatment with EGCG, Co^{2+}, Mo^{6+}, EGCG combined with Co^{2+} and EGCG combined with Mo^{6+}

5. Conclusion

Our results show that Ni^{2+} in combination with EGCG significantly increases damage to normal gingival fibroblasts and tongue squamous cancer cells, whereas the combination of EGCG and Co^{2+} increased damage only to gingival fibroblasts. In contrast, EGCG together with either Cr^{3+} or Mo^{6+} resulted in significantly less damage than produced by EGCG alone. Moreover, the cell cycle is arrested at G0/G1 and apoptosis after exposure to EGCG+Ni^{2+} is increased relative to that occurring after treatment with EGCG only. Combining EGCG+Co^{2+} significantly reduced the growth inhibitory effect caused by EGCG or Co^{2+} individually, and increased the percentage of cells in the G2/M phase. In contrast, no significant synergistic effect was seen with EGCG+Cr^{3+}/Mo^{6+}.

These results indicate that the toxicity of EGCG may be i) enhanced in the presence of Ni^{2+}, ii) diminished when given in combination with Cr^{3+} or Mo^{6+} or iii) partially inhibited by Co^{2+} (although this latter effect is seen only in normal fibroblasts).

Our studies have demonstrated interactions between EGCG and metal ions that affect cell cycle progression and apoptosis. However, more research is required to reveal the binding mode (s) of these substances and the potential mechanisms by which they affect normal and cancerous cells.

6. Acknowledgments

This work was supported by grants from National Natural Science Foundation of China (30840031, 30970726) and from Shanghai (0852nm03600, 11nm0504300, 114119a3700) and from Doctoral Fund of Ministry of Education of China (20110072110041).

7. References

Annabi, B.; Currie, JC. & Moghrabi, A. (2007). Inhibition of HuR and MMP-9 expression in macrophage-differentiated HL-60 myeloid leukemia cells by green tea polyphenol EGCg. Leukemia Research, Vol.31, No.9, (September 2007), pp. 1277-1284, ISSN 0145-2126

Albrecht, DS.; Clubbs, EA. & Ferruzzi, M. (2007). Epigallocatechin-3- gallate (EGCG)inhibits PC-3 prostate cancer cell proliferation via MEK-independent ERK1/2 activation. Chemico-Biological Interactions , Vol.171, No.1, (January 2008), pp. 89-95, ISSN 0009-2797

Azam, S.; Hadi, N.& Khan, NU. (2004). Prooxidant property of green tea polyphenols epicatechin and epigallocatechin-3-gallate: implications for anticancer properties. Toxicology In Vitro, Vol.18, No.5, (October 2004), pp. 555-561, ISSN 0887-2333

Elhabiri, M.; Carrer, C. & Marmolle, F. (2006). Complexation of iron (III) by catecholate-type polyphenols. *Inorganica Chimica Acta*, Vol.360, No.1, (January 2007), pp. 353-359, ISSN 0020-1693

Elshahawy, WM.; Watanabe I. & Kramer P. (2009). In vitro cytotoxicity evaluation of elemental ions released from different prosthodontic materials. *Dent Mater*, Vol.25, No.5, (December 2009), pp. 1551–1555, ISSN 0287-4547

Lü, X.; Bao, X. & Huang, Y. (2008). Mechanisms of cytotoxicity of nickel ions based on gene expression profiles. Biomaterials, Vol.30, No.2, (January 2009), pp. 141–148, ISSN 0142-9612

Neukam, K.; Pastor, N.& Cortés F. (2008). Tea flavanols inhibit cell growth and DNA topoisomerase II activity and induce endoreduplication in cultured Chinese hamster cells. Mutation Research, Vol.654, No.1, (January 2008), pp. 8–12, ISSN 0921-8262.

Noda, C.; He, JS. & Takano T. (2007). Induction of apoptosis by epigallocatechin -3-gallate in human lymphoblastoid B cells. *Biochem Biophs Res Commun*, Vol.362, No.4, (November 2007), pp. 951–957, ISSN 0006-291X

Park, SK,; Choi, SC. & Kim, YK. (2007). The rate of iron corrosion for different organic carbon sources during biofilm formation. Water Sci Technol. Vol.55, No. 8-9, (2007), pp. 489-497, ISSN 0273-0223

Qin, J.; Chen, HG. & Yan, Q. (2007). Protein phosphatase-2A is a target of epigallocatechin-3-gallate and modulates p53-Bak apoptotic pathway. *Cancer Res*, Vol.68, No. 11, (June 2007), pp. 4150-4162, ISSN 0008-5472

Su, JS.; Deng, ZY. & Shao L. (2005). Study of DNA damage of buccal mucosal cells after wearing casting alloy crowns. *West China journal of stomatology*, Vol.24, No. 1, (February 2006), pp. 21-25, ISSN 1000-1182

Su, JS.; Guo, LY. & Yu, YQ. (2005). Change of the apoptotic lymphocytes in peripheral venous blood after wearing casting alloy crowns. *Fudan Univ J Med Sci*, Vol.33, No. 3, (May 2006), pp. 315-319, ISSN 0257-8131

Su, JS.; Jia, S. & Qiao, GY. (2005). Expression of PCNA and Bcl-2 in Gingival Tissue After Wearing Casting Alloy Crowns. *J Tongji Univ (Nat Sci)*, Vol.34, No. 6, (July 2006), pp. 795-799, ISSN 0253-374X

Su, JS.; Tian, ZJ. & Guo, S. (2008). Study of released metal ions of three kinds of dental casting alloy crowns and DNA damage of mucosal cells in vitro. *Chin J Stomatol Res (Electronic Version)*, Vol.2, No.1, (2008), pp. 26-29, ISSN 1674-1366

Su, JS.; Zhang, ZW & Wan, SJ. (2008) Expression of IL-6 in gingival tissue after wearing casting alloy crowns. *Fudan Univ J Med Sci*, Vol.35, No.1, (2008), pp. 120-124, ISSN 0257-8131

Sungur, S.; Uzar, A. (2007). Investigation of complexes tannic acid and myricetin with Fe (III). Spectrochim Acta A Mol Biomol Spectrosc, Vol.69, No.1, (January 2008), pp. 225-229, ISSN 1386-1425

Umeda, D.; Yano, S. & Yamada, K. (2008) Involvement of 67-kDa laminin receptor-mediated myosin phosphatase activation in antiproliferative effect of epigallocatechin-3-O-gallate at a physiological concentration on Caco-2 colon cancer cells. *Biochem Biophs Res Commun*, Vol.371, No.1, (June 2008), pp. 172–176, ISSN 0006-291X

Yu, LF.; Su, JS. & Zou, DR. (2007) Assays of IL-8 content in gingival crevicular fluid for porclain teeth. *J Tongji Univ (Med Sci)*, Vol.28, No.3, (2007), pp. 45-47, ISSN 0257-716X

Yun, HJ.; Yoo, WH. & Han, MK. (2008). Epigallocatechin-3-gallate suppresses TNF-alpha-induced production of MMP-1 and -3 in rheumatoid arthritis synovial fibroblasts. Rheumatol Int, Vol.29, No.1, (November 2008), pp. 23-29, ISSN 0172-8172

Zhang, L.; Yu, H. & Sun, S. (2008). Investigations of the cytotoxicity of epigallocatechin-3-gallate against PC-3 cells in the presence of Cd2+ in vitro. *Toxicology in Vitro*, Vol.22, No.4, (June 2008), pp. 953–960, ISSN 0887-2333